FOOD FACTS & FALLACIES

FOOD FACTS & FALLACIES

The intelligent person's guide to nutrition and health by CARLTON FREDERICKS, Ph.D. and HERBERT BAILEY

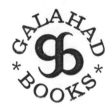

Galahad Books • New York City

Published by Galahad Books, New York, N.Y.
Copyright © 1965 by Dr. Carlton Fredericks and Herbert Bailey
This book reprinted with permission of the
Julian Press, Inc., New York
Library of Congress Catalog Card Number 73-75968
ISBN 0-88365-002-9
Manufactured in the United States of America

Both authors take pleasure in dedicating this book to the apostles of conformity—without whose punitive implementation of their determined opposition to freedom of thought in science, this text would never have been written.

The wise herd does not too severely punish its deviants—they are idiots, criminals, prophets, and discoverers.

BERTRAND RUSSELL
Nobel Prize acceptance speech

Contents

FOOD FACTS & FALLACIES

1. Why you need this book

The main purpose of this book is to help you achieve, through proper nutrition, a better life, both physically and mentally. We have several purposes in wishing to save you for a long, prosperous, and vigorous life by means of the information contained in our book. We like to see healthy people around us who really don't believe they should surrender to their so-called allotted life spans. We also like to see healthy persons of any age who defy the calendar and the clock, because we do not believe there is such a clock—except in the minds of those pessimists for whom it obviously *does* exist. We have other reasons for wanting you around and in vital health, reasons we will disclose later in this chapter.

To our knowledge, no one has heretofore attempted to bring together in one book, for the general public, the results of all the new research we shall describe. Perhaps a good reason is that most of it has had to face official disapproval. Yet any scientist worthy of the name would know after even a cursory examination of the evidence we present that it is sound. Most of it is based on hundreds—sometimes thousands—of cases, all authenticated beyond any serious question.

Now let us get down to specifics: Do you know that vitamin E helpfully treats—and very likely prevents—many forms of heart disease? That it is effective against many other serious ailments? Or do you know that intensive vitamin-mineral protein therapy either cures or alleviates symptoms in scores of diseases, including those of diabetes and arthritis? That in fact there are surprisingly few diseases in which vitamin treatments have not been helpful when properly administered? And do you know that there are definite indications that if you eat properly and fortify your body with the optimal amount of chemical substances it needs, the chances are you will have to worry less about disease in any form, mental or physical? Radical? Dr. Tom Spies promised more! [1]

If your body still has something to build on, you can and should enjoy radiant health for a very long time; in fact, much, much longer than you think. The authors of this book consider that a hundred years of good health should be man's natural birthright provided he follows certain simple rules of living—with special emphasis on a diet that meets the highly individual needs of the body—your body. If such an assertion annoys you, *you are sick.* If you don't want to live, to explore the universe, then you are not a true representative of Homo sapiens, because an alert, intelligent curiosity made us what we are.

The research findings described in this book could and should revolutionize medical treatments now in vogue. They could and should revolutionize *your* thinking about yourself, since they show you what you can do to obtain buoyant, vibrant health. Or normal health—the terms are synonymous. And all this without much trouble. No weird concoctions, no fad diets, no incantations uttered in the dark of the moon. Just use of plain, uncommon sense and application of the findings of scientific research that have largely been ignored and/or distorted up to the present. (We are not addressing ourselves to readers with so-called common sense. Common sense tells us the earth is flat. The reader with common sense is too inclined to accept the claims of authority.)

Many things you are going to read in this book will shock you, will make you ask "How could it happen?"—conditioned as you

[1] Dr. Spies operated the Hillman Clinic in Birmingham, Alabama. He was honored for his contributions to our knowledge of nutrition.

are to believe that science and medicine, having performed many miracles for mankind, are incapable of choking off promising new approaches. The answer, alas, is one that has been repeated, for one reason or another, since the beginnings of science. It is seldom the researcher or the true scientist who represses the new information; mainly, it is the medical politicians who "speak for" the scientists. Today, a considerable part of medical and nutritional information has fallen into the hands of those who possess "authority" and are in almost full control of all the various communications media, but who, because of self-interest, envy, economic motives, and other considerations, cling to the old concepts long after they have been scientifically invalidated. Powerful as these opinion-makers may be, they cannot prevent all scientific research, nor can they prevent all publication dealing with it, in medical journals and elsewhere. What they *can* do, unfortunately, is withhold the benefits of the research, through official denial or failure to accept the results. They can bury the information—prevent its acceptance by the average doctor or nutritionist, and therefore prevent it from ever reaching you.

An excellent example of the process is the American Medical Association's attempt to discredit over-the-counter sales of vitamins. The theme is: We don't need extra vitamins; it is foolish to take vitamins without a doctor's prescription. Yet while this campaign continues, in almost any issue of any medical journal you will find corroboration of the fact that extra vitamins *are* essential in both the prevention and the treatment of disease. And in these journals you will also find four-color advertisements for vitamin supplements! [2]

There has always been a time lag between research findings and their beneficial application to the public. A good example: Although Dr. Alexander Fleming discovered penicillin in 1929, not until 1939, under the great pressure of World War II, was any

[2] Note: The doctrine seems to be: Vitamins are wonderful—on prescription only. Why not a prescription for enriched bread?

attempt made to utilize it. Yet the full implication that the antibiotic would destroy disease germs had been evident ten years before.

Most other great scientific researchers have not been as fortunate in obtaining recognition for their discoveries in ten short years, and in addition to the time lag there is often a deliberate campaign to suppress or discredit. Take the case of Dr. Ignaz Semmelweis, who was driven insane after a lifetime of trying to convince his fellow doctors that childbed fever—in his day a raging disease that destroyed the lives of countless women and newborn babies—could be obliterated by the simple expedient of the obstetrician's scrubbing his hands. It took ninety years for that concept to penetrate the minds of the orthodox—and all the while women and babies continued to go to their deaths. Even though Semmelweis proved his point by lowering the death rate in his own hospital ward by more than 90 per cent, few doctors in his time were willing to test his simple method.

Again, the discoverers of ether anesthesia were bitterly assailed by their medical confrères. And almost everyone has heard of Louis Pasteur's tribulations in trying to convince the medical fraternity that invisible germs were associated with many diseases and that in many cases a disease could be successfully treated by eliminating the germs. Some of the old medical hierarchy never really forgave the upstart chemist for proving his thesis so dramatically that a new hierarchy of medical thought had to be established.

Or take the case of Dr. Emil Grubbé, the founder of X-ray therapy. Although Dr. Grubbé first used the rays against cancer in January 1896, only a few weeks after their discovery by Roentgen it was thirty-seven years before they were accepted by the American College of Surgeons as a potent anticancer agent. During those thirty-seven years, Dr. Grubbé was hounded and threatened by organized medicine, who finally almost totally ignored the pioneering genius who first harnessed the mysterious rays in the treatment of man's most feared disease. Today, of course, X-ray treatment is universally employed—by the sons and grandsons of the men who bitterly fought Dr. Grubbé.

It was not until 1951 that the junior author of this book, after interviewing the aging doctor and examining all the records, published a magazine article about him. The article was picked up by the wire services and radio and television. The combined coverage forced the organized medical groups to recognize Dr. Grubbé and his work, and he was then properly lauded. Today you will find him extolled in the newer medical books, now suddenly recognized as a great medical pioneer and a martyr to science and humanity.

Contributing to the cultural lag that intervenes in science between discovery and application—a lag particularly marked in the field of medicine—is an ancient axiom of the physician: Be not the first by whom the new is tried, nor yet the last to lay the old aside. This cautiousness has been justified on the grounds that the untried holds too many unknown dangers for the patient. While it is easy to demonstrate numerous valuable discoveries that were allowed to gather dust while lives were lost because of this spirit of caution, it is not as easy to demonstrate that the application of this philosophy has saved lives: the medical journals are filled with disaster and death caused by side reactions of modern medication. Certainly, the orthodox in medicine, frequent to cite Jenner as an example of the pioneering research of the physician that has contributed to man's well-being, will find it difficult to justify the door that was slammed in Jenner's face by his medical society, which for years refused to hear his paper on the subject of the new vaccine treatment for smallpox. Their grounds? The "consensus" said that this was quackery. Likewise, no axiom will justify the abuse heaped on Berger, whose invention of the electroencephalograph machine was denounced as electronic quackery that had no place in medicine. Inventors of steamboat and submarine had equal difficulty being accepted. It takes twenty-five years to persuade a farmer to accept a practice that will actually increase his income. This is human, and not strictly a medical problem. But the scientific training and the asserted altruism of the medical men should hasten their acceptance of the new, despite their "fear of harming the patient."

And so on. The process of ignoring or ridiculing the pioneers of science and medicine still exists in our day of highly organized mass communication; its force, as we shall see in this book, has become even more dictatorial. Today, therefore, it is harder than ever to win acceptance for a new concept or treatment that runs against the accepted viewpoint. Natural reluctance of man to change, arrogance of those in power who wish to maintain their power, pure malice toward those possessed of greater insight: These are some of the reasons. Scientists are not gods. They are men, and all their scientific training unfortunately does not condition out of them the old basic desires and drives of a creature fairly recently emerged from the caves.

Let us not leave out the economic motive. In nutrition, it plays a large part in widening the "cultural lag."

We want to spare you the spectacle of the tired old medical drama being replayed at length. For, by the time you come to the end of the drama (when you find the research in this book being officially accepted and practiced by your family physician), you may find that the point of no return has come for you.

In short, our purpose in publishing this book is to help as many people as possible NOW. We also hope—and are pretty well convinced—that the people we do aid will henceforward see through the veneer of the propaganda that today sometimes passes for medical science, and will help us establish a world built upon real truth-seeking, real science, devoid of any base pressures or motivations that obscure and deter the search.

2. So you think you are healthy

Do you believe this statement: "We Americans are the best-fed and therefore the healthiest people on the face of the earth, and while we do have some remaining medical problems, they do not compare with those of the poor, benighted natives of lesser countries, who in most cases die before reaching their fortieth year"?

It would be no disgrace to believe this, since in one form or another the message is constantly being presented to us. Like most sophisticated propaganda, it contains a small element of truth husked over by a very large amount of subtle untruths and half-truths. Interestingly enough, this propaganda admits that good nutrition *is* the key to good health and longevity.

It is true that two thirds of the world's population is underfed, suffers from infectious diseases, and dies early. But, in speaking of health, why should we be compared to peoples whose condition bears little if any resemblance to our own? Most of us do not die young of malnutrition or infectious diseases, but does this automatically mean that we are well fed and in good health? If you wish to compare a somewhat sick man with a dying man, then the analogy will serve. It will not serve if you know what will make the sick man well and refuse to prescribe it.

And if you do not believe that we are sick as a nation,[1] let us

[1] An examination of 1000 average Americans, ages 15 to 60, for 24 defects and disorders, revealed nearly 900 such deviations from health!

consider the well-publicized figures of the many prominent groups organized to "fight" our various sicknesses:

About sixteen million of us suffer from heart diseases—our Number One Killer, so-called.

Almost a million of us are under treatment for cancer—our most dreaded disease, with one out of four predicted to have it.

Eight million of us are arthritics. Some authorities say more, but let us take the conservative figure. Many of us are so badly crippled we have to spend our agonizing days and nights in bed, not even able to hobble around temporarily, as some can after cortisone injections.

Consider the diabetics—three million, though half do not yet know they have the disease. Chances are one in four, say the medical statisticians, that any one of us will become a victim. The same odds as are given for getting cancer.

And there are nearly three million Americans under treatment for mental diseases. Mental patients occupy about half the hospital beds in the country. And of course we all know about the numbers of persons who walk our streets but should be under treatment. The fact is suddenly and tragically apparent when innocent persons are brutally murdered by someone who is obviously insane and often has just been discharged from a mental hospital.

Let us continue our look at the woes afflicting the allegedly healthiest nation in the world. (The following statistics are from organized medical-publicity groups.)

Cerebral palsy accounts for 600,000. Multiple sclerosis for 250,-000. Muscular dystrophy for 200,000. Tuberculosis, which has been steadily declining since effective cures were found for it, still afflicts 400,000.

Five babies out of a hundred are born prematurely, and it has been estimated that one man out of six cannot father a child. One baby out of two hundred is born deformed, one out of a hundred is mentally retarded. There are many other lesser afflictions that one reads about, but perhaps with the major figures alone we have made our point. If you add up the known sick Americans and add to that number those who are half sick and therefore go unreported in the statistical evidence, you will realize that we Americans are not exactly the glossy, four-color picture of bursting, radiant health the magazine advertisements constantly portray.

Some medical authorities will say of these alarming statistics that most of the diseases mentioned are those of old age—heart diseases, cancer, and the like—and that it is natural for a person to die of some cause brought on by old age. Such authorities will deny that this vast disease incidence has anything to do with nutrition. "We were the first to observe that old people do not get proper nutrition," they will say. "The reason why we as a nation have so much cancer, heart disease, and so on, is because we are so healthy. That is, we live long enough to acquire the degenerative diseases."

At first this seems sound reasoning. But in fact, our life span has not actually increased very much when we recognize that the number of babies, children, and young adults who died by the million before the advent of antiseptic medicine and antibiotics now live, and live long enough to raise the total statistic of the "average" man. Any life-insurance actuary will tell you that we have not really increased the life span for adults now living; we have merely increased the *number* of those reaching seventy or beyond. This does not affect us as adults. In point of fact, the life expectancy has not materially been increased for adults forty-five years of age or older. A comparison of the life expectancies of a sixty-year-old man in the year 1850 and a sixty-year-old in the year 1960[2] will yield the reader a surprise.

Despite the medical authorities' assertions to the contrary, the so-called degenerative diseases are reaching steadily downward toward youth for their victims. Cancer, an "old-age" disease, is now a top killer of school children, according to the American Cancer Society. Heart and vascular diseases are taking a steadily

[2] Available from the actuarial statistics of the Metropolitan Life Insurance Company, New York.

increasing toll among the young. When the bodies of young Korean war casualties were autopsied, more than 90 per cent showed degenerative changes in their blood vessels sufficient to warrant predictions of forthcoming heart troubles—and these young men were the best the United States could send in her defense. They were the youngest and presumably the healthiest specimens of American manhood. They should not have had definite clogging of the arteries (arteriosclerosis and atherosclerosis) at age twenty-one and under.

Hard to explain away is the fact that nearly half the young men in the country today cannot pass the rather lax physical examination necessary for entry into the armed forces—even before a large proportion of the accepted men later showed these unmistakable signs of "old age." And today we see arthritis, considered another old-age disease, striking at younger and younger ages. The proved sterility of *young* persons can hardly be due to old-age degeneration.[3]

Now let us see how this incredible state of affairs may have come about.

When, decades ago, Sylvester Graham (originator of Graham Crackers) denounced the bread sold by Boston bakers, the outraged merchants made an unsuccessful attempt to hang Sylvester from the nearest lamp post. (Attack the man, not his ideas!) This tactic, which has been described as propping up the issue but not illuminating it, has its modern counterpart. Federal agencies join with trade organizations of the baking industry and others, in setting up a syllogism: "American bread is fine, nutritious bread. There is nothing wrong with it. Therefore, anyone who criticizes it has base motives, is misled and deluded, or is a food faddist." Perhaps hanging would be a more merciful technique to use upon the scientist who is attempting an objective appraisal of the American diet, for "faddism" is nearly an unanswerable charge. Be-

[3] Nor can their increased height be used to endorse modern food. It preceded modern nutrition, and has most markedly been influenced by the height of immigrants coming to America.

cause this book will find fault with the American diet, and very great fault with American bread, this discussion of faddism is necessary at the outset. It must be remembered that many of the pioneers in science were, by any definition, "faddists" when they made their initial contributions. We have seen this in the preceding chapter and we shall see more of it as we go along.

This deliberate use of social pressure against the educator in nutrition who refuses to carol "This is the best of all possible diets" in chorus with the vast army of home economists and dietitians brings to bear a powerful force.

In a pyschology classroom, some years ago, all members of the class but one were made aware of the conditions of an experiment that was being carried on. In the experiment, students were shown cards on which were straight lines of varying lengths. On the board, other lines had been chalked. The students were asked to select the line on the card corresponding most closely in length to one on the blackboard. The forewarned students deliberately selected a line unmistakably shorter. The one uninformed student, the "goat," at first made the correct selection. However, faced with the social pressure of the adverse vote of all other students in the classroom, the "goat" was observed to change his decision, and, denying the evidence of his own eyesight, to vote in favor of the erroneous line selected by the others.

It is this type of pressure that is inherent in the term "faddism" in nutrition. The same unrelenting pressure is applied to the innocent who select whole wheat bread, which 94 per cent of the public resolutely avoid. The user of vitamin concentrates is crushed under the term "hypochondriac." It is important that these opinion-forming devices be recognized for what they are. They are an expression of the popular belief that "190 million Americans can't be wrong." Make no mistake: There are faddists in nutrition, just as there are faddists in psychology, medicine, or any other field. There are those who have promised the public an extended life-span with practically eternal youth by the simple consumption of wheat germ smeared with blackstrap molasses. There are numerous gentry in and out of the professions who promise dietary cures for cancer and a hundred other diseases. Distinction should be made between the incompetent, on the one hand, and the scientists whose findings deviate from the comfortable conclusions of the complacent majority.

You, the reader, however, should learn to recognize when the accusation of faddism is a propaganda ploy rather than a scientific dissent. For instance, you will be called a food faddist if you end a meal with fruit which will give your gums and teeth cleansing and exercise; if you end with a sticky, gummy, gooey concoction of tooth-and-gum-destroying overprocessed starch and sugar, you are normal. If you drink vegetable juice, you are a faddist. If you rot your teeth with sugar-saturated cola drinks with the acidity of vinegar, you are normal. If you take vitamin supplements prophylactically, you are a faddist. If you are normal, you will wait until you are sick—and then take them by injection.

To use the general good health of Americans as an assurance of the adequacy of American diet is to ignore two important facts:

1. There has never been a large-scale survey of American diet which, by any standard whatsoever, has revealed us to be generally well fed. This includes surveys made by the very agencies that attest the worth of our diet by the triumphant announcement of our superb health.

2. There has never been a survey of American health that has revealed us to be a truly healthy people.

Apropos of diet surveys: years ago, the senior author undertook a study in depth of the dietary habits of his radio listeners as compared with those of a similar group selected at random from the general population. The listeners comprised a cross section of the American public, with two distinctive aspects. These were people interested in nturition (or they would not have been listening to broadcasts on nutrition); and they proved to be people who made an attempt to put into practice that to which they were listening.

As might have been anticipated, the listeners had a much better diet than the nonlisteners. Unanticipated, though, was the finding that the listeners' vitamin intake was better than that of the non-listeners' only by virtue of the more comprehensive use of vitamin concentrates and special purpose foods as supplements to the diet. When the values contributed by the concentrates were removed from the diet assays, the listeners' intake was about equal to the nonlisteners'. This occurred in a group of people conscious of food values, unusually selective in shopping for food and preparing menus, and unusually aware of the penalties for vitamin deficiency. What shall we say, then, about the dietary conduct of the general population?

In an experiment performed some years ago at the University of Pennsylvania Medical School, expectant mothers were divided into two groups of more than 1,000 each. One group was given personal instruction in nutrition, and also received vitamin supplements. The other did not receive this instruction and used supplements, if at all, on their own volition. In the instructed group there were fewer than a dozen premature births; in the uninstructed group the incidence of prematurity was five per cent, which is the American national average. In the properly nourished group, the incidence was 80 per cent lower than our national rate.

What shall we say about the adequacy of American diet in the face of all this specific evidence to the contrary? Since we are neither well nourished nor buoyantly healthy, it is more than time that we take an objective look at what we are eating and what it is doing to us. For that "look" we need a perspective that will carry us back more than two thousand centuries.

Man has not always eaten as he now does. Inconceivable as it may be, there was a time when the morning breaking of the night-long fast did not begin with a cereal snapping or crackling at the unwary eater. As a matter of fact, though the sugar-saturated public considers carbohydrates to be essential for energy, it is obvious that these were generously available to man only when he invented agriculture. Twenty-five thousand years ago—perhaps the date of the earliest agricultural artifacts—rice was nonexistent; wheat was a wild grass, inedible for man; corn, rye, and buckwheat were unexplored possibilities for the menu. Sugar, in the concentrated form in which we use it today, was unknown. To see man as he ate then, one need look only at the Eskimo of half a century ago. The diet of the huntsman and the herder did not and could not include bread, cake, macaroni, spaghetti, sugar, and other concentrated starches and sugars.

Probably man wearied of wandering with his flocks in search of their food, and so decided to plant grass to feed them. Our modern cereal foods come from this cultivated grass, and, like the man who ate the first oyster, the herder who decided to consume the grasses he had planted for his animals must have felt himself a truly courageous pioneer. His adventure must have been induced by simple arithmetic. It requires pounds of grain to produce a few ounces of animal meat. The portion that requires months of feeding to create satisfies a solitary human belly for just a few hours. The pounds of grain that helped to create it would fill many bellies.

Man is still exploring the consequences of this original dietary experiment. Its course is unpredictable. Are these concentrated carbohydrates suitable food for a creature who evolved largely on protein and fat, the present-day diet of many Eskimos? No one knows. One great man in the world of nutrition, E. V. McCollum, said: "We are engaged in the largest mass experiment in an untried system of diet, with unpredictable results, in the history of man."

So the American who consumes his "typical American meal," which is 50 per cent concentrated starch and sugar, is in the true sense of the word a faddist.

However, the experiment does not lie alone in the increasing consumption of carbohydrates. It is the form in which they come to the table that raises grave questions. The first tentative nibbling of starches was followed by centuries in which the principal food of the poor was bread. The comparatively recent introduction of sugar saw this sugar change from a rare, costly flavoring agent into a staple of the diet, now consumed in such unbelievable quantities that the average American is in effect eating a teaspoonful of sugar every 35 or 40 minutes, 24 hours a day, 365 days a year.

But there came a time when man could not rest content with feeding himself as he fed his animals. The Industrial Revolution brought with it the need for cheap nonperishable foods that could be safely stored to feed the ever-growing urban populations who were now no longer raising their own sustenance. How do you go about indefinitely storing foods, the values of which attract other forms of life: the fungus, the weevil, the mouse, the rat? There was a simple answer: remove from the food those factors which support life, and man's competitors will avoid it.

Techniques of processing were developed that did exactly this. The pure starch of the wheat was extracted. Some of the protein, much of the essential fatty acids, the minerals, the vitamins, and the hormone values were removed from this starch. To man went the starch; to farm animals, the life-sustaining factors. Incidentally, this was in keeping with the philosophy of a civilization that housed its farmers in ramshackle dwellings and its animals in immaculate barns.

Whether there were early voices raised in warning against the rising consumption of starch and sugar, we do not know. If there were, you can be sure that these Cassandras found themselves labeled faddists. There certainly were voices warning against the excessive processing of the cereal foods. In the 1850s a book was published entitled: *We Feed Our Hogs Better Than Our Children.* In 1950, an article with an identical title was published in a national magazine, in which, interestingly, appeared a large amount of advertising extolling the virtues of various types of these overprocessed cereals.

Now the experiment took full form: Man's diet became 50 per cent concentrated starch and sugar, practically all of which had been freed of the elements necessary to sustain life.

The warning voices belabored the milling and baking industries, pointing out that the loss of minerals alone in processed foodstuffs was a serious threat to human well-being. The industries did not bother to debate the point, but simply labeled the critics as quacks and faddists. (Attack the man, not his ideas! It works almost every time, though, unless one is familiar with the history of science, one doesn't expect it from scientists.)

Then, in 1912, vitamin B was discovered and named by Casimir Funk, and soon after it was recognized that the loss of vitamins in our bread, rice, and cereals was important. The milling industry reacted by pointing out, during a congressional hearing in Washington in the 1920s, that what is removed from a loaf of bread can be restored to the diet by a "teaspoonful of beef gravy."

Today, forty-five years later, the industry is boasting about the benefits to public health achieved by consumption of bread to which *a few* of the nutrients have been restored. Gone is the day when the public was told to count on a teaspoonful of beef gravy to replace deficits created by the processing machines. Gone are the cries of *"Faddist!"* against those who earlier had deplored the removal of these very nutrients from the bread. Today, the industry is busy defending itself against a new, small but potent group of critics who point out that the restoration of the lost nutrients is inadequate, that perhaps twenty factors are removed from bread and only three or five are restored. The industry, of course, has its time-honored method of dealing with such gadflies. They are—again—faddists.

Now let us consider the true food faddist: the average American sitting down at his table to consume a diet untried in the early history of man, from which, so far, can positively be traced the loss of his teeth. Many volumes have been dedicated to the proposition that moderately poor nutrition creates moderately poor health, and that the individual who is neither sick nor well may be eating a diet neither truly bad nor truly good. Were this our only thesis, this book would still have been worth the writing and reading, for the average person little understands the subtlety of the sabotage of personality and physiology by diets that fill the belly and starve the body. But drastic and specific effects of poor nutrition have not heretofore received proper examination by the public at large. Let us now begin to consider them.

The sugar industry is in a more fortunate position. It does not have to defend the inadequate restoration of nutrients removed from sugar—for one principal reason: Sugar does not contain many nutrients to begin with. Since sugar is a well-known cause of tooth decay, and reductions in tooth decay at least as good as those claimed for fluoridation can be effected by reducing the sugar intake, the naive sometimes wonder why there is so much pressure behind fluoridation. The explanation is simple: manufacturers of overprocessed breads, cakes, cookies, pies, flour, candy, and sugar long ago decided that the best defense is an offense. Instead of attempting to defend these foods against charges of their undeniable action in causing tooth decay, they promote the cause of fluoridation, which then becomes a license to continue eating foods which ostensibly will no longer attack the teeth but which continue to contribute to bad nutrition for the body. Ironically, these carbohydrates are a factor in periodontal disease— that group of disorders from pyorrhea to resorption of the jawbone—which cause more loss of teeth than tooth decay. That is why we have emphasized in this book the point that, thanks to fluorides, the teeth which loosen and fall out are more free of decay, even if cosmetically marred by fluorosis. The last—fluoride induced discoloration of teeth—is visible evidence of the interference with an enzyme process by this, one of the most potent enzyme inhibitors, so that "slight fluorosis" may be interpreted as "slight poisoning"—which appears in at least 15 per cent of the children raised in a fluoridated area. Whether or not the "slight" poisoning will be exhibited seems to depend on a constitutional factor, research indicating that the effect of fluoride on at least one important human enzyme is constitutionally determined—susceptibility ranging from marked, in one body type, to moderate to zero, in others.

Fluoridation, as rammed down the throats of millions of Americans, willy-nilly, therefore represents enforced conformity inflicted on bodies which (unfortunately for some) do not always enzymatically confirm the safety of the measure.

3. "My grandfather did all right without vitamins"

The ways of resistance to learning are subtle. Seldom in the fields of nutrition and medicine do we need the outright opposition of the old man who said that in his long lifetime he had seen many changes, and he had been "agin every one of 'em."

To realize why resistance to education in nutrition is a real but intangible entity with which every nutritionist must cope, consider the hazards peculiar to the dietitian's profession. The patient does not tell his physician how to write a prescription or instruct his dentist in the techniques of filling, capping, and crowning. But he meets a book on dietetics with an expression of distaste and pounds his fist upon it as he informs the dietitian that his grandfather lived to age ninety without the benefit of vitamin therapy and consideration of protein need.

Does he consider the nutritionist less qualified for his task than the medical man for his? We feel that the explanation is more simple: everyone eats, and so qualifies as an authority on eating. Then here comes this upstart nutritionist attempting to tell me—who have eaten forty thousand meals—how I *should* eat! The reasoning is reminiscent of that of the farmer who booted an agent of the Department of Agriculture off his premises, snorting indignantly: "He's going to tell *me* how to farm—me who has wore out *four* farms?"

Since you have read this far you obviously and happily aren't in this category.

Now let us consider objectively some of the many influences that shape our diet—and note the absence of an intelligent rationale for the selection of our food. Generally speaking, consideration of the needs of the body is always far secondary to the esthetic, cultural, and other conditioning influences that determine the content of the "average" housewife's market basket.

The strongest influence in a married man's diet will be the suggestions given to his bride, who sometimes specifically seeks them from her husband's mother. These influences are shaped by cultural considerations: Ants in an American picnic sandwich certainly mean a discarded sandwich and may mean an attack of nausea; in other parts of the world, ants are a staple and nutritious part of the human diet.

Religious influences also mold the diets of many: Millions of people would rather die than eat your breakfast bacon. Others will not touch the flesh of the cow. The Catholic and Hebrew dietary taboos need little comment, though the senior author has had many spirited debates with rabbis who cheerfully grant that the sick Jew may eat anything considered therapeutically necessary, but may not use these same foods to remain well.

Ethnic biases affect food selection probably even more than religious influences. The dietitian is familiar with the Italian family whose slender food budget does not permit sufficient milk for the children—although favorite Italian cheeses are regularly purchased at high prices.

Advertising conditioning also determines food selection to a formidable degree, a fact that will be denied by many people; but look at one of the many proofs: Remembering that concentrated sugar was unknown to the ancients (and relatively rare until our own century), consider the potency of the effect of advertising on someone who firmly believes that "sugar is necessary for energy." (Our teachers, indoctrinated, repeat this as axiomatic to our children.)

Since we have already given a hearing to the argument of the long-lived grandfather, let us face the corollary: Millions of men who might have been healthy grandfathers never reached that age.

Another typical rejection of rational food selection is heard in this statement: "I have eaten anything that would not bite back—and I have never been to a dentist, a physician, or a hospital." The serious nutritionist's reply is threefold:

1. What is the actual state of well-being of the individual who makes such a statement? Is he the uncomplaining sort who regards sinus trouble, post-nasal drip, frequent colds and sore throats, allergies, indigestion, constipation, neuritis, myositis, possibly a "touch of arthritis," as passable good health?

2. To what extent does this freedom from the need for professional attention imply that such an individual has skated on thin ice through the decades and never paused long enough to bring enough pressure to fall through?

3. What is the possibility that the speaker is one of those exasperating individuals who by virtue of heredity—the wise selection of vigorous forefathers—has come into the world from a "good" egg and so with some impunity can defy the fundamental principles of good nutrition? And, incidentally, thereby set a very poor example for us "bad" eggs, us "normal" eggs?

Other forms of resistance to nutrition education mimic the philosophy of the processing industries. They attack—as always—the man instead of the issue. The nutritionist may hear this kind of remark: "If you are such an expert in diet, why do you wear glasses?" Interestingly enough, this type of approach is not used with the medical man, who is permitted to have his attack of coronary thrombosis in peace and quiet, or the dentist, who can quietly wear his bridgework.

In part, the nutritionist is considered open to such attack because of the antics of cultists and faddists who have been willing to promise the public immunity from all defects and all illnesses if only they will nourish themselves perfectly—that is, according to the special rules of the particular cult.

The dietitian of the nineteenth century carefully compiled a "diet for arthritis" on the premise that arthritis is a disease with the same impact on all patients, who are essentially the same people. The same was true for diabetes and a host of other afflictions. Unfortunately, these concepts and diets have spilled over into our century.

Today some of us recognize that there exists not only the influence of a disease on a patient, but also the patient's influence on the disease. These influences create a unique problem in each instance, and no common denominator can be found that makes rational the endless duplication of irrational diets. In fact, an *ad hoc* committee appointed by the American Medical Association Council on Foods reported that *all* restricted diets prescribed for gastrointestinal disease are irrational. Their good effects, if any, they implied, come from ceremonial therapy (the power of suggestion). Moreover, the committee added, these diets cannot be made rational until we know more about the action of individual foods in the digestive tract. This confession of ignorance is refreshing when one considers that it is made by an organization constantly taking the position that its pronouncements on nutrition are definitive and authoritative, and dissenters thereby automatically food faddists.

Meanwhile, hundreds of thousands of patients emerge each year from physicians' offices with the very diets that the committee reported to be irrational. These are diets that accomplish nothing therapeutic for the patient's condition, but do invoke restrictions that may very well create dietary deficiencies. Very few diseases are helped by bad nutrition.

We can also extend this concept to the individual who is well. Human beings are all unique, to the extent that grafting so simple a tissue as skin from one individual to another—even from mother to child—is likely to provoke a violent rejection by the recipient of what is essentially alien tissue. The saliva of brothers and sisters is not alike; and the public is now aware of some of the hazards encountered in blood transfusions even when the blood is "matched."

Under these circumstances, it should not be surprising that no two individuals have the same dietary needs, quantitatively or qualitatively. Each of us comes into the world with unique nutritional needs, and it is quite possible for one to starve qualitatively on a diet that is perfectly adequate for another.

It is likewise possible that the diet adequate for you at a given time will be wholly inadequate under other circumstances. For example, a woman in her fifth month of pregnancy experiences heartburn. Her physician relieves it with injections of riboflavin (vitamin B_2). "Why did I need the vitamin?" she asks. "I am eating as well now as I was when I began pregnancy—and before." The answer is simple: The baby, in the fifth month, is drawing more heavily on the mother's reserves. Her own needs have increased, too. It is possible that the mother's diet was actually inadequate in riboflavin before pregnancy, but she was getting by.

This returns us to one of the questions asked of the individual who boasts that he has been free of the need for doctors through a lifetime of planless (and probably poor) eating. Was he fortunate in being born with an efficient physical organism whose nutritional requirements were easily met? Did he manage to escape conditioning factors that would raise his requirement beyond the level provided by his diet? And was he not fortunate in escaping any one of the common operations where the shock of anesthesia, blood loss, pre- and post-operative starvation (a technique now fortunately being discarded) would have raised his nutritional requirements and revealed his hidden weaknesses?

In the thousands of scientific reports that cross the desk of any professional man, there will be many, unfortunately, whose implications will be lost without careful study. Consider the observation made in a Southern hospital, where a baby's convulsions could be relieved only by the continued administration of quantities of pyridoxine (vitamin B_6) larger than those needed by most babies, well or sick. Investigation showed that the mother had suffered severely with pregnancy nausea. Unable to retain food, she aggravated a vitamin B_6 deficiency, which is likely to occur in most pregnant women, for there seems to be a universal disturbance in the utilization of this vitamin in the early months of pregnancy. So it may be that this caused her baby to come into the world the product of a uterine life in which a nutrient was not supplied in sufficient quantity. And the baby reacted with an inordinate and continuing need for the nutrient. Not enough vitamin B_6 was available; hence the convulsions, which can cause mental retardation.

A century ago, a baby might not have had a vitamin B_6 deficiency since mothers then fed babies in the old-fashioned way, and breast milk is a good source of the vitamin in a utilizable form. Should we dismiss the modern emphasis on dietetics by remarking that the baby of yesteryear grew up healthy in a period which knew nothing about vitamin B_6? Or shall we say that because grandfather lived a long lifetime without a great many advantages we should discard the advantages and knowledge the intervening time has made available to us?

There is another point involved. Does it not appear almost at once that the American pioneers were somewhat more vigorous stock then we are? Did they manage to survive their ignorance of hygiene and perhaps of proper nutrition by virtue of inherently greater stamina?

The point becomes a thesis: There is at work in us a subtly deteriorating influence—the American diet. When common versions of it are fed to animals, the stock indeed runs thin. The animals are plagued with the same illnesses which, afflicting humans, are responsible for the overcrowding of our medical offices and hospital wards. The animals become infertile, as we are infertile. They suffer with heart diseases and other "degenerative" afflictions. And the dietetic faults responsible for these debilitating influences on the animals are *not* recognized by the conventional authorities in human nutrition. But they are recognized by the authors, which is why you are reading this book. Further, we hope you still have your grandparent in perfect health, even though he may scoff at these "newfangled" ideas about eating. Let's face it, though: the risk is small in our expecting that you and your grandparents are well, if you are violating the concepts set forth in this book.

4. Heart Disease: What they don't tell you that may save your life

Approximately sixteen million of us are afflicted with some form of cardiovascular disease—disease of the heart itself and/or disorders of the circulatory system, the latter usually meaning ultimate involvement of the heart.

It is not the purpose of this book to offer conventional descriptions of heart diseases and conventional advice as to their treatment; we are principally interested here in showing how diseases can be prevented or treated by nutritional means. You will therefore not find the usual descriptions and cautions concerning the leading diseases—which you can obtain by the score from any magazine article or book on the subject—unless the disease can be prevented or treated by nutritional means, in which case the facts usually have been suppressed or ignored.

In this chapter, for instance, we will not spend time describing that wondrous organ that pumps many hundreds of gallons of blood through the circulatory system each day. Nor will we tell you to keep calm and not shovel snow. These points we assume you know or can easily learn any time the Heart Fund puts on a drive. Here we are interested only in what you (and your doctor) can do nutritionally to prevent cardiovascular disease.

As you probably know already, there are two major forms of disease of the blood vessels which lead to heart "failure." One is arteriosclerosis, a disease that causes the arteries to become brittle or like a pipestem and therefore easily broken. The second and much more common is atherosclerosis, in which the blood vessels become gradually choked up by a deposit of fatlike material and passage of the blood through them becomes a most laborious task —until finally the heart cannot manage the process. The heart is then said to "fail." Or, if a chunk of the fatlike material breaks off in the course of the blood's rushing through at high speed and high tension, it may form a dam or clot in the vessels that feed the heart itself. Then we have what is known as coronary thrombosis, the leading heart disease today, particularly among men, although women are by no means immune. It is believed that in the early process of atherosclerosis, the formerly smooth walls of the blood vessels become pitted with the fatty substance known as cholesterol (there's much more to it, though, as we shall see), and the break-off of some of this substance causes the thrombosis. It may also derive from a hemorrhage in the vessel walls. The tissue of the heart is fed by blood that moves through rather small vessels. When these are blocked, cutting the heart off from its nourishment, a certain amount of heart tissue dies. If the damage is too extensive, you do not recover. If you do, it is because you no longer have a clot or because your heart has managed to set up collateral circulation, which continues its nourishment even though the normal and main source may be partially blocked.

In practically all forms of heart disease there is a story so remarkable and so unbelievable that we hesitate to publish it in its entirety, because we realize what pressures will be put on you to keep you from believing it. What you are about to read is the history of vitamins in the treatment of heart disease—a history you are not likely to hear from the orthodox physician. His medical societies tell him, and he will tell you, that vitamin therapy for heart disease is practically worthless. He well knows that vitamin deficiency will cause heart disease in practically every animal subjected to test, but he has been marvelously persuaded that man is immune from this type of trouble originating in poor diet.

Before we begin our account, it should be remembered that

heart disease is too universal an ailment to be traced to a single cause, dietetic or any other. Failure of the heart is seen in vegetarian apes just as it is in meat-eating man and, all the assurances of the vegetarians to the contrary notwithstanding, there seems to be no particular diet that precludes failure of this organ—which begins its work even before it is fully formed in a developing baby and continues to the last breath of life.

However, in recent years, one study of coronary thrombosis—the incidence of which seems still to be rising—produced conclusions so diametrically opposed to current thinking that the paper on the subject appears to have been ignored only because it presented an ugly fact that seemed to contradict some very objective theories. You will recall that Dwight Eisenhower, among many other sufferers with coronary thrombosis, was treated with drugs intended to inhibit the clotting mechanism of the blood. This seems a logical approach, since the source of the difficulty obviously is the formation of a clot in the coronary artery, which feeds the heart. However, Dr. H. McGuire Doles asked himself an obvious question: Where does the clot come from? This question cannot be answered dogmatically in terms of vascular disease because coronary thrombosis has been known to occur in individuals who showed no signs of either arteriosclerosis or atherosclerosis. The physician, on the basis of information gained from autopsies, decided that the trouble in some patients originated with a hemorrhage within the wall of the coronary artery itself. Now, if one has a hemorrhage which is responsible for a clot, the problem can be attacked by dissolving the clot—which leaves us with the hope that the hemorrhage will stop—or one can approach the problem from the opposite direction, that of stopping the hemorrhage.

Orthodox medicine has chosen to attempt to dissolve the clot; Dr. Doles went back to the hemorrhage itself and tried to terminate it. He experimented with vitamin K—the blood-clotting vitamin.

Let's follow this experiment through: Two groups of patients with acute coronary attacks were given doses of vitamin K, a vitamin which is a direct antagonist of the substances with which thousands of coronary sufferers are regularly treated. The first group of patients was given small doses of vitamin K; the second group was given large doses. The mortality records of the two groups tell a significant story. In the group that received only small doses of vitamin K, the mortality rate was 38.5 per cent. In the group given large doses of vitamin K, the mortality rate was only 3.6 per cent. Stopping the hemorrhage apparently proved at least as fruitful as the orthodox attempts to dissolve the clot.

But even if the therapeutic results of vitamin K were no better than those of the anticlotting drugs, one would still have to vote in favor of the vitamin therapy for the simple reason that the anticlotting drugs are never safe. Even in a hospital, where frequent blood checks are practical, a patient who is being dosed with these substances may shift from a tendency toward excessive clotting to a tendency to hemorrhage within a matter of a few hours. If he is badly bruised, he may bleed to death.

The vote in favor of the vitamin therapy would also be weighted by another consideration. This invokes the authors' key axiom: "What nutrition cures, it ordinarily prevents." This would mean that the lifetime intake of vitamin K might become a formidable barrier toward hemorrhaging within the coronary artery and thereby act as the first line of defense against coronary thrombosis. Yet in spite of the evidence we have summarized, do you think vitamin-K therapy is in common usage for coronary thrombosis? No, indeed—dangerous drugs are still in common use. The vitamin K study has never received any attention.

But there is another story that is even more remarkable concerning the role of nutrition in the prevention and the treatment of heart disease. It is one that has probably never been told to the general public except in the broadcasts of the senior author.[1] This

1 And a book by Herbert Bailey, *Your Key to a Healthy Heart,* Chilton Company, Philadelphia.

is the story of vitamin E—a nutritional factor that has been neg-lected for several reasons, chief among which is the sex neurosis that prevails in this country.

The story of vitamin E becomes involved in a series of unbelievable points of confusion, beginning in the days when wheat-germ oil and vitamin E were considered synonymous. Actually they are not. Vitamin E is more richly provided by wheat-germ oil than by any other constituent of our food, but there are many other nutrients present in wheat-germ oil, including some hormone values. Nonetheless, at the beginning of nutrition research in this area, it was thought that *wheat-germ oil* and *vitamin E* were terms that could be interchanged.

Early experiments with wheat-germ oil were directed at investigation of its role in supporting fertility; it was found that animals deprived of the factors in wheat-germ oil became infertile, or at least their reproductive efficiency dropped. This action was attributed to the vitamin E in the wheat-germ oil, and the two substances, as we noted, were therefore considered identical. Subsequent researchers attempted to reproduce the results obtained in the early experiments; they used vitamin E. These investigators recorded triumphantly that the early experimenters who had used wheat-germ oil were obviously in error, since their results had not been duplicated with the use of vitamin E. Nevertheless, enough "information" had already leaked to the public for vitamin E to become linked with sex.

Out of such a scientific comedy of errors, our government agencies—also reflecting the sex neurosis—decided that manufacturers who made any particular claims for either vitamin E or wheat-germ oil would be attempting to capitalize upon the sexual implications of these "identical" substances.

Therefore, for a period of years vitamin E was known in this country as an antisterility factor. Ironically enough, while vitamins have a great deal to do with the ability of the male to father normal babies and a great deal to do with the ability of mothers to weather pregnancy without spontaneous miscarriage, stillbirth, and abortion, there is no particularly good reason for labeling vitamin E a sex factor, nor for calling it an antisterility factor. Yet it is now in the scientific books as such, and there it will probably remain for a long time. (The chemical name for vitamin E, tocopherol, means "child bearing.")

There was still another hazard vitamin E encountered in the course of its career in the field of nutrition. This one was based upon the peculiar reaction of the medical man to acceptance of the idea that a food chemical may conceivably be used in the treatment of a disease that he does not consider to be caused by deficiency.

It is interesting that the medical man is perfectly willing to accept the fact that digitalis, derived from the herb foxglove, is useful in the treatment of heart disease, but in the next breath he will deny the possibility that a vitamin might be at least helpful, if not equally beneficial. However, surrounding vitamins is an atmosphere that leads physicians to say, when pressed by patients on the point, "Well, you can take them; they can't do you any harm."

Let us now see how irrational is such an approach to the subject of vitamins, particularly vitamin E, in the treatment of heart disease; and let us see what we can learn in terms of prevention.

It has long been known by biochemists that vitamin E is involved in the processes—almost miraculous as they are—by which the heart derives energy from food. The actual chemistry has been set up at least on a hypothetical basis. The body produces a substance called adenylic acid, which has an affinity for phosphorus. The body then proceeds to form from adenylic acid three phosphorus compounds. These compounds are somewhat analogous to the phosphorus compounds formerly used in the manufacture of matches. Like the head of a match, they carry within them potential energy. The heart, by breaking down these phosphorus compounds, releases this latent energy, obtains the fuel it needs and proceeds to rebuild the compound. Some biochemists theorized that it is impossible for these phosphorus compounds to be manufactured from the adenylic acid unless two vitamins are present,

One of these is vitamin E; the other is inositol, a B-complex substance.

Understanding of the chemistry of vitamin E in the function of the heart muscle—which functions, of course, like any other muscle of the body—permits the conclusion that a vitamin-E deficiency obviously would interfere in many ways with the functioning of that organ.

Recent research has shown that there is a compound which seems to be involved in the very fundamentals of electron transport in the cells. This is called "ubiquinone." A spokesman for the American Medical Association said that an understanding of the functioning of this compound would probably give us a key to a great many degenerative diseases, including heart disease. His announcement carefully left out the observation that had been reported in the original research:[2] that vitamin E appears to be requisite to the formation of the ubiquinone compound. Such recognition would have collided head-on with the policy of downgrading the importance of vitamins—particularly the importance of a vitamin which, with the benign approval of the American Medical Association, the National Research Council, and the United States Food and Drug Administration is removed from the foods which comprise 50 per cent of the calories in the average diet: our starches and sugars (And anyone critical of this is by definition a faddist).

Therefore it is not surprising that just a few hours spent examining the literature of nutrition research reveals that vitamin-E deficiency has been found to cause various abnormalities of heart function—some of them resulting in death—in *every* mammalian species subjected to the test of a deficient diet. These disturbances have ranged from low voltage, revealed by the electrocardiogram in monkeys, to myocarditis (inflammation of the muscle of the heart wall) in cows.

Nevertheless, the attitude of American medicine, or at least of

[2] There is now a large body of papers on the subject of the ubiquinones. See *Proc. Soc. Biol. and Med.; Nutrition Reviews; Chemical Abstracts.*

the agency representing it, indicated that vitamin-E deficiency is not related to human heart disease, and from this it followed that vitamin-E treatment could be of no possible benefit in human heart disease. (This, incidentally, is a *non sequitur*. Digitalis is not given to correct a digitalis deficiency. Vitamin E—and many other nutrients—are often used to treat disorders *not* caused by poor diet.)

When confronted with evidence of favorable response to vitamin E therapy in thousands of cases of human heart disease, the comment of the American Medical Association was: "This is a reaction to ceremonial therapy!" This is a dignified way of indicating that sufferers with heart disease can feel better and their electrocardiograms can reveal a change toward the normal merely on the basis of the power of suggestion. If indeed this were a routine response to suggestion, it certainly would call for a throughgoing training in psychiatry for every cardiologist. Actually, suggestion may alter response to pain, but not an abnormal electrocardiogram.

However, the concept of vitamin E for useful treatment in heart disease did not begin with consideration for its chemistry in the heart muscle. True, that chemistry has been explored to the point where it can be said, as we previously noted, that the formation of the high-energy phosphorus compounds from which the heart derives its enormous energy is postulated to be possible *only* if vitamin E and inositol (both of which are removed from modern white bread and cereals) are present.

The theoretical chemistry, however, has been traced beyond this. It is supposed that somewhere in the intestinal tract, by virtue of enzyme action, vitamin E and inositol combine to form a new compound: an ether-condensation conjugate (jawbreaker, but bear with us). The failure of the body to manufacture this compound, incidentally, was once believed to be responsible for muscle dystrophy. The speculation is not too farfetched, not only because many diseases are known to result from the breakdown of enzyme chemistry in the body, but also because similar degenerative diseases of the muscles do develop in human beings and animals deprived of vitamin E.

But back to vitamin E and heart disease. Two Canadian physicians, William E. Shute and Evan V. Shute, observed that vitamin-E therapy seemed to give some benefits for bursitis. It happened that one of the patients with bursitis to whom vitamin E was given also had an attack of coronary thrombosis that had left him with angina—the painful disorder that signals the inability of the heart, because of damage or inadequate circulation, to meet the demands made upon it.

Dr. William E. Shute was surprised to find that the vitamin-E treatment had vastly increased the tolerance of the patient's heart to exercise and that his attacks of anginal pain were therefore reduced in frequency, severity, and duration.

Yet in spite of the fact that well over twenty thousand Canadian patients have been treated with vitamin E for heart disease, the Shutes' papers[3] on the subject have never been accepted by any major United States medical journal. This state of affairs—inasmuch as their papers have been published in other lands—might reasonably be called a conspiracy of silence.

Well, it is possible that the Canadian physicians may have deluded themselves, and it is theoretically possible that the improved electrocardiograms were altered by the power of suggestion—that the patients improved, not because of the vitamin therapy but because of their confidence in the treatment or in the physician administering it. To this the senior author replies that he has seen changes in the electrocardiogram toward the normal in human heart disease expedited as a response to vitamin E in cases in which the patient did not know he was being treated with the vitamin.

We have used the phrase *conspiracy of silence*. A favorite device of the cultist and the quack is the accusation that the medical

---

[3] See Bibliography, Vitamin E, National Vitamin Foundation, New York City, 1940-1960, also *Your Key to a Healthy Heart* by Herbert Bailey, Chilton Company, Philadelphia.

profession, on whom we rely for recovery from sickness, is con-
spiring for reasons of profit to deprive us of more helpful means.
This is nonsense. The conspiracy of silence does not originate with
the rank and file of practicing physicians. It stems from their sub-
servience to the medical opinion expressed by an official bureauc-
racy, ordinarily the only intermediary between the MD and the
public.

The fact is that the American Medical Association currently de-
nies the usefulness of vitamin E in heart disease and implements
this only by ignoring the evidence, which does not rest alone on
the work of the Shutes, but on hundreds of confirming reports.
This fact became apparent to the senior author in an interesting
incident that occurred in his office some ten years ago. There
came a knock at the door and a chubby little man sought entrance. He identified himself as a retired physician, occupied in
writing to earn a living. His retirement from medical practice had
been forced by a coronary thrombosis attack that left him with
angina so severe that merely walking from a warm room to the
cold outdoors, with the added burden that the change in temperature inflicted on the heart, was enough to bring on an attack. He
said that he had heard the author was aware of nutritional therapy that had been beneficial in angina. The files were turned over
to him; on the basis of what he read, the physician made an effort
to help himself with nutritional therapy involving large doses of
vitamin E accompanied by inositol (for the reasons we have seen)
and the entire vitamin-B complex in concentrated form.

The physician later wrote us three or four letters, the last of
which is as good an appraisal of the usefulness of vitamin-E therapy in human heart disease as any statement yet made. He said,
"My wife stopped me last night as I was running upstairs to remind me that I had heart disease!"

It was about a year later that a home medical advice book was
sent to the senior author for review. The book was edited by a
former high official of the AMA. In it was a chapter on heart disease, and one of its authors was the chubby little doctor who had

retired from practice because of his heart attack. The payoff? *Not one word in that chapter* hinted at the possibility that nutrition in any way is important to the sufferer from heart disease! Conspiracy of Silence, or concession to official dogma, or fear?

Another example: In the senior author's presence one spring day in 1955 a temperamental man collapsed with an attack of angina after an argument. This is no light matter: Hunter, who first described angina, remarked that any idiot could kill a sufferer by making him lose his temper.

This sufferer was under grave emotional stress because he had that day forgotten to take with him the nitroglycerin he used, as do most angina patients, to help restore circulation and eliminate the agonizing pain of the attacks.

The author called a physician who, forewarned, came with a supply of nitroglycerin tablets; after a little while the victim was feeling much better. At that point, the author asked whether his cardiologist had ever suggested that he supplement his diet with vitamins or use vitamin E therapeutically.

The patient replied in the negative, as might have been expected. It developed that his medical man was well known to us. With the patient's permission we called him, and with the doctor's consent the patient was placed on a regime of some hundreds of milligrams of vitamin E daily, accompanied by generous amounts of inositol and vitamin-B complex.

During the course of this therapy, begun in 1955, the patient has used nitroglycerin on only two occasions. One may evaluate his progress by comparison with his previous record: he had averaged five to seven nitroglycerins *a day*. Confronted with the necessity of climbing a flight of stairs, he took a nitroglycerin before starting, went up slowly with frequent rest, then took another before achieving the next landing.

When the patient asked his cardiologist to comment on his improvement, the medical man replied: "You are one of two in five patients with angina who responds to vitamin E." Said the patient with some bitterness, "How would you know? You routinely fail to give it to five in every five!"

Case histories could be given by the thousand, but let us examine the observations made by a German cardiologist[4] who spent a number of years studying both the objective and subjective effects of vitamin-E therapy on his heart patients.

It is difficult to evaluate a response when a patient says he feels better or that he has had fewer attacks. This is called subjective response. But is it easy at various times to measure exercise tolerance, evaluate cardiac reserve, and compare electrocardiograms. This cardiologist became so expert in reading electrocardiograms that he could distinguish between a patient given digitalis and a patient given vitamin E. He emerged from his research with the concept that the vitamin is indeed valuable in the treatment of certain types of heart disease, while in others it is not fully as valuable as the Canadian researchers suggested, but still helpful enough to warrant its routine administration.

An evaluation was made of the vitamin-E level in the blood and heart tissue in patients suffering from heart disease; similar evaluations were made from autopsies of persons who had died of cardiovascular disease. To the surprise of no competent nutritionist, low values of vitamin E were frequently encountered. But then, low values in other vitamins were also encountered—which brings up two very important observations:

First, not infrequently the sufferer with heart disease is placed on a restricted diet. There is the so-called low-salt diet, which is distinguished by the fact that good nutrition is most difficult when the sodium content is brought down to 2 grams a day. But nutrition becomes almost hopeless if the sodium content of the diet is brought to the level really effective—0.5 gram a day. Low values of vitamins in the heart muscles could therefore be a product of the "therapeutic" diet on which the patient has been placed. It likewise could be the result of a lifetime's deficiency—or a chronic

4 Dr. Wolfgang Seligmann, personal report to C.F.

deficiency of long enough duration to make the tissues less able to utilize the nutrients involved.

Such chronic deficiency is not at all unlikely, not only because of the bland diet with which many patients with heart disease are tortured, but also because the use of diuretics is customary in at least one type of heart disease, and any increase of the output of fluid is likely to result in a deficiency of the water-soluble vitamins. When increased output of these vitamins is superimposed on deficiency of intake, because of a diet inadequate owing to the restrictions upon the choice of foods, it is scarcely astonishing that there are cases of beriberi heart disease occurring in this country, in defiance of the eulogies of the adequacy of the American diet that we hear from the United States Food and Drug Administration, the American Medical Association, and similar agencies.

The second observation has to do with a vitamin already mentioned that is important to the human heart—and one which is also removed from the bread eaten by the public. This is vitamin B_6 (pyridoxine). There is an interesting story to be told about this vitamin—one that involves our old enemies, silence and adverse propaganda.

The bread industry will spend millions to defend its demonstrably inferior product and only thousands to improve it. Part of their defense is an offense in which critics are labeled cultists or faddists. This name-calling, however, does not originate with the industry itself. Some bread and flour manufacturers, for example, are clever enough to enlist the services of professors of nutrition at various universities.

Hence, we find Fredrick Stare, Professor of Nutrition at the Harvard University School of Public Health, stating that there are no significant differences between whole-wheat bread and white bread.

Of course, the statement that there are no *significant* differences between whole wheat bread and white bread does not mean that there are *no* differences, nor that the differences are not of great magnitude. The Professor of Nutrition at Harvard University

School of Public Health is as adept in employing deceptive phrases as he implies are the advertising gentry of Madison Avenue. The phrase "no significant differences" means that the professor anticipates that what is missing from white bread, and present in whole wheat—or more adequately supplied by the latter—will in the "average diet" (hopefully) be supplied by other foods. Unfortunately, the public accepts this statement of "no significant differences" as meaning that enriched white bread and whole wheat are nutritionally equal. They are not. In fact, Borsook[5] recently suggested what the senior author proposed twenty years ago—that the inadequacy of enriched white bread in vitamin B_6 must be rectified by adding vitamin B_6 to the enrichment vitamins. Whole wheat bread has about four times as much of this vitamin factor.

The senior author wrote to Stare, out of curiosity, to ask if he theoretically ignored the facts that (1) whole wheat is a good source of vitamin B_6 while white flour is not, and (2) vitamin B_6 deficiency has been found to be damaging to the efficiency of the human heart. Dr. Stare replied that he would very much like to see any scientific evidence from any reputable source to indicate that deficiency in vitamin B_6 harms the human heart. To this the senior author replied that such a report had been carried in *Science Service,* a publication widely known by both scientists and laymen. It dealt with the loss of efficiency of the hearts of ducks placed on a diet low in vitamin B_6. To forestall the inevitable comment that this research involved ducks rather than humans, he also pointed out that the author of the report specifically drew from this experiment definite implications for the human heart. The source? Harvard University. The report was signed by Fredrick Stare.

We think it relevant to point out here that this man, whose public eulogies of overprocessed flour always identify him as a Harvard University Professor of Nutrition, also wears another hat.

[5] Dr. Henry Borsook, a pioneer nutrition researcher who helped to develop the M.P.F. program, at a symposium on nutrition.

He is one of the editors of *Nutrition Reviews*, published by the Nutrition Foundation, which is subsidized by General Mills, Pillsbury, and other major producers of white-flour and other highly processed products.[6]

Interestingly enough, the white-flour industry has been growing a little sensitive to pressures such as those indicated here, and is now talking about adding pyridoxine to the enrichment program.

For many years the authorities have refused to recognize vitamin E as a nutritional requirement of the human being. Through those years many nutritionists, including the senior author, have prophesied that this arbitrary attitude would ultimately change, because the evidence indicating the vital role of vitamin E in human metabolism was mounting too high to be ignored.

The FDA *had* embarrassed the industry by recognizing the human requirement for vitamin B_6. The evidence was too overwhelming. This naturally made the industry uncomfortable, because it was busy insisting that what is not restored in enrichment is not essential to human beings. Now, vitamin B_6, the content of which in white flour is very much lower that that of whole wheat, suddenly received an official blessing that made its absence from the enrichment tablet conspicuous. It is still absent.

It is noteworthy that our press time for *Food Facts and Fallacies* coincided almost exactly with recognition by the U.S. Pharmacopeia of a substantial human need for vitamin E, implemented by including generous amounts of vitamin E in their recommendation for a "standard" multiple vitamin capsule.

Official recognition of the human need for vitamin E was even more embarrassing (bread should be one of our good stable sources of the vitamin, and white bread is not), for what is not removed in the milling of the flour is largely destroyed in the bleaching.

The FDA's recognition of vitamin E was a grudging conces-

[6] Oddly enough, this organization, which fought the Delaney bill to give FDA control of food additives and derided Rachel Carson, is depicted as a source of scientifically impeccable, commercially untainted, and objective information. (The publicity denouncing Rachel Carson was paid for by the pesticide industry.)

sion, we gather, from the explanation and warning that accompanied the official announcement. It said, in effect: "Despite the fact that vitamin E has been recognized to be required by human beings, deficiency in it is impossible, because it is contained in such a wide variety of easily available foods." This, of course, is completely misleading. But it comforted the white bread and cereal industries.

For instance, vitamin K is available in dozens of easily obtained foods, and yet thousands of babies died during or after birth because of hemorrhages attributable to vitamin-K deficiency. If deficiency in a vitamin is impossible when it is widely available, why then does the obstetrician almost routinely administer small amounts of vitamin K to pregnant women?

The mischief of the official statement goes beyond this. It is quite true that vitamin E in many forms is available in a large number of foods. It is, however, also true that only one form of vitamin E is truly potent and active in the human organism. That form, alpha tocopherol, is *not* found richly in a wide variety of foods. The grains are the best source when not degerminated—which they regularly are—and wheat is the best of the grains as a source of this potent form of the vitamin.

However, when you eat fruits and vegetables harvested prematurely and ripened in transport; when your grains, cereals, and flours are degerminated—as 94 per cent of them are—it is difficult to obtain truly protective amounts of vitamin E (alpha tocopherol). Therefore, it is our advice that vitamin E should be added to the diet in supplementary form each day. Deficiency in this vitamin is easy to incur, and the diet may be more universally inadequate in this factor than in any other single vitamin, with the possible exception of vitamin B_6—national deficiency of which has been postulated; and vitamin D, which is therefore widely added to common foods. The recent medical obsession with polyunsaturated fat, which is an excellent example of faddism at the medical level of the type that the medical man condemns in the public (for there is not yet significant evidence to support this obsession), may have caused a great deal of vitamin E deficiency because the only popular vegetable oil supplying enough vitamin E to offset the antivitamin-E action of the polyunsaturated fats is cottonseed oil. It is quite possible to cause vitamin-E deficiency by an excessive intake of polyunsaturated fat, if the fat does not supply enough of the vitamin in the active form, and many fats do not. In fact, at least one death (in a sick baby being fed large quantities of polyunsaturated fat) has been directly attributed to vitamin-E deficiency caused in this manner.

The junior author can bear personal testimony to vitamin E's efficacy in heart disorders. Several years ago he suffered a heart block with congestive heart failure resulting from overexertion. He was told by his physician (a personal friend and an excellent practitioner) that he had had a very close call and that absolute bed rest for a period of weeks would be essential in addition to the usual drugs, digitalis and nitroglycerin.

While in bed, he happened to tune in the senior author's broadcasts. On one of them the role of vitamin E in heart disease was discussed. Although a medical writer for many years, he was unaware of vitamin E in this relation. (So was his doctor, proving again the close blackout of official medical information.)

The junior author obtained a medical book by Drs. William and Evan Shute and other cardiac specialists.[7] He became more convinced by the evidence contained therein, and began large doses of vitamin E. His improvement was so rapid as to be amazing. Soon he was chopping wood and digging clams again (his favorite leisure pursuits) without a sign of his heart "failure." Today, as souvenirs, he still has part of his original supply of nitroglycerin and digitalis.

In any discussion of heart disease, the subject of cholesterol invariably comes up. A few years ago, when it was fashionable to blame cholesterol for hardening of the arteries, some doctors were writing and saying: "If you don't want to drop dead from heart failure, don't eat eggs or animal fat." While there are doctors who

[7] *Alpha Tocopherol (Vitamin E) in Cardiovascular Disease.* Ryerson Press, 299 Queen St. West, Toronto, Canada.

still parrot this line, research doctors and official medicine today display much more caution.

In the first place, it is now recognized that cholesterol is a vitally needed substance and that if the body doesn't get enough of it, it will manufacture its own. But it now has been found that if the body has enough of the substances called phospholipids, they act in dynamic equilibrium with cholesterol to maintain the integrity of each cell. (The phospholipids have many other functions as well.)

Eggs contain both cholesterol and its antagonistic-yet-synergistic phospholipid partner, lecithin, in abundant amounts; therefore, never let anyone persuade you not to eat them. Eggs are probably the most nutritious staple food available to man. (Milk is second.)

The medical profession is probably just as guilty of faddism as the wildest of those it denounces. But few indeed are the medical voices raised in protest when the profession itself pursues senseless fads. A classic example of such medical faddism in nutrition is the flood of dietary attacks on hardening of the arteries recommended by medical men during the past few years.

The whole tale of the effort to control hardening of the arteries and heart disease by regulating the cholesterol content of the blood through restriction of the diet represents a typical example of the medical penchant for negative dietetics and linear thinking. The full meaning of these terms will become painfully apparent as we explore the picture of cholesterol and fat in hardening of the arteries—as envisioned by the medical profession.

Our story begins with the observation that cholesterol clogs our human plumbing. To this problem the profession applied its standard thinking: "If thine eye offend thee, pluck it out"—if cholesterol is deposited in hardened arteries, get rid of it by the simple expedient of avoiding the foods that contain it. As we have already noted, this method ignores the fact that cholesterol is both essential to life and manufactured within the body. Likewise ignored is the fact that the electron microscope has taught us that the initial invader of the artery wall may not be cholesterol but an abnormal sugar-protein molecule. It is on a plaque of these abnormal molecules that cholesterol begins to deposit. However, eager to find and indict a culprit for heart disease, the medical profession ignored the evidence and rushed advocacy to the low-cholesterol diet (no eggs, butter, milk, and countless other valuable foods). Meanwhile, heart disease continued to take its toll.

The medical profession has had other unhappy experiences with negative dietetics, for instance, in its diet for diabetics in the pre-insulin days. The oversimplified approach here said: Diabetics do not properly metabolize sugars and starches, therefore feed them only fat and protein. The simple theory encountered the ugly reality that the diabetic cannot get along without metabolizing sugar and starch, and insisted upon going into coma and dying for want of the insulin effect on carbohydrate metabolism.

The proposal to avoid cholesterol in the diet ignores both the fact that we cannot live without a supply of it, and the fact that the stuff is impossible to exclude without the risk of arriving at a nutrition so poor it may not support life long enough to allow the arteries to harden! And the proposal is made despite the fact that nobody has yet proved that a reduction of the cholesterol in the blood offers any protection whatsoever against hardening of the arteries. How silly can you get? Persons with normal blood cholesterol can and do develop hardening of the arteries and heart disease, while those with high cholesterol may—and often do—escape. In any event, a reduction in blood cholesterol does not mean a reduction in tissue cholesterol—and if the substance should be harmful, the tissue content is quite as meaningful as the blood content.

Those obsessed with the avoidance theory have assembled formidable supportive evidence. They cite the relative freedom from hardening of the arteries and heart disease in countries where the diet is low in cholesterol, and the opposite picture in countries where it is high. To do this effectively, however, they must ignore both the countries where cholesterol in the diet is low and yet heart disease and hardening of the arteries are major problems and the countries where the diet is high in the factor but circulatory and heart troubles represent no great problem.

If the memory of the public were not short, there would be a wave of popular indignation against the professional men who have so dogmatically espoused the low-cholesterol diet. Factually, those most responsible have shifted their positions diametrically in the last six or seven years. They began with the low-cholesterol or no-cholesterol diet. When this thesis was shot full of holes, the medical men reversed themselves and announced that cholesterol is not itself the mischief-maker, unless it is accompanied by too much fat. But it was apparent that there are cultures where cholesterol is accompanied by a great deal of fat and yet the people are not unduly troubled with hardening of the arteries and heart disease. In his book *Cancer: Disease of Civilization?* the noted explorer and anthropologist Vilhjalmur Stefansson presents convincing evidence that heart disease, cancer, diabetes, and tooth decay are all diseases of modern civilization and were unknown among the Eskimos until their contamination with the white man's food around 1900—and are still unknown among certain remote peoples. The Eskimos eat large amounts of animal fats and were, until recently, free of our top killers.

Weighing such evidence, the medical men reversed themselves again. It is not the cholesterol, they announced; it is not the amount of fat; it is the *kind* of fat accompanying the cholesterol that determined whether or not it will make trouble. Vegetable fats, they say now—with the same dogmatic authority that marked the earlier pronouncements—are protective; animal fats are dangerous. What an amazing collection of contradictory assertions! Are we entitled to reject them as unsupported dogma? Let us see by examining a particular case.

The director of the nutrition department of the Board of Health in a major city, after research with a low-cholesterol diet on seven patients for a period of about six months, made headlines from coast to coast with the suggestion that American women should stop killing their husbands by feeding them eggs. If he *had* been justified on the basis of adequate scientific documentation—which of course could not have been obtained with so small a sample in so short a period of time—did he have the moral right to release such a pronouncement to the public? The same investigator subsequently published a paper on a long-term observation of a group of patients on a diet with a high content of the vegetable type of fat. Although he is enthusiastic about the virtues of this new procedure, it is a matter of scientific fact that the drop in blood cholesterol which he cites is so small as to be without significance even if it should be proved that lower blood cholesterol really offers some protection against cardiovascular disorders.

Now let us examine some more of the complex facts surrounding cholesterol. Cholesterol in the blood rises when the body is under stress. This suggests the possibility that the elevated level performs some kind of protective function. Such a protective function in dogs in fact was reported about ten years ago in the *Bulletin* of Mt. Sinai Hospital in New York City—a report that, predictably, is certain to be ignored by those who are obsessed with the campaign against cholesterol.

A beautiful example of ugly facts ignored because they contradicted beautiful theory is found in the story of Rosetta, Pennsylvania. Here is a community of Italians, many of them overweight, all of them laden with fats taken in high-calorie diets, replete with saturated fat and cholesterol, where the incidence of heart disease in men is so low that Rosetta is perhaps the only community in the United States where there are as many widowers as there are widows. The happy population of Rosetta is being solemnly studied by medical men, and the whole thing studiously ignored by physicians busy prescribing low cholesterol and low animal fat diets. Note: When these Rosetta men move to other cities, they lose their immunity!

The rest of the story is a sorry recital of contradictions ignored, dangers treated contumaciously, and opposing evidence contemptuously brushed to one side. The patent fact of hale-and-hearty eighty-year-olds who have eaten freely of butter and eggs throughout their lives is ignored.[8] So are the implications of the experiment that started this whole scientific circus. A researcher fed cholesterol to rabbits, which then developed hardening of the arteries. Three important observations must be made about this experiment:

1. Rabbits, being vegetarian animals, do not eat cholesterol and are apparently not able to handle it. (Vegetarians, both animal and human, may indeed develop hardening of the arteries, even though their cholesterol-free diets are solely supplied with vegetable fats.)

2. The condition the rabbits developed resembled, but was not the same as, hardening of the human arteries.

3. The *quantity* of cholesterol fed the animals was tremendous, the equivalent of what a human being would receive by eating fifty eggs a day.

The reasonable conclusions, as one considers this experiment, are: Rabbits should not eat the equivalent of fifty eggs a day, and neither should human beings.

At the height of the low-cholesterol fad, a physician wrote to the *Journal* of the American Medical Association suggesting seriously that the public be instructed to boil all its food for four hours. We wondered why he omitted suggesting that the diet then be dipped into a solvent to extract the last milligram of cholesterol.

Another physician wrote to the senior author, who of course had continued to include eggs as part of the pattern of good nutrition in his broadcasts, demanding to know: "Why are you trying to murder the public?"

Here we ought to take a good look at eggs, which, being rich in cholesterol, became an early target of this medical faddism. It happens that eggs are rich in the very type of fat which, we are now told, prevents cholesterol from working the mischief it is supposed (but not proved) to create in the arteries. Eggs are also

[8] At least we know where they obtained their Vitamin A—sans supplements.

rich in choline, inositol, pyridoxine, and lecithin. These factors have been used successfully in the medical treatment of hardening of the arteries. Therefore, the deletion of eggs from the diet deprives the eater of the cholesterol-controlling factors but not of his supply of cholesterol—because it is contained in many other foods and, as we have noted, it is synthesized within the body itself.

Even the objections to butter are not justified. If cholesterol were proved to be the mischief-maker, if animal fat were proved to be the co-acting factor, no one would have the right to ban butter from the diet on the ground that a pound of it contains about 1200 milligrams of cholesterol. Normal human beings do not eat butter by the pound but by the pat, and a pat contains only 17 milligrams of cholesterol.

When the emphasis on cholesterol shifted to emphasis on the amount of fat in the diet, and then to the kind of fat, an interesting syllogism was offered to justify this kaleidoscopic change of emphasis. The anticholesterol men set up the thesis that we are eating more fat than our ancestors ate, particularly more saturated fat. (At the risk of oversimplification, the terms *saturated* and *hydrogenated* are considered to be equivalent to animal fats as opposed to vegetable fats.) They pointed to the introduction of the hydrogenated shortenings to justify the statement that we are eating more saturated fats. Since we are allegedly having more trouble with hardening of the arteries and heart disease than did our ancestors, they could now arrive at their Q.E.D.: Increase in fat intake, particularly saturated fats, has created this cardiovascular Sword of Damocles. The only trouble with the syllogism is the complete falsity of the premise and the inconsistencies of the conclusion. First of all, we do not know that we are having *more* cases of heart disease and hardening of the arteries than did our ancestors. Even in the limited number of cases today in which autopsies are actually performed, we have learned that 15 per cent of our death certificates reflect an error in diagnosis of the cause of death. How much more erroneous were the diagnoses in the past? Second, we do not know that we are eating more fat of any kind than our ancestors did. In point of fact, a glance at an old-time menu will indicate that our forefathers were very much less concerned with calories than are we—and indulged themselves in sauces, gravies, and pastries laden with fat on a scale that modern girdles and insurance companies forbid to us. The supposed rise in consumption of the type of saturated fat attributed to the introduction of hydrogenated shortenings is likewise a myth, for these have simply been substituted for similar fats of animal origin previously used. As a matter of fact, we cannot even accurately estimate the amount of fat the American public eats. We can estimate the fat content in the amount of meat we know the public *buys*, but we certainly do not know whether your wife trims her lamb chops or cooks them as they come from the butcher.

The current drive, calmly presented as absolute fact by those who until a short time ago presented opposing theories, is toward a completely unjustified and possibly dangerous substitution of vegetable fat for animal fat in the diet. This might result in a housewife's deciding to use, let us say, peanut oil in place of butter or margarine in her frying recipes. But no one has yet bothered to tell the public that when seeds are soaked in peanut oil, their genes and chromosomes are affected, causing mutations. This is a phenomenon that may need to be investigated in terms of possible cancer-causing activity on the part of this oil. The medical men who are busy prescribing pills filled with concentrated vegetable fat, recommending margarine, in which this type of fat has not been fully hydrogenated, and extolling substitution of vegetable oils for animal fats in the over-all diet seem now to be blissfully unaware of what they learned in biochemistry: that fats are stored in the cells of the body. There they can grow "rancid," not in the exact sense of the term but exact enough to produce the damage that rancidity causes. Vegetable fats are prone to rancidity, and when there are rancid fats in the cells, the human body can develop a vitamin E deficiency that can start a collagen disease for which medicine will have little explanation and as little valid

treatment as it does for arteriosclerosis. The only common vegetable oils self-protected by an adequate content of vitamin E are
cottonseed [9] and wheat-germ oil.

Survey the picture now. Here are Eskimos, filled with both
types of fats and cholesterol, and certainly having no more difficulty with hardening of the arteries and heart disease than we do.
Here are Thailanders, filled with cholesterol and animal fat, and
suffering far less difficulty with arteriosclerosis and heart disease
than the Japanese—who are not eating much cholesterol and are
addicted to vegetable fats. Here is a disease supposedly attributable to cholesterol in the diet but which develops in purely vegetarian animals that have never tasted cholesterol. How do we inject
the vitamin called uncommon sense into this saturnalia of emotion
and prejudice masquerading as objective thinking? And how do
we give our professional people enough moral stamina for them to
withstand the social pressure of the bandwagon tendency in science? Let the professional man remember these eight points:

1. Correlation does not guarantee causation. Example of this
fact, which any Ph.D. had to recognize or he would not have obtained his degree: A physician notes that all his women patients
over sixty walk pigeon-toed. Is he entitled to write a paper on a
phenomenon, a change in stance exhibited only in older women?
He is not so entitled. One likely cause might be that these women
were educated at a time when such a position of the feet in walking was regarded as "proper" for women.

Second example: A statistician notes that whenever feminine
fashion calls for short skirts, we often have a business depression.
Are we allowed to conjecture that short skirts distract the busi-
nessman's attention from the proper operation of his business? Or
shall we deal with the possibility that in times of depression a
reduction in the amount of material in a skirt enables a manufacturer to reduce the retail price to meet the needs of a financially
depressed feminine public?

[9] Margarine made from cottonseed oil would therefore be preferable. The
preferred cooking and salad oil would be cottonseed.

Third example: High blood cholesterol is found in some but not all cases of hardened arteries. Are we entitled to cite this as cause and effect?

2. It has been shown that blood cholesterol rises, even in the presence of a low-cholesterol diet rich or poor in vegetable fats, if the individual is placed under tension.

3. We must remember that cholesterol in the tissues is quite as much or as little a consideration as cholesterol in the blood. A drop in blood cholesterol does not necessarily mean a tissue drop. Further, the thyroid gland to a goodly extent controls blood cholesterol and influences tissue cholesterol. The efficacy of old-fashioned cod-liver oil in reducing blood cholesterol has been traced, not to its unsaturated fatty acid content but to the iodine it supplies to the thyroid gland. Since an underactive thyroid will raise the blood cholesterol, it should also be remembered that a chronic mild deficiency of vitamin B_1—so easily possible in a sugar-saturated public—can cause thyroid underactivity and consequent elevation of blood cholesterol.

4. There is ineluctable evidence that exercise plays a role. The Dutch[10] ride bicycles rather than drive cars. The Dutch are full of animal fat and cholesterol, but they are not full of hardened arteries and heart disease. On the other hand, exercise is no panacea—some athletes develop these disorders, and laborers statistically die younger than white collar workers.

5. Some attention should be paid to the factors in the diet that help us metabolize fats, including cholesterol. For instance, cholesterol intake has little effect on the arteries of monkeys unless they are deprived of vitamin B_6. Consider the fact that vitamin B_6 and lipotropic factors such as lecithin, which help us to utilize fats, are removed from white bread and not restored. Remember that the foods rich in fat and cholesterol are very often rich in the

10 While Dr. Paul Dudley White popularizes the bicycle, as a leading exponent of the role of exercise in reducing blood cholesterol, any life insurance actuary can tell you that blacksmiths and others engaged in occupations which call for increased physical activity tend to die younger than the more sedentary members of the male population.

"antidotes"—for example, eggs, with their high content of the very factors recommended for possible prevention and treatment of hardening of the arteries.

6. It is impossible to eliminate cholesterol from the diet, even if it eventually is demonstrated that such an elimination is desirable and beneficial. The body is of course able to convert vegetable fat into the animal type and can make cholesterol from starch, sugar, and any kind of fat. Further, the body can manufacture fat from sugar—women's hips testify to this. Moreover, the kind of fat manufactured from sugar is the saturated animal type. If, therefore, any usefulness is ever found, without danger, for a rise in the intake of the vegetable type of fat, it will become necessary for us to restrict sharply our sugar intake. Incidentally, while we cannot corroborate the theory that we are eating more fats than our ancestors did, we are definitely eating more sugar. Moreover, there are several papers which indicate that the kind and amounts of starch and sugar in the diet may be more relevant to the problem of hardening of the arteries than is the quantity of the chemistry of fats.

7. It is a little inconsistent to place the responsibility for hardening of the arteries primarily upon the diet, when husband and wife share the same breakfast and dinner menus, and yet arteriosclerosis and coronary thrombosis are by a considerable margin more the husband's problem. Surely the medical man should not ignore the fact that surgical sterilization of women significantly increases their incidence of hardening of the arteries. In short, the female ovary, like the thyroid gland, is very much part of the picture of diet versus hardening of the arteries. It is interesting that Vitamin E has certain effects resembling those of the estrogenic hormone.

8. And finally, if animal fat, cholesterol, and tension promote arteriosclerosis, and exercise is an effective antidote, what are we supposed to conclude from a study of hard-working Trappist monks, abstaining from all animal fats except milk and minute amounts of cheese; living a placid, frugal, life in their monastery

—and yet showing more cardiovascular degeneration and arterial hypertension than men of the same age in the general population?

After almost a decade of watching medical mental gymnastics in dealing with diet versus hardening of the arteries, the senior author has been driven to the conclusion that while the American diet requires a great deal of change, there is no justification whatever for arbitrary exclusion of good foods from the dining table, in the hope of evading or mitigating hardening of the arteries. Moreover, there is some reason to believe that the nutrients supplied by some high-cholesterol foods such as liver, eggs, and others, may be quite important in that effort. They are certainly important to well-being. Avoiding over eating would be the only sane conclusion.

5. Conception: Why so many sterile marriages?

Any diet should be judged by the answers to three basic questions:

1. Will it support reproduction?
2. Will it support growth?
3. Will it support maintenance of the adult organism and a normal life span?

All three questions must be answered, for it is entirely possible that a selection of food will meet two of these requirements and fail to satisfy the third.

When these criteria are applied to the ordinary American diet today, we are in trouble immediately, for the American diet does *not* support efficient reproduction. You may find this hard to believe, in view of the number of baby carriages that crowd our parks, but by being impressed with the number of women who can have babies, you are in much the position of the drunkard who, with Limburger cheese on his mustache, is able confidently to state that the entire world is malodorous. What you are not evaluating is the number of homes with a climate of heartbreak because conception cannot be achieved or healthy babies born. It is estimated that one conception in every four does not result in a live baby.

Yet medical help for the infertile is still woefully deficient. The first question the veterinarian will ask the owner of an infertile animal concerns its diet. This is too seldom asked of the human would-be mother. If her problem appears to be the birth of defective children, aside from a more-or-less cursory inspection of the husband's sperm little attention is paid to the possibility that the husband's nutrition and well-being—or lack of them—may be a factor. The popular medical treatment of the infertile woman currently revolves around dosages of hormones, usually administered without regard to the couple's nutritional status. We may liken this to fertilizing a field without regard to the quality of seed to be sown.

Aside from the obvious contribution to medical diffidence about nutrition that comes from the absence of this kind of instruction in the medical curriculum, the professional man's failure to consider his patient's nutrition as a possible contribution to her infertility rests upon his acceptance of the biological "all-or-nothing" concept. This likens the role of diet in fertility to the functioning of the common light switch: You may turn the light on or off, but you cannot halt midway for lessened illumination; it is all or nothing.

So, for many years, the medical view of diet in fertility could have been expressed in these simple terms: Either a diet is good enough to support reproduction or it will cause complete sterility. In this concept, there can be no twilight zone of nutrition, where the diet may be good enough to pemit conception but still poor enough to bring about infertility, miscarriage, spontaneous abortion, stillbirth, or a defective baby. This conviction was furthered by a widely read book, the work of a United Nations investigator, who pointed out that the birth rate is highest in countries where the diet is poorest. This amounts to arguing that to achieve fertility one should eat garbage, and is a type of thinking that ignores two highly relevant points. In the nations thus underprivileged in diet, intercourse is one of the few inexpensive pastimes available, and the law of averages will permit many conceptions, with a goodly number (if a low percentage) of survivals. After all, the ability to procreate once a year is all that is necessary. Second, the more relevant, the organism tends to adapt to consistently poor nutrition, and the undernourished populations develop a smaller body, thereby conserving limited nutritional resources that are directed toward the reproductive processes.

But in the United States (and these statements might well be applied to the civilized world generally) we are not lacking in quantity of food, and the human organism has therefore not been forced to adapt in size. Indeed, the more abundant quantity of food produces a more abundant quantity of body—through not necessarily a more healthy one.

But do we have evidence that the type of therapy applied by the veterinarian to the infertile cow is deserved by the infertile woman? Do we have evidence that mothers who have known spontaneous abortion, miscarriage, stillbirth, prematurity, and the birth of defective babies might have avoided a sizable percentage of these events if they had been fed as intelligently as our thoroughbred horses and pedigreed dogs? Do we have evidence that a father's diet before conception has any influence on the baby? The answer to all these questions is *yes*.

You will recall the experiment described in Chapter 2 which showed that properly nourished women will bear 80 per cent fewer premature babies than the American average. Since nutritional deficiencies and prematurities are well correlated, it is useful here to remember that the premature baby is handicapped. To what extent he catches up with a full-term infant is still a subject of debate among progressive pediatricians. The Biblical axiom might be rewritten: *The nutritional sins of the mother set the children's teeth on edge.*

However, let us not delay facing the most bitter problem: The lament of the woman who has never been able to achieve conception—the woman who has been given the battery of tests and examinations, who has undergone surgery for a retroversed uterus, who has been plied with hormones (one of them suspected of contributing to cancer). Since there is a 50 per cent chance in an infertile marriage that the problem originates with the husband, her husband's sperm may also have been examined. It is estimated that 16 per cent of men up to the age of twenty-five—the most fertile group—are infertile, and the expectation of infertility rises beyond that age.

After years of fruitless endeavor our typically "infertile" wife submits to artificial insemination, which, if it originates with a donor other than her husband, plunges her into a twilight zone of the law. It is a fact that divorce suits have been based on artificial insemination. At best, when it involves an unknown donor, the procedure places the woman in a precarious emotional relationship with her husband.

All this has failed, let us assume, and nowhere in her wanderings has our unhappy wife encountered anyone who has asked the simple question: "What do you eat?"

How significant is the question? The senior author has in his files a collection of Christmas cards that supplies the answer. They were sent him by a family with four children. The mother married at sixteen. At twenty-one she still had not achieved a successful pregnancy. Three conceptions aborted; no others eventuated. She had endured the gamut of endocrine therapy, "opening of the tubes," and uterine surgery—although of the latter her mother, a registered nurse, remarked: "I don't know—I have seen an awful lot of babies spill out of a tilted uterus."

The girl had had gray hair since age fifteen. This was regarded as a family trait; her mother had also been gray as a young girl. When the patient's doctor consulted the senior author, this early graying of the hair and the shape of the girl's palate suggested a pituitary gland possibly not functioning at full efficiency. The girl was placed on a high-protein, low-sugar, low-starch, medium-fat diet. A percentage of the fats were derived from vegetable oils rich in unsaturated fatty acids. The diet was supplemented with vitamin-mineral concentrates. Just as pituitary- and adrenal-stimulating factors had been emphasized in the diet, so were they emphasized in the supplements, with particular emphasis on para-amino-benzoic acid, pantothenic acid, and vitamin E. Probably the patient would have been amused to know that one of the supplements she was taking contained wheat-germ oil, which is used to stimulate fertility in animals.

The physician was instructed to watch the girl's hair for signs of recoloring. This was described not as a positive clue to a pituitary response, but a possible one. Recoloring of the gray hair appeared in due course, and when the process was well on its way, the patient was instructed again to attempt conception.

The result? The first Christmas card sent to the author showed a picture of the happy mother and father with their first baby. The fourth Christmas card, with a picture of four babies, carried a terse query from the proud husband: "How do you turn if off?"

At this point many an orthodox medical man will say "coincidence," or "spontaneous remission." Both are favorite terms in medicine. Typical comments would be: "How do you know that any of these vitamins played any role in this recovery from infertility? How do you know that babies would not have eventuated anyway, without nutritional treatment? How do you know that the previous hormone therapy did not bear delayed fruit?"

Let the skeptic go back in the literature to the work of Benjamin Sieve, M. D.,[1] a rare combination of endocrinologist and medical nutritionist. He gave para-amino-benzoic acid to a group of twenty-two infertile mothers, judged by five years or more of unsuccessful attempts at conception. Twelve of the group bore healthy babies within a period of two years! There are numerous other reports, of course, on stimulation of reproductive efficiency through improved nutrition.

One interesting point is that fact that Sieve gave a substance, paba, which is a constituent of all good foods containing vitamin-B complex, but which is processed out of most of our concentrated carbohydrates. A second point is the fact that our government agencies that regulate the advertising claims of food products

[1] *Vitamins and Hormones,* Vol. 2, Academic Press, 1944, p. 225.

stanchly refuse to admit that para-amino-benzoic acid is a vitamin[2] —this despite the fact that every human body contains the factor and notwithstanding the fact that it is a component of folic acid, which itself is recognized to be an essential vitamin.

What evidence have we to support the heretical belief that the father's diet prior to conception may influence the baby? That this *is* heresy is apparent when we realize that only comparatively recently has science accepted the folklore belief that the *mother's* diets affects the baby. You may think this is a well-established principle. Not so. Only in recent years has research shown that grading of the mother's diet will permit prophesies of the well-being or lack of it for the forthcoming baby. Obviously, then, when one postulates a relationship between the father's nutrition and the baby's welfare, the area entered is full of skepticism. Actually, only two investigations have yet been done on this subject, but they lend some credibility to the thesis.

One of these was an experiment by Dr. Weston Price,[3] in which he mated four female dogs with four males, all the dogs being in good health. The result was four litters of normal puppies. Then he placed the four male dogs on poor nutrition. Subsequent matings produced litters of sickly puppies with deformities of the type which, in human babies, have been described as birth defects. Interestingly when the sickly puppies were given good nutrition and later mated with the same females, their issue was entirely normal.

The other research project was conducted by Dr. W. E. Shute, of whom we have already spoken for his work with vitamin E. His subjects were a group of mothers who had previously borne defective babies one or more times. Any medical statistician will tell you that the chances of such a disaster for a first baby are about two in a hundred; but where there is a previous history of such

[2] Why regulatory agencies court the favor of our food processors is a subject to be explored by the senior author in a book now being written.
[3] *Nutrition and Physical Degeneration*, Weston Price, D.D.S., Lee Foundation.

babies in the family, the statistical odds against a normal baby increase astronomically.

Shute administered vitamin E to the fathers in these families prior to the next conceptions. According to ordinary medical statistics, there was an expectation of seventeen abnormal babies in this group of pregnancies. As it turned out, *there was only one.*

The possibility of such an improved record occurring by mere chance is remote. One does not have to work out research projects with mothers who have previously given birth to deformed babies, nor is one compelled to research the literature on dog-feeding to support the thesis that the repoductive efficiency of American women would be vastly improved if somebody paid attention to what they eat, not only during pregnancy but before. Part of the blame devolves on the mother herself. It is very easy to be critical of the obstetrician's failings, but it should be remembered that pregnancy is not the time to begin to repair the nutritional errors of a lifetime. The pregnant woman who attempts this is asking of her diet that it correct the effects of her past mistakes, fulfill the needs of her baby, and care for her own body at the same time. No diet can accomplish this much during the limited period of a pregnancy.

It is all very well for the authorities to say, as they do, that the "normal woman" (however they may be able to isolate one of these) does not need super amounts of nutrients in pregnancy, but such a generalization operates on the premise that we are dealing with healthy, well-fed women on whom pregnancy imposes but a slight extra nutritional burden. Such a generalization is more than reckless when drawn into it are girls barely out of a teenage of hot fudge sundaes, their teeth rotted by carbohydrates —starches and sugars—which in processing have lost their content of pituitary- and adrenal-supporting nutrients.

A view of the history of diet in pregnancy offers an interesting vantage point from which to appraise current "advances," and the smugness of the declaration that super nutrition is of no advantage to the pregnant woman or her baby. There was a time when "one child, one tooth" reflected the inadequacy of nutritional knowledge. There was a time when puffiness of the face and ankles—today regarded as the price for protein deficiency in pregnancy—was considered normal. To this day "stretch marks" are accepted as normal, despite the fact that these marks often appear before there has been any stretching and are often a sign of a pituitary-adrenal system not able to assume its proper load. And to this day, varicose veins are sometimes described as the price for the extra weight a pregnant woman carries, the presumable corollary being that, since all pregnant women carry extra weight, those who escape varicose veins are somehow abnormal. And the phrase "The baby's normal loss of weight after birth" reflects the enduring concept that babies must be born hydrated, so that in the first week of life the child will lose about one ounce for each pound of body weight.

The last observation brings us into the area of stress. Being born, some pediatricians say, is the greatest stress many of us will ever suffer. In response to this physiological pressure, the baby's adrenal glands produce large amounts of cortisone—and, just as large doses of cortisone often affect adults—the hormone carries sad effects for the baby, in the form of retention of fluid. Such a reaction is not normal, and reflects an inadequate capacity of the child's endocrine system to respond to the emergency. The first week's "normal" weight drop of half a pound is, of course, the loss of fluid in tissues hydrated by shock. The fact that this is really an abnormal situation is demonstrated by the thousands of babies who have emerged from pregnancies supported by supernutrition, with a generous supply of the gland-supporting nutrients. These babies, having no tissue load of water to eliminate, defy the textbooks by gaining at once.

The senior author's five children, born of two different mothers, are typical examples. Their weights remained constant for the first forty-eight hours, after which they proceeded to gain in the normal fashion. Moral: A pituitary-adrenal system that is properly formed and properly nourished is not driven into hyperactivity by stress—in this case the stress of birth.

If you are still inclined to underestimate the importance of the uterine nutritional environment, we might note that a doctorate thesis done at Columbia University a few years ago reported the finding that pregnancies nourished with an adequate supply of vitamin B_1 produced babies with higher I.Q.'s than those with inadequate supplies of this vitamin.

In thousands of pregnancies followed by the senior author, where optimal nutrition (pregnancy diet with a generous cushion) was fed, few stretch marks have ever been reported, and varicose veins are a very infrequent complication. The drop in the incidence of varicosities is not a unique observation; more than twenty years ago our good friend, Dr. William Coda Martin, published the observation that pregnant women generously supplied with vitamin C were much less susceptible to varicose veins during and after pregnancy.[4] His paper supports the thesis that the difficulty arises not from the weight gain or the stress of pregnancy, but the superimposition of such factors on a blood vessel weakened by an inadequate diet. This is at least one contributory factor.

It is known that the output of female hormone in pregnancy is high, and that this hormone affects the blood vessels. It has been established by Dr. Morton Biskind that a well-balanced diet helps the mother to control the activity of this hormone. (Thus, nutrition may well become a weapon against those types of malignancies in women that are believed to arise from excessive activity of, or excessive sensitivity to, female hormone.)

It is probable that elevation of the output of this hormone during pregnancy bears directly upon the problem of varicose veins. Since the output can be controlled nutritionally, it is also probable that the well- fed mother will escape or have minimal varicosities,

[4] "Report on the Relation of Vitamin C Deficiency to Varicose Veins," *Western Journal of Surgery, Obstetrics, and Gynecology*, Vol. 50, 1942.

not only because her blood vessels are better supplied with vitamin C and vitamin E, but because her circulatory system will not be attacked by excessive female hormone activity.

In the authors' view, prospective mothers should not have to be placed on a specific diet for pregnancy. They should be eating practically the same diet during pregnancy as before and after—which is another way of saying the diet for pregnancy should begin when the girl is an infant, so that she never confronts her obstetrician with a request for nutrition that will compensate for a lifetime of error while meeting the suddenly increased demands of mother and her unborn.

However, we know this is wishful thinking on our part, for the present, at least. Therefore, we present the following diet for reproduction with the hope that both would-be parents will employ it at least six months (preferably a year) before conception is undertaken. The diet and its supplements should also help the infertile (both male and female) as well as those with impaired reproductive efficiency (both male and female), as evidenced by miscarriage, stillbirth, spontaneous abortion, or the birth of defective babies. Before adopting the diet, the mother-to-be should of course discuss it with her doctor.

DIET FOR REPRODUCTION (FOR BOTH SEXES)

The use of vitamin-mineral concentrates with this diet is mandatory, not optional. The purpose of the diet is to inhibit weight gain in the pregnant woman to sixteen pounds, which helps to shorten labor. Because the diet is restricted in caloric value, it is automatically restricted in vitamin-mineral values, and for this reason the supplements—which are calorie free—must be used. Below is a listing of the daily food requirements, vitamin supplements, and a listing of foods to be restricted.

Foods, daily requirements
    Bread: Whole wheat or whole rye, four slices.
    Butter and Margarine: Three pats.
    Cereals: Cooked Ralston, oatmeal, cooked whole wheat, or similar whole grain cereals, one serving.

Eggs: Two.

Juice: Orange or grapefruit, one eight-ounce glass.

Fresh Fruit: One serving.

Vegetables: Two cups, cooked.

Salad: Dark-leafed vegetables, with a dressing of cottonseed oil plus vinegar or any other condiments, one cup.

Meats: Lean meat, fish, or fowl, with emphasis on liver, kidneys, sweetbreads, tripe, etc., six ounces.

Milk: Whole milk, five glasses.

Dessert: Whole gelatin, junket, custard, stewed fruit, fresh fruit, or fruit whips.

(Brewer's yeast, wheat germ, dried skimmed milk, and soy flour can be added to appropriate recipes.)

Foods, restrictions

No pastries, ice cream, nuts, or candy.

Not more than one and one-half tablespoons of potatoes, spaghetti, rice, corn, lima beans, or dried beans.

Not more than eight glasses of liquids of all kinds in twenty-four hours.

Salt is restricted and salty foods minimized. (The use of salt substitutes is sometimes recommended by the physician where the ankles swell during pregnancy.)

Vitamin supplements

Multiple vitamins.

Vitamin-B complex syrup.

Multiple mineral concentrate.

Concentrated vitamin E.

Wheat-germ oil.

Bio-flavonoids.

To anticipate the scientific questions raised by the overlapping of some of these vitamin supplements the following should be considered:

1. Vitamin-B complex syrup is used in addition to the multiple vitamin capsules, though some of their values overlap, because the natural vitamin-B complex contains factors not yet synthesized; and therefore, not yet available in capsule form.

2. A multiple mineral capsule is used because salt is being restricted, and with it the intake of iodine, and because, for example, vitamin B_1 cannot function in the absence of zinc.

3. Wheat-germ oil is used in addition to concentrated vitamin E

because there are factors in wheat-germ oil, other than vitamin E, which help to prevent spontaneous abortions. The wheat germ may be administered by the teaspoonful, or can be added in appropriate quantity to the salad oil specified in the diet.

This is not intended to be a complete survey of technical reasons for the use of such supplements. However, a diet so arranged and so supplemented should reduce by 35 per cent the number of babies born dead: should diminish by 15 per cent the number of baby deaths in the first few weeks; will reduce prematurities by as much as 70 per cent; and may cut pregnancy toxemia by 50 per cent or more.

If the diet and the use of the supplements are instituted prior to pregnancy, the incidence of pregnancy nausea (morning sickness) may also be sharply diminished. If pregnancy nausea does appear, the obstetrician can have substantial potency of vitamin B_6 added to the vitamin-B complex syrup. If excessive swelling of the ankles or other tissue occurs, the obstetrician can at will increase the protein foods: eggs, meat, fish, or fowl. The increase can be in the magnitude of five additional ounces of meat daily. Where the appetite is finicky, and such swelling occurs, strained baby meats may be stirred into the allotted milk, and appropriately flavored.

The weight gain with this diet should aggregate three pounds in the first three months, ten pounds in the next three, and three pounds in the final three months, for a total of sixteen pounds.

6. Woman: Her unique problems
menstrual—reproductive—menopausal

While workers in nutrition may sometimes be justly accused of undue enthusiasm, they are never as ecstatic about the benefits of modern nutrition as is the woman who has been freed of premenstrual tension by control of diet.

Dr. Morton Biskind, whose work on diet and female hormones has been cited in advanced medical circles for some time, opened the door to a problem which is all too common. Women themselves, by coining the phrase "the curse," reveal their belief that pain associated with the menstrual cycle is a normal price for being feminine.

Biskind showed that control of female hormone metabolism by the well-fed liver is the key to quick "return of the organs to normal" after childbirth, to greater freedom from premenstrual tension and distress and menstrual pain and discomfort, to resistance to cystic mastitis and fibroid tumors. He demonstrated that the dietary supply of vitamin-B complex and protein is the *sine qua non* for proper liver control of female hormone. Deficiencies in these factors not great enough to cause other symptoms may interfere with the ability of the liver to break down excess quantities of female hormone, which then accumulate in the body to cause mischief associated with the reproductive tract and the secondary sexual organs in women.

Prior to Biskind's nutritional research, folklore indicated that diet might play some role in controlling premenstural disturbances and menstrual pain. In Europe to this day, women so troubled are advised to drink dark beer. Modern science attributed any possible helpfulness of this treatment to the hops, and at least one patent medicine alleged to be helpful for this condition contained hops as one of its ingredients. Brewer's yeast, being a source of high protein and vitamin-B complex, may have been another factor. (Sad to say, today's beer contains little or no yeast. As with many other foods, the good qualities are processed out.)

In the early 1950s the senior author was teaching nutrition at a coed university. There we assembled a group of young women whose premenstrual week and early days of the menstrual cycle were accompanied by so much pain, tension, irritability, bloating, and backache that they frequently absented themselves from school at this time. Because of the possibility that power of suggestion would be a factor in the experiment, the girls were not told why they had been selected for the experimental group. They were told merely that we were interested in possibly helping them to improve their complexions, nails, and hair. The selection of foods was aimed at increasing the intake of the lipotropic (fat-controlling) factors. These included choline, inositol, vitamin B_6, thiamin, and lecithin—virtually a description of eggs, among other good foods.

In some instances, the small miracle was achieved merely by persuading the girls to eat breakfast, something a number had rarely done before—and it proved effective even when the total change in the diet was confined to the addition of two eggs to breakfast. Faster responses were obtained when moderately potent B-complex supplements were used.

After six months of this improved diet, 38 per cent of the group *voluntarily* reported significant lessening of premenstrual and menstrual disturbances. In some cases, the relief was complete—to the extent that one girl, who had described herself as previously "climbing walls" in the premenstrual week and the first week of the period, remarked that now she knew her period was arriving when it actually arrived.

You see, therefore, that "the curse" need not be that at all. The difference is often the difference between improper and proper nutrition.

"THE PILL—FOR GOOD OR ILL"

People toss about the term "population explosion" so freely that one wonders if the phrase has meaning in reality for them. Perhaps this will define it: if we do not put a brake on man's capacity for reproduction, in the foreseeable—and near—future, there will be one square foot of land for each human being to stand upon, while he starves to death.

It is this grim reality that is bringing sweeping changes in outmoded laws interfering with dissemination of birth control information. It is this that is subtly altering the opposition of the religions to birth control. It is this that has made THE PILL a focus of hope—and controversy.

Stated simply, all birth control pills represent a glandular key to a simulated pregnancy. Since nature does not permit reimpregnation while pregnancy is in process, these hormones are practically foolproof guarantees of contraception. Moreover, it is clear that they do not permanently impair fertility. Indeed, if anything, the evidence argues for a rebound phenomenon, in which fertility—as though Nature were determined not to be cheated—seems to increase when the medication is abandoned.

Some medical men attribute to birth control pills another virtue: they say they prevent cancer. Fewer cases of cancer have appeared in women taking the medication than might be expected in a random sample of the female population, over the same period of time.

With this, though, there are arguments. Estrogenic hormone is one of the ingredients of birth control pills; and estrogen is labeled carcinogenic by some experts. Among these is Dr. Roy Hertz, endocrinologist of the National Cancer Institute, who flatly says that any woman who takes estrogens—for any purpose—is "playing with fire." [1] Dr. Hertz has his antagonists. Dr. J. Ernest Ayre, to name one, an eminent research figure with the Cytology Foundation of America, disagrees. He does not argue that estrogens are intrinsically innocent of cancer-causing properties. He claims that the progestin hormone, also an ingredient of the birth control pill, "neutralizes" the effect of the estrogen.

A wise judge once remarked, in admitting evidence from unsavory characters, that "wise men profit when rogues fall out." When scientists fall out, the public does not profit—particularly when the issue is one of life and death; and there are those—the senior author included—who feel that the only choice that can be sensibly made by the layman, when science cannot make a firm decision, is the pathway of safety.

The allegation of carcinogenic action by the estrogenic hormone is not the only possible "side reaction" attributed to the birth control formulae. Still unanswered is the question: Do the pills increase the risk of abnormal blood clotting of coronary thrombosis? One can find scientists or equal competence and fame on each side of that controversy. Less controversial is the effect of the birth control pills in decreasing tolerance for carbohydrates—so sharply that a state of "pre-diabetes" in a woman may be disclosed by her reaction to this medication. This has been described as being useful in eliciting signs of a hidden disease. But that type of reasoning seems a little specious. It smacks of the rationalization one medical man used in trying to dispel the public's fear of cancer from the birth control pills. "After all," said the doctor, "the use of the pills will require that women come in for a checkup—and this might even let us catch some cancers we ordinarily would not have had the chance to observe so early."

Less acrid criticism—though pointed—has been made by some

[1] The FDA remarked, apropos of Dr. Hertz' warning, that a "slight statistical risk of cancer does not justify banning the birth control pill"!

thoughtful medical observers, who point out that these pills inhibit the pituitary gland, and say that no one can prophesy what effects this may have, over a period of twenty-five or thirty years.

Alternate suggestions have been made by competent medical men who are wary of the pills. These include sterilization of the male, a simple operation which can even be performed under a local anaesthetic; and surgical sterilization of the female, by a technique that will not interfere with the menstrual cycle or the libido or the figure, but which does result in permanent sterility. So far as present knowledge goes, there are no side reactions and no risks in either of these procedures. But there are risks in the plastic devices that are inserted vaginally, for foreign body reactions have been known to occur; accidental conception does take place; and in a number of women, the "Pap" smears have changed toward the precancerous when these devices have been worn for a number of months. (This has also happened with the birth-control pills.) On the assumption that, not withstanding speculation on carcinogenic action, thrombophlebitis, and diabetes as possible by-products of actions of the birth control pill, the average woman will be using it, we should like to remind the reader of the discussion in Chapter 7 of dietary control of excessive estrogenic hormone activity. Here is one factor of possible safety: the action of the liver, encouraged by a generous intake of vitamin-B complex and protein, in destroying excess amounts of estrogen. This action may help to protect a woman against undesirable effects of the female hormone, whether self-produced, administered for menopause, or taken for contraceptive purpose.

DIET VERSUS THE LIBIDO

Long before Shakespeare observed that alcohol giveth and taketh, strengthening the male's desire while lessening his ability, the search for aphrodisiacs has denoted man's effort to close the gap between his sexual ability to give, and woman's to receive. The problem is very obviously rooted in the difference between psyche and physiology of the two sexes, and not in the tensions of civilization alone, for even among primitives there is a folk-lore (and a collection of jests) dealing with impotency.

Any reference to aphrodisiac actions of diet or nutrients will immediately meet the condemnation of the orthodox, and with some justification. Notwithstanding the American myth about oysters and such, the evidence is clear that para-amino-benzoic acid alone, of a list of more than 50 nutrients required by man, exercises any stimulating effect on the libido and the ability of the male. It has already been pointed out that this B-complex vitamin rarely has such effect on the female, but frequently will stimulate her fertility.

There is no doubt that male impotence is by far a more common problem than its female counterpart, frigidity. Nor is there any pat remedy for either. Female frigidity, like the counterpart problem in the male, is very often purely an emotional problem, and one which in the woman may require intensive psychotherapy (or the right man). Impotence in the male has within it an emotional vicious circle, for tension and fatigue can cause failure; and failure breeds renewed tension and fatigue.

Overlooked very often is the fact that the tide of sex operates within the will to live; and the fact that the very will to live is depressed when nutrition is poor. It has been pointed out that the primitive term for severe vitamin-B deficiency is "beriberi," which means "I can not." This negative climate must extend to the sexual relationship; and it is obviously present when the diet is merely poor, rather than atrocious. This is to say that the libido in both sexes is depressed by poor nutrition, by borderline vitamin deficiencies, by pituitary dysfunction based on subclinical vitamin and mineral inadequacies, by any nutritional environment which does not allow the organism to function at its maximum potential.

Only in this way can the senior author explain that which he has observed: a renascence of sexual desire and potency in both sexes, when rescued from the doldrums of diet neither truly good nor truly bad, producing "health" which is neither truly sick nor truly well. It is pertinent here again to remind the psychologically oriented that the patient under psychotherapy or analysis does *not* ordinarily eat well; some of the benefits attributed to emotional reorientation alone derive in part from a renewed zest for enjoyable eating that accrues as psychological healing progresses.

The flame of sexual desire is a slender one in many men (and women). It requires more than the fuel of proximity and opportunity. It may be upset by undesirable attitudes, odors, tensions, or incompatibilities. Is there any reason to suppose that the great force that sustains brain, glands, nerves, muscles, and tissues, nutrition, can be ignored in this relationship?

The type of diet frequently recommended in this text—frequent small meals, high in protein, moderately high in fat, low in processed carbohydrate, and supplemented with vitamin-mineral concentrates is the nutritional pathway to heightened well-being. When that is achieved, one's diet will no longer operate to dampen the sexual drive.

MENOPAUSE: IT NEED NOT BE DREADED

All this means that physiological events should be physiological. They should not bring with them the symptoms of pathology. In other words, normal things should be normal. For example, we should not gasp in amazement at the primitive woman who has her baby and is soon back at work in the fields. This is normal. Indeed, in our hospitals we are just beginning to realize the advantages of early ambulation. Human beings were not intended to stay in bed, and no nutritionist can possibly catch up with the serious disturbances in protein and calcium metabolism that come to the bedridden.

Why, then, should the menopause, another normal physiological event, be equated with undeniable old age? The nervous, irritable, anxiety-ridden menopausal woman, perspiring without provocation and afflicted with hot flashes is today given sedation, tranquilizers, and injections of female hormone. This treatment, even with our still limited knowledge of the change of life, fails to take advantage of two emerging sciences: psychology and nutrition. It certainly does not recognize the physical harm that tranquilizers can cause, the psychological help, badly needed, that they do not give, or the risk that persistent dosage with female hormone represents. When you hear the administration of the synthetic hormone defended, as it sometimes is, on the grounds that "the roulette wheel is crooked but it's the only one in town," you might reflect on the information given in our chapter on cancer and wonder whether such gambling is wise.

To what extent menopausal symptoms lie in the area of the psychosomatic may be debatable, but no one is likely to quarrel with the basic fact that the woman who has been anxious and insecure all her life is not going to improve during the menopause. The change of life serves as a magnifying glass that brings preexisting anxieties into sharp focus as the woman realizes that she is now parting with her biological birthright of having children and as she comprehends, no matter what she had told other persons about her age—no matter what she has told herself about being young—that biology has finally caught up with her.

The very "success" of female hormone therapy against symptoms of the menopause argues for a strong psychosomatic influence. When this hormone first became available, it was derived from the urine of pregnant mares (its origin naturally was not discussed with many menopausal women). Injections of the substance produced prompt relief from sweats, flushes, and hot flashes in a substantial percentage of the women treated. But the material then available was not highly concentrated, and we now realize that the early injections could not possibly have had any genuine therapeutic effect. The evidence for this is the fact that today's dosage, now that the synthetic hormone is available, is very much greater.

To what, then, were those early menopausal women responding? Obviously to their confidence in their physicians, or to the therapeutic ritual of an injection? The well-known placebo ("mind over body") effect may show improvements in patients' conditions running as high as 40 per cent. The difference between the placebo effect and that of a genuine therapy is that the placebo is usually temporary in its benefit, especially in more serious disorders. Thus, the power of the human mind can rarely exert a lasting effect on cancer or heart disease.

When, however, it is remembered that the female hormone may be cancer-producing, and when one also remembers the psychological response of recipients of the inffective dosages of the 1930s, the possible gains of hormone therapy do not appear to outweigh the risk.

A menopausal woman, when truly emotionally disturbed, needs and deserves psychological therapy. It may not only be her lifetime of insecurity and anxiety, being intensified by the physiological stresses of the change of life. It should be remembered that this period is one of tremendous emotional stress, which must make its mark even on the woman who is a well-adjusted, balanced personality. Loss of the ability to have children for many women represents a direct challenge to their right to call themselves women, and in our culture women are as protective of their womanhood as men are uneasy about their masculinity.

Many women erroneously consider the menopause to represent an end to physical love. Many think of it as definite parting with youth, unaware that, with the nutritional resources of today, they are really entering the prime of life. And many are unaware that lifetime nutrition, as well as special nutritional measures undertaken during the menopause, will bear strongly on the degree to which the experience shakes them.

How the pituitary gland knows that it is time for the menopause, no one knows. We do know that as life goes on, the active cells of that gland are replaced by minute particles of inert material sometimes called "sand." When this process has gone far enough, the pituitary, the master gland of the body, issues chemical orders that begin to diminish the production of certain hormones.

The theory behind female hormone therapy rests on the premise that the drop in estrogenic (female) hormone activity is responsible for the disturbances of the change of life. This drop does occur, and, interestingly, it is often much more severe when the menopause has been surgically induced by total hysterectomy.

Parenthetically, it may be that the some two hundred thousand hysterectomies performed yearly, with all their tragic sequelae, reflect a great deal of unnecessary surgery. Some of it could have been avoided by competent examination. Our sources for this statement? Well, the percentage of normal organs, so identified after pathological examinations, was so high in one series of operations that the Journal of the American Medical Association published an editorial which posed the question: "Hysterectomy—A Surgical Necessity or Therapeutic Racket?" In that series, some 400 sets of organs removed in a series of 1100 hysterectomies were found to be normal to a degree indicating that mere digital examination should have ruled out the surgery.

Some portion of such surgical defeminization of American women might be avoided, too, if the authorities would cease to feed the American public the soothing syrup of their statement that we are supremely well fed. Research in nutrition indicates that it may be feasible to prevent or to control the growth of fibroid tumors—a major indication for hysterectomies—by nutritional means. We will illustrate the point with a case history.

Gloria, thirty-two years of age, was suffering from fibroid tumors of the uterus that were causing constant hemorrhage. The senior author, consulted by her gynecologist, felt that her previous history of hypoglycemia (low blood sugar) and cystic mastitis indicated the possibility that disturbed liver function was allowing accumulation of female hormone, and had contributed as much to the fibroid tumors as it had to the cystic mastitis. Appropriate nutritional therapy not only stopped the hemorrhaging but brought the growth of the tumors to a stand-still. At the moment of writing, they have remained in *status quo* for some five years.

But let us return to the menopausal woman. Other than in the recognized deficiency diseases, it is rare in nutrition that we find so specific an action as that of vitamin E in the menopause. It is no more a panacea than the estrogenic hormone therapy, but it is effective for many women, and presents none of the hazards inherent in female hormone treatment.

Relatively small doses of vitamin E have quieted the anxiety, alleviated the irritability, and in many cases completely eliminated the attacks of unprovoked perspiration and sensations of heat. Since what nutrition cures it ordinarily prevents, such responses must inevitably make one wonder whether the woman who is genuinely well fed all her life—and well supplied with vitamin E—might not have a much less stormy course in menopause.

Indeed, the effect of vitamin-E therapy on personality and mental function in menopausal patients has been so dramatic that trial of the vitamin was suggested in the treatment of mental disease. In one such experiment, patients who had not responded to shock treatments were given the vitamin. A substantial percentage responded so well that the experimenting psychiatrists concluded that while they would not consider the vitamin to be a substitute for shock therapy, it would be a worthwhile treatment for those who do not respond to the more violent method. (How many mental hospitals followed up on this significant finding? None, to our knowledge.)

The quieting effects of vitamin E, of the vitamin-B complex, of calcium, and of lecithin supplements, are as demonstrable in the menopausal woman as they are in other disorders. If the use of these supplements is coupled with administration of a high-protein, high-fat, low-carbohydrate diet, the patient often will respond in a degree that would make anyone wonder why the regime of sedatives, tranquilizers, and female hormone is ever prescribed for anyone.

Two special dietary requirements are encountered frequently enough in the menopausal woman to deserve mention. Eating habits *are* habits, and the woman who becomes less active during the menopausal years yet continues to eat in her accustomed way is likely to gain undesired weight. For her, reducing is often necessary in terms of the total symptoms of the menopause, but only if special steps are taken to make sure that the diet does not contribute to low blood sugar, which is the second special problem of some menopausal women.

In a reducing regimen for a woman at this time, therefore, the use of protein supplements[2] between meals—just as they are recommended for low blood sugar—helps her to refrain from nibbling, sustains her nutritionally so as to minimize her periods of weakness, and gives her a nutritional basis to help in maintaining the characteristics of youth, which is the great promise of good nutrition.

Where low blood sugar is present, the hypoglycemia diet described in Chapter 11 is to be employed. If the two conditions coexist—if the overweight woman has low blood sugar—the reducing regimen, coupled with protein and other supplements, should be arranged in the form of frequent small meals; these will prevent sudden changes in the blood-sugar levels while still contributing to loss of weight.

Apropos of retaining the characteristics of youth, there is no need for the menopause to usher in drastic changes in the skin, nails, and hair to which the "average" woman thinks she must surrender as the inevitable price for the aging process. Gray hair has sometimes been darkened nutritionally, and may be delayed nutritionally. Enough research has been done to show that changes in the hair coloring and the condition of the skin and hair are not caused by age alone. Time is not toxic, and the readiest proof lies in the examination of the seventy-year-olds who are not gray, not wrinkled, and whose hair still retains youthful sheen and texture. In Chapter 18 we review the full application of nutrition in reversing or preventing changes blamed on age. Much of the information given there can be applied preventively to the menopausal woman.

[2] Nonfat milk is a cheap and effective protein supplement.

7. Cancer: Can you prevent it?

Some years ago the senior author received *unofficial* notification that his radio broadcasts were to be cited by the American Cancer Society. The award, it was indicated, would recognize the service rendered by the broadcasts in persuading listeners to undergo preventive examinations for cancer. A few days later came word that the award would not be made. It was said that the ACS had discovered that the broadcasts were guilty of creating false hope by virtue of talks on the subject of nutrition versus cancer.

The change of mind was puzzling, since it happened that the supposedly objectionable information in the broadcasts originated entirely from a monograph on the subject of nutrition in cancer published by the New York Academy of Sciences, a group affiliated with the most respected scientific body in the country, the American Association for the Advancement of Science. To us, the whole affair is a classic example of the neglect nutrition suffers in the thinking of orthodox workers in the field of cancer, at the same time that chemical therapy receives vast overemphasis. The nutritional implications of the virus theory of cancer are unperceived or discarded without adequate scientific examination.

Indeed, only recently an officer of the American Cancer Society declared that while nutritional deficiencies caused cancer in Bantu tribesmen, diets so signally bad are simply not found in America, so that poor nutrition can be completely absolved of responsibility for even a small part of the cancer incidence in this country. One would never guess from this official's statement that *no* survey of American diet reveals us to be a well-fed people, nor would one possibly imagine that it has been shown in research, subsidized by the American Cancer Society itself, that certain dietary deficiencies which *do* occur in America can directly lead to cancer.

Let us examine a few findings by official agencies in medicine, which, when taken together, show unmistakably that dietary deficiency of a type not uncommon in this country can and does cause cancer.

The American Medical Association once remarked in its nutrition handbook that the deficiencies likely to be most frequent in the American diet are in protein and vitamin-B complex. Any nutritionist or dietitian can tell you that this is the kind of deficiency which, when severe, causes pellagra. In the early 1940s, workers[1] in the New York Skin and Cancer Hospital noticed a striking similarity between lesions (injuries) of the soft tissues of the mouth labeled as "precancerous" and lesions which commonly appear in sufferers with pellagra. The similarity was so great that they decided to treat patients with such precancerous lesions *as if they had pellagra.* The patients were given a diet generously supplied with protein and the B complex vitamins. The researchers reported a triumph: *The precancerous lesions disappeared.*

Here, then, was concrete evidence that deficiency in these dietary factors themselves occurs in this country, as the American Medical Association said it does, and that such deficiency can contribute to precancerous changes in tissue. Nor is this the only such report to be found in the medical literature.

At the same time that the American Medical Association was discouraging the public from the use of vitamin supplements, it reported the case of a man with precancerous changes of the membranes of the throat, which yielded to large doses of vitamin A.

There is even clearer proof of B-vitamin deficiency's association

[1] Martin and Koop.

with cancer. We are all aware, from recent news stories, that certain food additives, including sprays and processing materials, have been shown to be cancer-causing. Some of these chemicals produce, among other things, an oxygen deficiency in the cells, and it has been established that a cellular oxygen deficiency will help produce cancer. While it is significant that oxygen deficiency in the cells is linked to cancer, it is even more significant that a deficiency in the B vitamins and vitamin E is perhaps the most direct way to interfere with the utilization of oxygen in the living cell.

The great promise of nutrition in the fight against cancer lies in a phenomenon which is discussed elsewhere in this book: the interaction between the diet and the ability of the body to control the activity of certain of the hormones. Let us review this point in the context of cancer. For years, the United States Food and Drug Administration permitted the chicken and cattle industries to speed the marketing of their meat by administering to the fowl and animals quantities of stilbesterol, a synthetic form of female hormone. Certain medical men and certain of us in public health education were convinced that stilbesterol is capable of causing cancer. It has long been known that male chemists occupied in synthesizing this hormone are apt to develop cancer of the breast, an extremely rare occurrence in men. The cancer is probably caused by exposure to the stilbesterol dust in the laboratory.

Nevertheless, for voicing our apprehension at the systematic addition of stilbesterol to our national meat diet, we were called —once again—"food faddists." For a period American mothers continued to feed their babies the hormone-dosed chicken. Then, under public pressure, the Food and Drug Administration reversed its stand. It announced that the cancer-causing action of the hormone made its use in the chicken industry unsafe, though the ruling still allowed the beef producer to employ the substance. There were, of course no apologies or even acknowledgments to the "food faddists" who had directly and indirectly forced the belated change.

Certain physicians have now protested against the use of stilbesterol in medical practice. One medical man wrote to the American Medical Association seriously suggesting that on every box of ampules of female hormone the warning in large letters should appear: "Doctor: are you sure that your patient does not have cancer?" The suggestion was based on the realization that the hormone can cause pre-existing cancer to flare up. It brings up pertinent questions about the estrogen content of all birth control pills.

Just how potent this substance is you will realize when you learn that mink breeders who fed their animals chick heads and necks found the animals becoming sterile. The hormone implant was ordinarily made in the neck area of the chicken.

But more important to us, our beef continues to originate with animals that are so treated; and physicians are still administering the hormone to menopausal women—although vitamin E, which carries no cancer-producing action, is at least as useful in relieving many menopausal symptoms. Such is the glory of modern medicine!

For you to appreciate the probability that nutrition offers in the prevention of a common type of cancer in women, we must go back to World War II. American fighting men confined in Japanese prisoner-of-war camps barely existed on the starvation diet provided by their captors. In one of these camps, two physicians were among the prisoners. As the months dragged on, they noted certain changes in the famished men that suggested a change toward the feminine: loss of libido or sexual interest, which, in the American G. I., certainly represents something pathological;[2] less frequent need for shaving, and in some cases, enlargement of the breasts. They suspected the symptoms were produced in some way by the starvation diet, but could not reconcile that concept with another observation: When Red Cross packages were delivered to the camp, and the men enjoyed a period of good nutrition,

[2] The diabetic male also frequently complains of impotence, infertility, and loss of libido. These symptoms can sometimes be traced to the same dietetic process that occurred in the American prisoner of war, which is described more fully, later.

the feminine symptoms became more pronounced, rather than less.

The mystery was not unraveled until the war's end, when the report written by the prison-camp physicians was reviewed in the light of Dr. Morton Biskind's research.[3] Biskind had shown that the liver, which deals with many toxic and potentially toxic substances either entering the body or metabolically produced, was responsible for destroying any excess of female hormone. He was able to demonstrate that a malnourished liver loses this ability, and he showed that deficiency in protein and vitamin-B complex was the specific pattern of deficiency that would impede the ability of the liver to inactivate this hormone.

The bizarre effects of the prison-camp diet could now be viewed in context. The male produces female hormone, though in a lesser quantity than the female; under starvation conditions the hormone tends to accumulate, since it is not being destroyed by the liver. It has long been known that an accumulation of female hormone in men will produce certain female characteristics. It can cause enlargement of the male breast, and most certainly can lead to loss of sexual interest in the opposite sex.

Flare-up of symptoms when the Red Cross packages were available was easily explained. The temporary period of good nutrition stimulated hormone production (including female hormone), but the good diet did not last long enough to permit the liver to recapture its ability to cope with the hormone. Therefore, in the brief periods of good diet, the hormone accumulation actually increased, and with it, the symptoms.

This research threw interesting light on certain characteristics of alcoholics. Men who have damaged their livers by substituting alcohol for needed food will, as the liver damage proceeds, lose the hair on their chest—an evidence of feminization. Abundant scalp hair—sometimes considered a female characteristic—is fre-

[3] Many papers by the Biskinds—particularly Morton and Leonard—will be found listed in the *Index Medicus,* beginning in the late 1940s and continuing to appear over a period of ten years.

quently observed among alcoholic derelicts completely innocent of any scalp sanitation. And finally, it is axiomatic that many male alcoholics are devoid of interest in the opposite sex.

Biskind's research stirred Canadian medical thinking. At one of the fine Canadian medical schools, two researchers[4] decided to compare a group of women suffering from cancer of the reproductive tract with a group of women of the same ages who were free of cancer. The investigation was to answer three questions:

How did the two groups compare in the production of female hormone? How did their dietary intakes compare, with special reference to vitamin-B complex and protein? How did their blood levels of vitamin-B complex and protein compare?

A striking difference was discovered between the two groups. Of the women with cancer, 94.5 per cent showed an elevated output of female hormone, dietary shortage in vitamin-B complex and protein, and blood levels of the vitamins, as one might suppose, similarly low. Exactly the same percentage of the women free of cancer showed a diametrically opposite picture: Normal or low output of female hormone, diets well supplied with vitamin-B complex and protein, and therefore blood levels within normal range. Is this not a most significant evidence of the effect of diet on cancer? One wonders how the orthodox can continue to ignore it.

Now let us turn to other evidence which indicates that careful selection of food may arm us against cancer. We shall consider cystic mastitis, the disease in which there are multiple obstructions of the milk-producing tubules of the breast. The disorder often appears after pregnancy, when output of female hormone is elevated; it also tends to worsen as a woman goes through that state of her menstrual cycle when female hormone production is elevated. So specific is this relationship that application to the face of a cosmetic cream containing a concentration of female hormone has, we have observed, caused chronic cystic mastitis to worsen.

[4] Ayre and Bauld.

The disease is regarded as precancerous, inasmuch as a group of women with cystic mastitis statistically may expect more cases of breast cancer than may be anticipated in a group of women free of this disorder. In research with his medical colleagues, the senior author has been able to bring cystic mastitis under control by dietetic and vitamin therapy alone, with emphasis on protein and vitamin-B complex.

The literature is replete with references indicating clearly that the ordinary human diet contributes to cancer. From the many that could be described, we choose the following example because of its convincing simplicity and incontrovertible result.

In a British hospital, animals were fed the hospital's table scraps—an "average" diet but low in protein and vitamins. A second group of animals was given the same diet, with a supplement of brewer's yeast, which is rich in protein and vitamin-B complex. The incidence of cancer of this group was much lower than in the first.

Regardless of its effect on cancer, we still recommend a type of diet that carries known benefits. As we have already explained, such a diet, high in the B vitamins and protein, has been shown to relieve markedly the distressing physical and emotional symptoms of the menstrual woman. It may also heighten resistance to varicose veins, fibroid uterine tumor, and cystic mastitis. So even if all the cancer research we have mentioned is in error or meaningless —an almost inconceivable proposition—our recommended diet carries with it no harm and confers much benefit. These benefits will be apparent even in types of cancer that bear no direct relationship to nutrition, for one can be sure that, whatever therapy is employed in cancer and ultimately found successful, the response in the better-nourished individual will always be better.

Of course, this is not the full story of nutrition versus cancer. Vitamin E, for instance, reduces the need of the tissues for oxygen and might be expected thereby to offer some protection against toxic influences that initiate the first steps toward cancer by interfering with the chemistry of oxygen in the cells. It is conceivable, too, that vitamin C, intimately concerned with the permeability of the cells, vitamin B_1, and the bio-flavonoids, which have a similar action, may help bar the entrance to the cell of viruses capable of causing cancer.

These are speculations that the researchers of tomorrow will surely investigate. But today, you, the female reader of this book, and perhaps the male reader as well, have a possible weapon against cancer. Whether you use it or not will depend on your dietary habits. If you buy the foods most popular with American housewives, you will be depriving yourself of some of the B-complex vitamins. However, if your diet is planned to include the organ meats and whole grains; if you use to full advantage the special-purpose foods which are rich in protein and vitamin-B complex (wheat germ and brewer's yeast); if you supplement your diet with a generous amount of the B vitamins, your health dividends may accrue in the form of what does *not* happen—and among these dividends is likely to be the cancer that never begins.

The United States Food and Drug Administration has willfully described broadcasts and publications of the senior author as offering a dietary treatment for cancer. It may very well be that someday some type of diet may be found that will prove useful as an adjunct in the treatment of cancer. We do not believe such a diet has yet been devised, and certainly the senior author has never presented one. This outright lie by a government agency was reprinted, nonetheless, in such newspapers as *The New York Times*. When the senior author reproached *The New York Times* for lending its support to an obvious effort to damn dissident opinion in nutritional science, *The New York Times* reporter replied that releases with a Washington dateline are ordinarily "not investigated." This policy has vastly implemented the efforts of this government agency to portray as quacks those who do not subscribe to the nutritional philosophy of the Food and Drug Administration. It will interest the reader to know that this government agency has recently attempted to assume complete editorial control of all nutritional publications—in magazines, newspapers, books, television, and radio. Although such an attempt did not meet favor in the Federal court, it nonetheless exemplifies the philosophy of the agency: Those who disagree with us are not only wrong, not only quacks, but criminals. If the reader is not aware that differing with the consensus, as expressed in Food and Drug Administration regulations, can include penalties up to jail sentences, he is not unique.

8. Diabetes: Do you have it without knowing?

Some three million Americans, half of them unaware of it, have diabetes, and according to the American Medical Association, one in every four Americans has a tendency toward diabetes.

The disorder is today often coupled with a classic example of negative dietetics—the kind of dietetic advice that tells you what not to eat. As we have already seen in the discussion of the low-cholesterol diet, negative dietetics is almost routinely productive of poor nutrition.

If we go back to the early days of medicine's struggle with diabetes, we find the patient the victim of a simple but deadly philosophy. Diabetes, the thinking ran, is a disorder in which the body is not able to manage starches and sugars. The suggested remedy was simple: Do not eat starches and sugars. There was only one unfortunate complication. Deprived of the metabolism of starches and sugars, the patient went into a coma and died.

We now know that diabetes is not a disease of sugar and starch chemistry. It is not even just the failure of the pancreas to secrete enough insulin to "burn" sugar, as many medical men believed. It is a disorder in which the utilization of *food* is disturbed—from water to vitamins to minerals to proteins to sugars and starches. Yet even today the attention of most therapists is concentrated on the carbohydrates—the starches and sugars. Years ago the level of sugar in the blood became the all-important index. Hence the early attempts to place diabetics on a sugar-free diet. Hence the loud acclaim for the discovery of insulin, which "saved" the diabetic. Saved him for what? For cataracts, hardening of the arteries, kidney involvement, cancer—to all of which he is prone?

The discovery of insulin was in part a tragedy, for it stifled further research and yet it did not solve the problem of diabetes. Nearly twenty years ago it was observed that certain sulfa drugs lower blood sugar. This unleashed on the diabetic, as one specialist put it, a "horse race" in the sale of oral diabetic drugs that at best lower blood sugar, but in some instances lower it unphysiologically (artificially, interfering with normal body processes) and with harmful side effects. Meanwhile, let us remember that the blood sugar of a diabetic is but one aspect of his problem, and neither insulin nor the oral drugs cope with his other troubles. This would not be so bad if the unilateral action of the hormone and the drugs were recognized as such—if the control of blood sugar were not carelessly hailed as the control of diabetes.

This carefree and fractionated viewpoint on diabetes is matched by another. It is only a few years ago that a leading specialist in the field announced that the properly controlled diabetic does not encounter complications. "Properly controlled" is of course an elastic phrase—any diabetic developing complications could automatically be labeled as not having been "properly controlled." Nonetheless, at the time of that announcement and through to the present date, any practicing physician could have displayed for the specialist numerous "controlled" diabetics replete with complications. These collateral disorders have been labeled by one authority in the field as being the product of the treatment rather than of the disease. Somogyi[1] has pointed out that insulin dosage can never be so accurately controlled that there are not occasions when the blood sugar of the diabetic is dropped below the normal for him as a person. When this occurs, there is an immediate compensatory reaction of the pituitary and the adrenal glands in an effort to raise the blood sugar to normal.

[1] *Bulletin,* St. Louis Jewish Hospital in early 1950s.

It appears that the body can stand elevated blood sugar better than it can tolerate low blood sugar. There is therefore a running fight between the pituitary and adrenal glands, on the one hand, and the insulin hypodermic on the other—a struggle which is likely to be won by the hypo, since the resources of the laboratory are greater than those of the body. There therefore comes the time when the adrenal gland is overworked and hypertrophies (overgrows). At this point, complications begin which actually represent stress adaptation disease, as described by Selye.[2] Somogyi's suggestion for preventing these complications therefore is addressed to the physician, who is urged to *minimize* the dosages of insulin.

There are vitamin factors that improve carbohydrate tolerance, which is a scientific way of saying that they work with insulin. Such factors would permit reduction of dosage of insulin, if competently prescribed. However, official medicine has adopted the propaganda line that all Americans are well fed, that vitamin deficiencies occur only in alcoholics, and that prescription of vitamin supplements is therefore unnecessary. In this negative climate the medical man who might be inclined to give his diabetic patient the benefit of brewer's yeast[3] and vitamin-B complex concentrates may very well hesitate for fear of being denominated as a "faddist." He will maintain medical rectitude, however, if he treats his patient only with insulin or the oral drugs and diet, and later heroically medicates the patient with vitamins and hormones in the attempted control of hemorrhagic retinitis, kidney complications, hardening of the arteries, and other "complications of diabetes."

Parenthetically, it should be made plain that the new oral drugs for diabetes represent a tragic exploitation of the ignorance of patient and general practitioner. (The diabetic specialist knows better what he is doing when he prescribes such drugs.) Bitter criticism was directed against the senior author for dispens-

---

[2] Hans Selye, *Stress*, Grune and Stratton, 1951. (Original volume and supplements.)
[3] Used in diabetes for a century.

ing "misinformation" on the subject of these drugs in his broadcasts. The author's remarks, however, were entirely based on papers read at a meeting of the American Diabetic Association in
the late 1950s. These papers were invidiously critical of many of
the new oral drugs, and in these criticisms we may learn a lesson
in control of a very common type of diabetes: the type which
strikes late in life, frequently without symptoms, and is often discovered on a routine checkup of the unsuspecting sufferer. For, it
was pointed out, these drugs are useful in control of the blood
sugar *only* in this type of diabetic, and since he can usually be
brought under control with diet and diet alone, it seems pointless
to give him possibly toxic drugs with possible side reactions which
act unphysiologically.

The unphysiological aspect of their action is as disturbing to
contemplate as is the claim that any drug or hormone that controls blood sugar is controlling diabetes.

Insulin is a two-edged weapon for the body. It helps sugar to
enter the cells to be used as fuel, and it helps the body to draw
upon reserves of glycogen (sugar) in the liver as it is needed to
replenish the supply in the blood. Some of the oral drugs do not
help the cells to obtain sugar; indeed, they interfere with the supply because they act by interfering with the ability of the body to
draw upon the reserves of sugar in the liver. Thus they set up a
block to the recycling of the fuel supply and lend no aid to its
combustion. Certainly the blood sugar levels fall with the new
oral drugs in *some* patients. They fall for the same reason that
produces the side reaction of weakness: because the patient is
being chemically prevented from drawing on his reserve food
supply. This action is quite different from the physiological action
of insulin, production of which some of these drugs are claimed to
stimulate. However, it is noteworthy that proper dosage of insulin
is very rarely accompanied by the "side reactions" encountered
with the oral drugs in some people.

The side reactions also include muscular weakness, for the reason that the drugs likewise upset the utilization of sugar in the

muscles, which heavily depend on this fuel. Add to this, allergic reactions, sudden hypoglycemia, granulomas, cirrhosis of the liver, and other disasters in patients taking oral drugs for diabetes (those studied on autopsy), and one can see that these drug "discoveries" might better have remained in the limbo of the undiscovered.

Ironically, the new drugs cannot be used for juvenile diabetics, who are too "unstable," and they are therefore being prescribed primarily for the group who encounter the disease in middle age —the very group most amenable to treatment by diet alone. For this latter group, therapeutic nutrition holds a promise via an action of certain nutrients. These nutrients are useful to diabetics of any age, juvenile or middle aged.

One must be careful in evaluating any treatment for diabetes, for the patient usually has an obliging way of responding beautifully to diet, insulin, oral drugs, or, for that matter, vitamins, for the first few months. Yet vitamin therapy (despite the fact that it is scornfully discounted by orthodox authorities) coupled with controlled diet, holds long-lasting and substantial benefits for diabetics.

Let us examine the claim. Some years ago, the senior author was called by a physician who was faced with an unusual problem. His patient, a diabetic, was a woman weighing more than 300 pounds, and she had every intention of remaining at that weight, for she refused to cooperate in reducing. Her diabetic condition, under these circumstances, was obviously most difficult to control, since she had a virtual mania for the very foods she had no right to eat. Her blood sugar was over the 200 level—very high—and her urine showed a maximum in excreted sugar. The physician had attempted to give her insulin, only to discover that she was allergic to it in all forms.

The foregoing explains his initial remark: "I thought," he said, "this would be a wonderful case for the vitamin therapy that you described to me."

What he was discussing was theory, rather than fact. After

some six months' work in a medical library, the senior author had drastically revised his concept of diabetes. He had begun by thinking of diabetes as a disorder of food metabolism, the first symptom of which was a rise in blood sugar caused by underproduction of insulin—a deficit customarily rectified, and the disease controlled by an appropriate, well-balanced diet, supplemented (where necessary) with injections of insulin.

The papers in the medical library revealed quite a different picture. Many diabetics *show no sign* of inadequate production of insulin. At least, on autopsy their pancreata show a normal or even an elevated content of the hormone. This is true of about 50 per cent of all diabetics examined. The same percentage—though not necessarily the same individuals—do show signs of a liver disturbance.

Furthermore, the incidence of diabetes is not, as the senior author had originally supposed, linked alone to the intake of sugar and starch. It is the nations that eat the most fat and processed carbohydrates that show the most diabetes.

On this slender premise the author wondered whether diabetes might not be a disease involving the liver, that organ having been insulted by a burden of fat it could not handle. Further, he wondered whether deficiencies in fat-metabolizing nutrients, such as are removed from white flour in processing, contribute to this liver disfunction.

The physician with the uncooperative patient proceeded to test the theory by giving her copious dosage of a vitamin-B complex concentrate rich in the lipotropes (fat-utilizing factors such as choline, inositol, pyridoxine, and lecithin), and well supplied with other crystalline vitamins of the B complex, and fortified with vitamin B_{12}.

At the outset the doctor remarked to the senior author that the procedure made sense, even if it had no influence on the faulty metabolism of starches and sugars. As he pointed out, many of these B vitamins are used in the treatment of certain disorders to which diabetics are prone: neurological disturbances, hardening of the arteries, and liver disease.

The diabetic "rebel" responded with a fall in her blood sugar—*this without change in diet*—from over 200 to approximately 110. Excreted sugar in the urine disappeared. Her vision, obfuscated by cataract, had been 3-300, or very poor. It improved to 3-25.

Such a dramatic response would not impress a diabetic specialist, for, as has been pointed out previously, diabetics respond to almost any new treatment in the first few months. What was impressive to us was the realization that this response was obtained with physiological substances—substances normal to the body—and that these factors might well arm the diabetic with more resistance to some of the degenerative disorders spoken of as complications of the disease, but which actually are part of the diabetic process.

Let us illustrate this point. Diabetics are prone to neurological disturbances, which are painful, and have been treated with more or less success with vitamin B_{12}. Some five years before the disturbance of the nerves becomes overt and painful, careful examination with a tuning fork will reveal areas of the diabetic's body where he does not feel the vibration. This insensitivity is a warning sign. Is it not better for the diabetic to receive his extra supplies of vitamin B_{12} *prior* to the development of the numbness and insensitivity? And before he is agonized with the intense pain of a diabetic neuritis?[4]

Shall we wait for hardening of the arteries to strike the diabetic, knowing that he is prone to it, and then give him massive doses of choline, inositol, B_{12}, and pyridoxine (B_6)? These were the nutrients given to this woman—nutrients removed from white bread—the very bread distinctly specified in many standard diabetic diets. (Why white bread is specified, we have never understood. The carbohydrate content of white bread is practically identical

[4] When vitamin B_{12} will then be administered under duress, in huge doses—and often too late for success.

with that of whole wheat so that calorie-wise there is no point in specifying the less nutritious bread, which lowers the diabetic's intake of these protective factors.)

Following our success with the overweight patient, a long series of diabetics were given the vitamin therapy with striking results attested to by the patients' physicians. One physician commented:

This patient is sixty years old. She gives a history of suffering from Diabetes Mellitus, or true diabetes, for the past fifteen years and has been taking thirty units of globin insulin for control of the diabetes. Her last record of a blood sugar that she can remember is 183 mg. per cent. Examination reveals an adult white female who does not appear acutely or chronically ill. The examination was essentially within normal limits except for the blood sugar which, when taken two months after her remembered record, was 142 mg. per cent. She has been taking thirty units of insulin since this examination. I placed her on the following regimen: (1.) high choline-inositol, vitamin-B complex syrup daily; (2.) mixed tocopherols twice daily; (3.) multiple vitamin-mineral supplements supplying zinc, three times daily; (4.) vitamin C, 250 mg. daily, plus a diabetic diet of 2,000 calories together with B complex injections once weekly. She continued to show sugar in the urine but to a lesser concentration for the next three weeks. On the fourth week, the urine was entirely negative for four daily samples. The insulin was dropped to 10 units daily. However, the following week showed ¾ of 1 per cent sugar in the urine and the insulin was raised to 15 units daily. After one week of 15 units, she was placed on 10 units and the urine remained free from sugar. For the next three weeks, the insulin was reduced to five units per week until, at the present writing, she is not receiving any insulin and the urine remains negative. A blood sugar taken three months after the first examination was 148 mg. per cent and no urinary sugar.

In summation, this is a sixty-year-old white female with a history of known diabetes for fifteen years who is placed on vitamins and vitamin supplements as recommended by Carlton Fredericks, and who is able to maintain herself on a 2,000-caloric diet without the use of insulin after having required as much as thirty units of globin insulin daily. This is an example of control of a metabolic disease with the use of vitamins and vitamin supplements.—(Name deleted) M.D.

In a disease marked by improper utilization of every fraction of food, it seems reasonable that those vitamins important to the utilization of food should be offered in generous amounts. Yet does the standard diabetic diet do so? Pick up any orthodox text or any diabetic manual issued by any of the large clinics or pharmaceutical companies, and you will find them recommending the overprocessed carbohydrates, in filling the carbohydrates allowance of the diet. Is this rational?

Thus the diabetic is informed how much he may eat of rice cereal, of white bread, and of the other overprocessed carbohydrates which in processing are deprived of the very nutrients that might help to control his diabetes and might help to mitigate, if not to avoid, the "complication of the disease."

After a *few hundred* diabetics had been treated with vitamin therapy with *significant* results, the senior author wrote to a great diabetic clinic with an offer phrased this way:

> If I, as a Ph.D., publish this research, it will have little influence upon your profession. I suggest, therefore, that you take the protocols, study them; and if you feel it justified, continue the work. If it proves to be valid, or for that matter invalid, publish it. In the event that it is valid, you need give me no credit—I am merely anxious that this information reach those who are treating diabetics.

The response was—remember, now, from the largest and probably the richest diabetic clinic in the world—"We have no facilities for such research."

Do you need more proof that the iron fist of orthodoxy is tightly clamped around medical research? And that the only way it can be loosened is by an enlightened and aroused public?

9. Diet: You are an individual

THE FUNCTIONS OF FOOD

As levels of income may vary from the inadequate to that which offers reserves for any emergency, so are there levels of "adequacy" in nutrition. Exactly as the person on an inadequate income will attempt to adapt to it by restricting his purchases, so does the body attempt to adapt to inadequate nutrition. This explains the short stature of the Japanese on their native diet, and the fact that their children grow taller in America. Here, protein is the limiting factor.

Thus the fact that you have survived on your diet is not necessarily a testimonial to its adequacy. It may instead be a signal pointing to the body's capacity for survival. Sometimes, the survival on a poor diet is earned at a price. One exists, rather than lives. And one then rationalizes by calling an accumulation of a half hundred minor disorders "average health," instead of recognizing it to be a state of incipient disaster, triggered by a wretched diet that offers no reserves. To the avoidance of this twilight zone of nutrition—where the diet is neither good enough to support optimal health nor bad enough to cause major illness—at least immediately, these notes are dedicated.

CALORIES

In bygone years, calories were much emphasized, and it was considered that ideal nutrition consisted of a diet which would supply enough caloric value or energy value to meet the needs of the body, which in this context was viewed as a furnace.

However, it became obvious that the *sources* of the energy value were important, because animals lavishly supplied with calories insisted on dying—though the addition of a little milk to such a diet converted it into one which would support life. Since none of the known constituents of milk would make this difference, it became obvious to the scientists of that day that there was something wrong with this concept of the body as a mere furnace, and something very wrong with the concept that a diet adequate in calories would be adequate to support good health.

Science then decided that the source of the calories—protein, such as meat; fat, such as butter; or sugar and starch made a difference. But when purified protein, fat, sugar, and starch were fed in adequate amounts to meet the energy needs of the body, the animals still died—and milk still rescued them. This fixed the attention of the scientists on minerals, but no combination of minerals conceivably needed by the body would convert any of these purified diets into one capable of supporting life, much less health. This was the starting point of the search for what Casimir Funk ultimately named "vitamins."

As research progressed, it became obvious that the calorie theory itself had something wrong with it. It was for many years accepted that your relationship to calories was much like that of Mr. Micawber to financial income. You will remember that he said that when the income and the outgo balanced or left a small reserve, this spelled happiness. When the outgo exceeded the income, this was unhappiness. If you substitute calories for income in that axiom, you have the concept of weight gain which for many years governed nutrition. In other words, if your diet supplied the exact number of calories you expended in the form of energy, your weight would remain constant. If you had an excess supply of calories, you would gain weight; if you had an inadequate intake of calories, then you would withdraw the deficit from your reserves of body fat—or in a thin person, from the protein structure of the body, and wind up losing weight. Unfortunately, there were some persons who insisted upon gaining weight on a calorie intake that was by every standard inadequate. There were those who did not lose weight on a calorie intake so low that a deficit necessarily had to be created. This led to the discovery of the new kind of calorie equation, invoked in the low-carbohydrate diet, where individuals fed rather large amounts of food, virtually excluding sugar and starch, managed to lose weight while seemingly eating enough for weight gain.

The discovery of the vitamins made it possible for us to explain how the body manages to burn food at 99 degrees, where in the laboratory identical oxidation of foods would require hundreds of degrees. This was made possible by the action of vitamins as part of enzyme systems. Perhaps the best analogy is to suggest that the reader experiment with a lump of sugar, a substance which the body manages to burn (release energy from) at 99 degrees. The reader will find it impossible to ignite a lump of sugar with a match flame, which is much hotter than the body. If cigarette ashes are placed on the sugar, the ashes will act as a wick, and the sugar will catch fire. In the body, the wick is a group of vitamins making possible low-temperature oxidation. This explains how it is possible to starve to death with the stomach filled—if the food is not accompanied by the necessary vitamin "wicks."

The interrelationship between food intake and vitamin requirement is one which in modern civilization presents certain problems. We set a ceiling on calorie intake, because under ordinary circumstances there is a limit on the amount of food a person can and should eat. We also set a floor on calorie intake, because however good the selection of food is, it is obvious that there is a minimal amount of food that must be consumed in order to achieve qualitative adequacy in all the nutrients which food supplies. In modern civilization, the floor under calorie intake and the ceiling over it may tend to become mutually exclusive. This is to say that in a button-pushing civilization, man may not be active enough to warrant his eating enough food to obtain an optimal intake of the minor nutrients—vitamins, minerals, and the like. This obviously calls for food concentrated in vitamins and minerals and low in calories. However, the direction of food processing is opposite: it tends to concentrate calories at the expense of the trace nutrients. Thus, for instance, in manufacturing sugar and white flour, the vitamin-mineral content is drastically reduced; the calories of the carbohydrate, however, are more or less concentrated.

THE VITAMINS

There are but a few teaspoonfuls of vitamins in the seventy tons of food you eat in a lifetime—which is a terrible figure and may give you one. The amount of vitamins in food may vary tremendously, being subject to inimical influences that begin with cultivation, and act in storage, transportation, processing, and cooking, and tend to lower the vitamin potency of food. The talk of vitamins being "destroyed" would seem to imply that they are alive. Actually they are chemicals, and some of them are highly susceptible to destruction by alkalies or oxygen—which, in changing them chemically, converts them into substances that do not have vitamin action.

The reader will find in the Appendix a list of the known vitamins, with an approximation of optimal intake to be achieved from diet or from diet plus supplements. The term "approximation" is needed: vitamin requirements may vary by a factor of eight or nine to one from one individual to the next, even in the same family.

The requirement for vitamins may range from daily quantity weighing no more than the weight of a period made with a lead pencil to one required by the teaspoonful. Generally speaking, these are factors needed in minute amounts, the absence of which from the diet will cause death and a partial deficiency of which will interfere with function.

Generally speaking, vitamins tend to be concentrated in foods that are unpopular with the public. They are more generously supplied by whole wheat than by white flour; by brown rice than by white rice; by organ meats than by muscle meats; by dark green leafy vegetables such as escarole rather than the lighter ones such as lettuce; and by such unpopular foods as wheat germ and brewer's yeast.

A distinction has been made between natural and synthetic vitamins, which appears to exist only in the minds of those who are engaged in the marketing of the "natural" type. The thiamine found in whole wheat and that manufactured by man are, atom for atom and molecule for molecule, identical. Indeed, before a vitamin synthesizer is permitted to call his product a vitamin, he must initially demonstrate its capacity for curing all the symptoms of a deficiency in that factor, with the same efficiency and in the same period of time as the "natural." There are, however, vitamin factors not yet isolated, which have not yet thereby been identified chemically, and which are therefore not yet synthesized. It is thereby not possible with synthetic vitamin C completely to duplicate the action of orange juice, for the very good reason that in citrus juices there is another vitamin factor—the bio-flavonoids—which work with vitamin C, protect it from oxidation in the body, and have some actions of their own. Commercial marketers of "natural" vitamin concentrates have made much of the distinction between the action of a vitamin C tablet and that of orange juice, without explaining to the public that, when synthetic vitamin C is administered together with the bio-flavonoids, there is then no distinction between the action of this combination and the effect of the same factors in the form of citrus juice. In fact, in a number of studies synthetic versus natural vitamins have been the variables, in which it has never been possible to demonstrate any difference—significant or insignificant—between their actions, so long as comparable products were being compared. However, since we do not yet know all the vitamins, and cannot make them all synthetically, it is obvious that a supplement is a supplement—which is to say that it is not a substitute for food, nor a license for improper eating. Moreover, when the crystalline vitamins are employed as supplements, they should be accompanied by a natural source of the vitamin-B complex—since in such a natural source there will be many vitamins not yet made synthetically. This is the rationale for using, together with a multiple vitamin and mineral supplement, a B-complex concentrate that contains liver or some similar source of the unknown or unsynthesized vitamins in addition to the synthetic ones. Liver is the best source of these unknown factors.

THE "I" IN DIET—THE "U" IN MENU

Let us now appraise *your* diet, first acknowledging that no such appraisal is really possible. Although the scientific literature is replete with methods for testing the state of an individual's nutrition, these tests are predicted upon a concept of an average person. But you are an individual, with individual needs. What is good for the average person may not be helpful at all for you.

Let us suppose that we have determined the amount of vitamin B_1 in your blood. What does this tell us? To the average dietitian, to the medical nutritionist, this might mean that your blood content of this vitamin falls within a range considered average or normal. But this equating of average and normal is fallacious. Suppose, for instance, we were to establish our normal range by an assumption about the blood content of vitamin B_1 in a group of twelfth-century French peasants. These people ate several pounds of black bread daily—bread that, not yet "improved" by today's processing, provided a substantial amount of vitamin B_1 in each loaf. This was a period when bread truly was the staff of life; an individual's daily consumption of the food was measured in pounds. On such a diet, the peasants would have *exhibited* high levels of vitamin B_1. (It is interesting to note that Biskind attributes to the very high intake of vitamin B by peasants for whom bread was the staff of life, the early recovery of peasant women from childbirth, so that they were able to return to work in the fields. He specifically notes that a diet high in vitamin-B complex allows earlier involution of the uterus, which the public would describe as "the return of the organs to normal." He also notes that the heavy menstruation experienced by modern women in the first few menstruals after childbirth is also prevented by such high intake of the vitamin-B complex.)

The range of the values, it might be expected, would be narrower than that encountered in blood samples from twentieth-century men and women. Who is to say what constitutes the norm in this picture? Were the peasants oversupplied, or are you, with twentieth-century average blood levels, undersupplied? To us, this approach is directly related to the problem of determining if a thousand dollars a week can be considered a munificent income. For you and us, quite possibly it would be. But would it be for a Rockefeller?

In addition to tests that establish the "normal" blood levels of a vitamin, there is a more elaborate approach to the question: the depletion test. In this, an individual is deprived of a vitamin until the excretion of the vitamin in the urine drops. Then the vitamin is fed.

At the point at which excretion begins to increase, the tester considers that the individual has reached a level of intake beyond the body's basic requirement.

Surprisingly, although the concept seems foolproof, it is misleading. In repeated experiments, numbering hundreds of thousands, research scientists have been able to show that, between the body's basic minimum requirement for a nutrient and the level that is ideal, there is an enormous difference; and in that difference may lie the distinction between minimal health and buoyant health. Obviously, the depletion concept does not include consideration of the role of nutrition in helping us to reach buoyant health.

Dr. H. C. Sherman, for instance, in research that has become classic, has shown that an intake of calcium or certain vitamins, far beyond the minimum requirements of the body, confers upon the animal health, a prolonged prime of life, and superior longevity. The depletion or excretion test, which purports to establish requirements for endurance, actually only establishes the minimal intakes that will keep the flesh from parting with the skeleton. Yet these minimal intakes are what the American Medical Association and other groups tell us are *all* that are needed for good health. Everything else, because it is finally excreted, is, they say, of no value.

Let us return to our analogy in which the adequacy of a given income is problematical until you know the circumstances of the spender. It is conceivable that an individual might have a million dollars held in trust for him, and so be in need of money. It is not only conceivable but an actuality that the amount of vitamin B_1 in the blood gives no indication whatsoever of its availability to the individual. To be utilized in the body, this vitamin—and this is true of many other nutrients—must be combined with phosphorus. (Phosphorus is needed by the body in regular amounts to perform complex biochemical functions, as yet little understood. It is known to be, along with calcium, vital in bone formation, and plays an important role in the function of vitamin B_1 and others.) Some nutrients require further linkages with other substances to form enzyme systems. (Enzymes function as catalysts; that is, they assist and speed up almost every activity of the body from digestion to thought.) The amount of vitamin B_1 in the blood does not tell us how successful you are in *phosphorylating* (combining with phosphorus) the vitamin. It does not tell us whether your body is efficient in forming the particular enzyme system in which vitamin B_1 is a necessary component.

It is again not only conceivable but an actuality that there are individuals who show signs of deficiency in the presence of "adequate" (average) intake of a vitamin and high "normal" blood levels of the factor. The classical, if exaggerated, example of this type of fault, it is believed, is found in muscular dystrophy, where the muscles are starving for vitamin E because the enzyme is lacking that would permit the muscles to utilize vitamin E—this, despite the rich supply of the vitamin in the blood.

Poor nutrition is part of an inevitable cycle. At the outset it debilitates the pituitary gland. This gland influences the enzyme systems through which nutrients are utilized. Thus, as deficiency lowers the efficiency of the gland, digestion, absorption, utilization, and formation of enzyme systems will, in parallel degree, suffer impairment. Now, the very nutrients needed to stimulate the pituitary are utilized with steadily decreasing effectiveness, and the gland in turn continues to go downhill. An individual suffering from this condition frequently refuses to respond to the therapeutic dosages of the nutrients he apparently needs. What, then, would be the significance and the usefulness of classifying his blood levels?

Parenthetically, this interplay between the functioning of the glands and the worth of the diet, largely unexplored in American scientific research and largely unappreciated by American endocrinologists, requires study. It offers, for one thing the opportunity to escape via the glandular system from the inflexible and purportedly immutable dictates of heredity. (See Chapter 13 for a detailed discussion of this point.)

Unfortunately, there is no blood test that will define an individual's unique inherited nutritional requirements. In Chapter 12 we point out that deficits in prenatal nutrition may be reflected in the individual's later life by an exaggerated need for a particular nutrient. Dr. Roger Williams has demonstrated that deficiencies incurred by an individual's exaggerated need for certain nutrients may take the form of symptoms apparently far removed from nutritional causes. In his book *Free and Unequal* he gives the example of a chemist with migraine headache that disappeared when his thiamin (B_1) intake was raised to seven times the estimated normal requirement.[1]

In the senior author's experience, likewise, there are many indi-

[1] The senior author has observed a similar response in a stammerer.

viduals in the population whose qualitative diet needs are sharply different from those of the mythical "average person" whose chemistry has been made the authorities' yardstick. Perhaps the most striking response to more than the recommended normal intake of a nutrient occurs in those individuals ranging from the mentally retarded to the so-called normal. Heightened mental alertness, rises in IQ, less difficulty in concentration, prolonged memory span, even changes in the neurotic personality toward the norm have been the results of even a comparatively small increase in glutamic acid intake.

Glutamic acid is a protein substance. It is abundant in protein foods; milk casein is more than 20 per cent glutamic acid. Furthermore, it is believed that the acid is synthesized in the body. But despite the apparent generosity of the supply, a small rise in the intake—perhaps a tablespoon or so daily—has been found to yield improvement in mental performance, social adaptability, and personality structure, which is another way of saying what we said before. But we cannot overemphasize our point. How are we to explain such responses unless we conclude, since all individuals do not respond in this way, that there are some of us in this world who need and would profit by larger than "average" or "normal" intakes of beneficial nutritional substances? Yet the American Medical Association maintains that a "normal" person, eating a "normal" diet, does not need glutamic acid or any other supplement.[2]

While we have shown that blood assays offer no help in this area, it has been suggested that depletion tests have another usefulness. Surely, it is argued, we can gain some idea of the individual's nutritional needs by how long a poor diet must continue before signs of a deficiency appear. If anything, this method of testing—both drastic and possibly dangerous—will do nothing except to fortify the key concept of this chapter: that each of us has unique nutritional needs. The human organism exhibits a remark-

[2] One physician, outraged by AMA dogma on the "uselessness" of food supplements, asked how they can generalize about 190,000,000 diets.

able ability to adapt itself to unfavorable environment, internally and externally, and the duration of survival or the duration of the maintenance of good health or freedom from signs of deficiency on a poor diet tests nothing more than the capacity of that individual body to resist punishment.

We have already had such tests on a grand scale. There were individuals who were carried out of the concentration camps of World War I in the terminal stages of beriberi, pellagra, and other deficiency diseases. There were those who, though emaciated, managed to totter out, and there were those who showed no sign of deficiency other than loss of body fat. What shall we conclude from this massive "test"? Only this, that individuals have individual nutritional requirements, and that norms computed on the basis of averages constitute no proper yardstick by which to appraise the dietary needs of a mass population.

There are other fallacies in the biochemical attempts to measure nutritional needs. For one thing, the quantitative estimation of blood nutrients faces resolutely toward the past and gives us no estimate of future needs. Take the case of the woman whose heartburn in the fifth month of pregnancy is relieved by riboflavin injections. A blood assay done before her pregnancy began would probably have shown her to be reasonably well supplied with the vitamins, but would have offered no basis for prophecy when, as in this case, her body was faced with the steadily growing, parasitic demand of the baby. All that we can say is that conditioning factors exist: factors which, coming into play at a given moment, may raise nutritional requirements far beyond the level of those supplied by the "average" diet yielding the "average" requirement.

We will anticipate some of the discussion to come via a "typical" teenager who will also exemplify the points already made in this chapter. Let us consider a fifteen-year-old girl. She is a very feminine person, with a rounded body, with strictly feminine distribution of body hair—underarm and pubic—and no noticeable amount of hair elsewhere. Her structure and certain characteristics of her biochemistry indicate that she is what she is by virtue of a strong dominance of female hormones (estrogens) over male hormones (androgens). All human beings, male or female, manufacture both these factors, but the ratios differ, and so we sometimes encounter masculine women and feminine men, as well as the "'real'" man or "real" woman. Our example is intensely feminine.

We know that very large production of female hormone, at its peaks in the glandular cycle, may result in truly incapacitating menstruals, preceded by disturbances in the premenstrual week. In that period there will be perhaps a craving for sweets, a feeling of shaking or actual tremor, a sensation of being bloated abdominally and in the breast; and pain in the back, thighs, and bosom. We have reason to believe, as we explained in another chapter, that this high output of female hormone may contribute to varicose veins and may precede the development of cystic mastitis—a disease of the breast which in turn has been known to precede cancer of the breast.

Now the nutritionist knows that there is a regulatory system in the body to prevent the excessive accumulation of female hormones. Manufacture does not drop; but the hormone is destroyed by a well-nourished liver. Furthermore, the factors needed to aid the liver in destruction of the female hormone are known; they comprise certain B-complex vitamins, and complete protein.

Should the nutritionist call for assays of the blood chemistry of this girl? Or should he recognize that nutrient levels falling well within the "normal" range may fail to protect her against an excessive accumulation of female hormone? This teenager has a conditioning factor at work, and one that makes the concept of the "well-balanced diet" too indefinite and too generic to be useful. Her output of estrogenic hormone is such that she requires unusually high intake of certain dietary factors so that her liver may cope with the situation. Is it not the obligation of the nutritionist, then, to institute for this girl a standard of protein and vitamin-B complex intake that ignores completely the minimum

daily requirements set by the authorities on the basis of a mythical "average" woman?

We could multiply similar examples until they obscured the issue. Instead, let us pursue our thesis. We know that no two individuals have exactly the same *quantitative* dietary requirements.
Qualitatively we all need the same things; but *our* need for vitamin C and our teenagers' are things apart. We know also that
there are circumstances that may raise (and conceivably, those
that will lower) dietary requirements very sharply. If you show us
a diet and ask whether it is adequate, our reply must come in
terms of you as a person, and our reply, tempered by consideration of only one factor, might be this: "This diet will keep you out
of trouble if you stay in bed, but if you are working under either
physical or emotional pressure, it may not be adequate."

Apropos of this point, years ago the senior author received a
telephone call from a group of interns of a large municipal hospital. They were engaging in an experiment in an attempt to define
the level of vitamin C intake (or deficiency) at which signs of
scurvy would appear. They described the experiment. They were
to stay in bed (an experimental condition that will always be of
interest to overworked interns) and consume a diet devoid of vitamin C. The author prophesied that probably no signs of deficiency would appear until they left their beds and undertook
some kind of active labor. The young medical men accepted this
view reluctantly, since it did not fit their preconception of the
situation. The author's forecast, however, was firmly grounded.
Few medical men are familiar enough with medical history. If
their knowledge of it were greater, they might be more wary than
they are of making dogmatic statements.

In medieval times, when salad foods were grown for cows, and
oranges and tomatoes were considered dangerous for human consumption, signs of deficiency in vitamin C tended to exhibit themselves in the organs or the systems of the body where stress made
its impact. Blacksmiths of old, for example, complained of a hem-

orrhage condition then called "blacksmith's arm." Soldiers complained of "soldier's leg," and sailors had similar complaints.

For years it was supposed that newborn babies had reserves of vitamin C or manufactured the substance—for even upon the vitamin C-deficient formulas masquerading as substitutes for mother's milk (which is adequate in vitamin C) the babies, to the age of five months, did not develop signs of scurvy. It was later realized that babies up to the age of five months are relatively inactive—and deficiency, once again, tends more to exhibit itself in the presence of and in organs subjected to stress.

There are conditioning factors within the diet itself, even where the identity of the eater is not a variable which must be considered. Contemplate, for instance, the nineteen-year-old who presented himself at a dentist's office with a complaint which turned out to be gingivitis of the fourth grade: the worst form. The grading is predicated on the ease with which the gums bleed. Obviously, gums that bleed when faced with the challenge of a celery sandwich on rye crisp are in better health than those that bleed spontaneously. When a person awakens in the morning to find his pillow slip blood-stained, that is spontaneous bleeding.

In this latter category the teenager fell. The dentist, a specialist in nutrition, recognized what appeared to be a classical vitamin C deficiency, but this evaluation collided head-on with an analysis of the diet, which showed an average intake of distinctly more than the "minimum daily requirement" of vitamin C at the age level.

Investigation revealed that the young man was employed in a bakery and, as part of his remuneration, he had the privilege of taking home what he chose from the day's leftovers. This privilege he exercised by consuming from a dozen to two dozen sweet buns daily, an item he had neglected to list in his menu report.

The intake of starch and sugar and the need for vitamin C (B_1 as well) are correlated. Rising consumption of foods such as sweet buns brings with it an increased need for the vitamin not supplied by the buns. Moreover, a youngster stuffed with cake is not likely to feel the impulse to consume fruit, so that the circumstance gives us a perfect example of what is meant when we call sugar and processed flour "displacing foods."

Before the dentist discovered that the young man was in the habit of stuffing himself with buns, he tried the experiment of raising the vitamin C intake. Not until he elevated the dosage to a figure twenty times the "minimum daily requirement" did the bleeding stop. It is not uncommon in therapeutic use of nutritional factors to find that dosages far beyond "requirements" are necessary, but this level of need seemed fantastic. Accordingly, the practitioner searched for factors that might have raised the vitamin C requirement, and ultimately the buns were indicated.[3]

But there is another important point in such a case as this: While such a conditioning factor appears to exist within the framework of the diet itself, the personal equation must still be considered, for there are individuals in whom similarly exaggerated intake of processed sugar and starch might produce no demonstrable effects at all.

It may be seen from this case that the adequacy of a given diet may seriously be shaken by changes that would not alter the superficial compliance of the diet with minimum daily requirement. Consider the dentist's patient. We can assume that his menus in his pre-bun days gave him the proteins, the vitamins, the minerals, the fats, and the calories deemed essential to well-being. The addition of the buns might create a superfluity of calories. It would also create a relative deficiency of vitamin C, for the absolute intake of the vitamins would not have changed.

Would you like more evidence? Colloid goiter develops in cows fed a diet deficient in iodine. This relationship between nutrient and gland function has long been recognized. Less known is the observation that the colloid goiter resulting from iodine deficiency in cows may be reduced by administration of vitamin B_1. Does

[3] Even here, the consensus disagrees: it does not recognize a relationship between sugar intake and vitamin C requirement.

the amount of vitamin B_1 in the diet affect the need for iodine?

A drug used to treat the overactive thyroid, a thiourea derivative, was originally found in cabbage. Since it had been noticed that persons eating large amounts of cabbage as a principal constituent of the diet—which was therefore unbalanced—suffered from goiters, it seemed logical to administer the drug in an effort to reduce the activity of the *overactive* gland. Now, in addition to suppressing thyroid activity, thiourea reduces oxidation. One packer of frozen apricots, fully appreciating the commercial value of the drug, added it to his fruit to keep the fruit from darkening, until the authorities intervened. Presumably, the consumer would always have the privilege of adding thyroid hormone to his fruit cocktail, as an antidote. Few of us realize that there is a possibility that our choice of foods—in this instance, of the cabbage family—may increase the need for critical nutrients such as iodine and vitamin B_1, to protect the thyroid.

If you are not alarmed that a principle found in cabbage may interfere with thyroid action, it may also not panic you to know that carotene, vegetable vitamin A, in large quantities has the same effect. This is an occupational risk of overenthusiastic vegetarianism, and a penalty not appreciated by those who consume tremendous quantities of vegetable juices at "health food" bars. Liver also contains an antithyroid principle, though it should be pointed out that it functions only when the intake of the meat is truly very large; thus, we are not here limiting the consumption of liver once or twice a week. (In fact, eat plenty of it if you can; it's an excellent food.)

A vitamin that has been used in an attempt to recolor gray hair —successfully, in some instances, despite the derision of the gray-haired authorities—para-amino-benzoic acid (paba), is also an antithyroid factor in high dosage, and has been used successfully in the treatment of hyperthyroidism. This is not the only instance in which para-amino-benzoic acid plays a role in glandular function. Its action in gray hair, it seems to us, should be credited to a stimulating effect on pituitary and adrenal function. Any scientist voicing this latter statement would find himself under fire in a conclave of nutritionists, yet it happens to be solidly based on observations already reported. For instance, the dosage of an adrenal hormone, cortisone, needed to benefit an arthritic, may be cut if para-amino-benzoic acid is given simultaneously. Thus, an individual with low adrenal activity may need more paba—as he needs, for the same reason, more salt.

Still another factor in nutrition displays an interesting action when the thyroid is overactive. When the functioning of the gland is so excessive that a toxic state develops, in the course of which the sufferer exhibits intense nervousness and intense anxiety, vitamin E has been found helpful as a tranquilizing agent. This condition also increases the need for the vitamin-B complex.

Turning now from our discussion of diet content, let us dwell for a moment on *when* to eat.

It has been estimated that 10 per cent of us suffer with low blood sugar, and that 10 per cent of American men have stomach ulcers. These disorders call for frequent small meals rather than infrequent large meals. We do not know what percentage of us have the body structure that is accompanied by a fast-emptying stomach needing frequent refueling. The chances are, however, that millions of Americans would profit by escape from the meal schedule dictated by the exigencies of commuting. Meals should meet the demands of one's constitution rather than those of the clock.

Primitive people who eat whenever they are hungry escape the dyspepsia, heartburn, gas, and indigestion that constantly trouble civilized people. It has also been found, though the reasons are not yet understood, that animals maintained on frequent small feedings are more resistant to hardening of the arteries, a ratio of something like seven to one, than animals fed the same diet in the ordinary manner. This raises the question, is it not possible that the body metabolizes less efficiently when food is ingested in smaller amounts? That this is true of human beings has been demonstrated. Cholesterol does not rise as high on a given diet if it is fed in frequent small meals rather than the usual three squares. It is lower when the diet is low in sugar—even in the presence of saturated fat and cholesterol in the diet.

These notes should give you pause for thought when you turn to the diet for low blood sugar (Chapter 11). That diet is not only for sufferers from hypoglycemia. It is essentially a very good diet, presented in the pattern of frequent small meals which is a useful pattern for a great many people. Such a diet, supplemented with generous amounts of brewer's yeast, wheat germ, and liver, would constitute ideal treatment for those who must recover from severe nutritional deficiencies. In the form in which it is present in this text, the hypoglycemia diet may be conducive for some people to a relative freedom from digestive disorders and malfunction in the utilization of food.

However, the very subject of this chapter will warn the reader that no dogmatic statement of a "well-balanced diet" will be found here. There are those, perhaps, who have adapted to the large carbohydrate intake of modern man. There are those who have less successfully adapted and who thereby would profit greatly by a return to man's earlier diet—fat and protein, minus the processed carbohydrates and largely devoid even of the unprocessed varieties. There are those who will do perfectly well on a diet devoid of any concern for the nutritional niceties. These are the individuals who, as we have remarked, have such a good heredity—derived from such good eggs—that they can ignore the rules of hygiene and good nutrition.

Actually, at this point the authors may seem to be abdicating their nutritional responsibility to you, because of the individuality of the dietary equation. It is impossible to say what percentage of you would find tremendous profit by placing yourselves on the diet for hypoglycemia. Certainly no person in normal health would be harmed by such a diet; and many individuals would find heightened well-being. It is likewise true that there are readers who will profit by the diet for pregnancy given in this text, whether or not they are bringing children into the world. Such a diet represents a more conventional "well balanced," and happily exceeds the "minimum daily requirements" which have been inflicted upon the public, as though requirements are stereotyped. The reader must therefore seek out his own nutritional destiny. The effort is worthwhile.

Regardless of the dietary pathway chosen, it is necessary to know in a practical and realistic way how to shop for the right kinds of food. This information you will find in Chapter 19. The proper vitamin-mineral food supplements are described in Chapter 15.

10. Reducing: Don't fall for the fads

As we write this, a sizable number of the American public (perhaps you?) are attempting to reduce by consuming daily four glasses of a prepared liquid diet with a 900-calorie value for the day. This fad, like many others, will ultimately disappear as, unfortunately, the excess weight *will not*—for any system of reducing that does not establish a new pattern of eating habits will inevitably be followed by the reacquisition of weight.

There are many misconceptions concerning individuals who need to lose weight and the manner in which weight should be lost. The public has been persuaded that, by some process of biochemical prestidigitation, the calories of protein flit through the system, gaily yielding energy but refusing to thicken the hips. The public believes that fats are fattening, and that unwanted curves can be "vibrated" out of existence.

Untold fortunes have been made by exploitation of these bizarre ideas. Quack physicians have retired in wealth after "inventing" injections that are supposed to make you slim while you are eating like a pig.[1] Reducing salons with a full panoply of machines of many types have earned fortunes for their promoters. Milk farms have waxed prosperous by instituting starvation procedures that could have been pursued more conveniently and less

[1] There appears to be genuine merit in the chorionic gonadotrophic injections of Dr. A. T. W. Simeons, but he also employs a low-calorie diet.

expensively at home. Psychiatrists and psychologists have occupied their valuable time in dealing with emotional causes, real or fancied, for overeating and excess weight.

Perhaps it is pointless to throw the white light of truth on this tangled situation, for it is in the area of reducing that the public (sometimes knowingly, we are afraid) indulges its penchant for seeking the bizarre and the exotic in dietary fadism. Nor is the truth easy to elicit, for, as the Lama observed in *Lost Horizon*, there are many pathways to the truth and we moderately believe in all of them.

Let's first pick a quarrel with our omnipresent friends, the psychoanalysts. Although some doctrinaire analysts would not agree with our statement, it is manifestly ridiculous to suppose that every fat person represents a suitable subject for the couch, just as it is ridiculous to assume that eight or ten pounds of excess weight necessarily means that the person is eating to express a need for missing affection, feelings of insecurity or inadequacy, or a requirement for the building of a fat blanket as a shield against a cruel world. In short, we are justified in assuming that a fat person is a normal person carrying some excess weight—at least, until some other explanation is proved.

We recognize that some individuals do eat compulsively, reverting to the pattern of infancy where acute distress could be alleviated by warm milk or any other kind of oral diversion. In fact, the senior author had a remarkable experience in this area with an entertainer who weighed 300 pounds at the age of twelve and never dropped far below that level throughout his adult life. He had been assured that his problem was purely glandular, since in puberty there was a milky secretion from his breasts. He had also been assured that the only remedy for his obesity was surgical removal of the fat. This suggestion resembles the "cure" offered by the use of the 900-calorie beverages: aside from some magnificent surgical scars it would leave the individual without dietary re-education, and thereby almost inevitably disposed to return to the dietary habits that initially created the excess weight.

We suggested to the troubled entertainer the possibility that his 125 pounds of excess fat answered some kind of psychological need for him. Under much prodding he went to a psychiatrist. Within seven months he had discovered the emotional basis for his lifelong gargantuan appetite. Now that he had the knowledge that could preclude the recurrence of his trouble, we proceeded to remove his 125 pounds of excess weight, without surgery, *without glandular medication,* without continued psychotherapy, and *without drugs* to depress the appetite. The diet we used is given at the end of this chapter. It is designed to provide 1200 calories daily: not the starvation level of the 900-calorie preparations, which constitute a cause of weakness, hunger, and deficiencies that can often produce serious effects. Certainly, death certificates have indicated excessively rapid reducing as the prime cause, but more often the death is attributed to some other sickness, following a period of rapid reduction. The certificate honors the aggravation rather than the real cause.

Here two points arise that will interest you. They should interest the medical profession as well. The entertainer was reduced by a technique that *distributed the weight loss evenly.* This method, devised by the senior author and a medical colleague, partially solves a problem that has particularly plagued a great many women. It is usually expressed: "When I reduce, I lose weight, but not where I want to," or, "When I reduce my face looks ghastly, but my midriff and hips do not shrink." The other point concerns the statement that 900 calories a day constitutes a kind of starvation. This requires explanation: Many of the products sold for use as the basis for a 900-calories diet bear the promise that they provide all the nutrients essential for good health. Such a claim reminds one of the clerk who resigned from the Patent Office in 1895, on the grounds that his job had no future: everything that could be invented already had been.

Yet in nutrition, without waiting for future discoveries, we are aware of a number of factors in food that have not been isolated and identified. There is, for instance, an antithyroid factor in liver.

But in the same food there is an antifatigue factor so effective that the addition of liver to the diet prolongs the endurance of animals violently exercising by more than 300 per cent; an effect that *cannot* be obtained with any known vitamin or nutrient. A factor in carrots, as yet not identified, reduces the need of the body for oxygen.

There are undoubtedly new vitamins to be discovered and there is no way of knowing whether a mixture of cottonseed oil, soy flour, and nonfat milk fortified with the *known* vitamins and a few minerals (these are the common ingredients of the 900-calorie wonder diet) will include these unknown factors, any more than we know which of these unknowns will turn out to be essential to the human organism. It is therefore possible that these products will cause types of deficiency we are not yet qualified to recognize. But if you insist upon using them, we suggest that an evening meal, with a normal menu, be substituted for one of the "liquid meal" servings. If there are no deficiencies created by these products, at least the additional food will help to avoid the constipation created in many persons by a liquid diet.

A second kind of deficiency is created by the liquid diets and this is not in the realm of conjecture. You may recall the Berlin Airlift. Understandably, the Air Force wanted to cut to the minimum the food allotment for each inhabitant of Berlin in order to reduce the demand upon pilots and planes. That minimum was determined to be 1600 calories a day. Below this, the diet was considered to represent starvation for working people.

Likewise, experiments at the University of Minnesota on controlled starvation found that the subjects became weak, apathetic, irritable, and asocial, lost interest in the opposite sex, developed circulatory disorders, and became obsessed with thoughts of food to the point that all other activities were relegated to a secondary place. Were these conditions caused by a diet of 900 calories? Far from it: the diet allowed 1500. It is also true that the subjects remained on the diet for six months; it is also true that most persons do not use the new liquid preparations for so long a period. Let it also be remembered, though, that good nutrition, continued for at least as long a period as the starvation regime, did not bring about complete psychological recovery in the subjects of the starvation experiment. In other words, despite the fact that they were volunteers in the research, the men who underwent this experiment were left with lasting scars.

So we find neither scientific rhyme nor psychologic reason in the 900-calorie foods. Weight is not ordinarily accumulated rapidly; it should not be removed rapidly. A reducing diet should be a *miniature* of the normal diet, so framed that expansion of the size of the portions will permit the diet to be used *after* weight loss has been stopped.

The belief that the calories of protein "stick to the ribs" has been the basis for exploiting the ignorance of the public, and has made fortunes for bakers who market "reducing breads." There is no such thing as a reducing bread: nothing that you eat reduces you; and there is *no such thing as a calorie that confines itself to the production of energy.* Excess calories will usually be stored—alas!—where they can be seen.

When a bread is advertised as a "protein bread," the baker does not have to make misleading claims, because the misconception has already been planted in the public's mind. Though protein yields approximately 4 calories to the gram, 120 to the ounce, the identical value of *sugar and starch*, the average person not only believes that protein calories are *not fattening*, but that with such food he is consuming lower calorie value than comes from starches and sugars. In advertising the calorie value of such a bread as low, the baker plunges boldly into half-truth. Since protein has the same caloric value as starch and sugar, and since bread contains practically no fat, it is obvious that for any loaf (of equal weight) of bread to be lower in calories than any other loaf, part of it would need to be sawdust. Since this material is not employed, the baker evades outright mis-statement by a simple device: He gives the calorie value of a *slice*—and the public seizes upon this because the value given for the caloric value of a slice of reducing bread may be as little as half the value of a slice of ordinary bread. The explanation is simple. Ordinary bread is sliced in 1-ounce units; the slices of reducing bread are thinner and weigh less. Weight for weight, all bread will have the same caloric value. Still another device is used to create the illusion of low calorie value in bread: the bakers employ more yeast food, rendering the leavening more effective, to create more air in the loaf.

The public's faith in protein, which the baker capitalizes upon in protein reducing breads, happens to be based on a germ of truth. Though calories from protein are the same as any other kind of calories, the term merely being a measurement of heat or energy value, a substantial proportion of the calories from protein are converted into glycogen. This is a carbohydrate. However, unlike *preformed* carbohydrates, starches and sugars, which are absorbed and digested quickly, as the discussion on low blood sugar indicates, the calories yielded by the glycogen formed from protein become available to the body slowly. This is the technical explanation behind the public's belief that "protein sticks to the ribs." It explains why a breakfast of starch and sugar permits mid-morning fatigue, and why one high in protein lends support to the body that is evident even through lunch hour. Likewise, it explains why a high-protein, high-fat diet is helpful to reducers. Calories are calories, but the energy value of protein is available to the body over a longer period, which is another way of saying that protein tends to keep the blood sugar elevated for a longer period of time, calorie for calorie, than will starch and sugar. Since a drop in blood sugar tends to trigger appetite, it is obvious that a high protein diet helps to keep the reducer from feeling weak and tends to control his desire to nibble.

The reader will inevitably want to know about the "Calories Don't Count" theory that a diet high in fat[2] and protein and almost totally devoid of carbohydrate promotes reduction more effectively. It is true that Dr. Taller was the target for vicious

[2] With a proportion of the fat unsaturated.

slander by the American Medical Association, Dr. Frederick Stare of Harvard University, and the United States Food and Drug Administration. It is also true that the latter agency seized upon one of Dr. Taller's alleged commercial associations to make him the target for a criminal charge. It is, however, not true (*a*) that Dr. Taller originated this theory; or (*b*) that the theory is invalid and an example of food faddism.

The realization that some persons will reduce more effectively when starches and sugars are left out of the diet was first reported by a layman named Banting, hundreds of years ago. The theory was also put into practice in the so-called Salisbury diets, which were designed for the Earl of Salisbury, and from which book, entitled the *Mahda Diets,* we derive the term "Salisbury steak." The Salisbury or Mahda diets were simply high-protein, high-fat diets without much carbohydrate. Pennington then experimented with the diets, and found them effective; and Taller capitalized upon the thesis in his book, *Calories Don't Count.* It is true that calories do count, but it is obvious that Taller was simply striving for a catchy title. It is likewise true that there are statements in the book that cannot scientifically be justified. But the attack on Dr. Taller in the main was also not justified, for a diet of this type *is* successful in promoting reduction where the same diet with part of its calories derived from starch and sugar may not *for some individuals.* The fact of the matter is that Dr. Taller appears to have been penalized because he was not a member of "the club." This is demonstrated in a publication by the *Journal of the American Medical Association,* in October, 1963, of the Gordon diet, which was so meticulous in excluding carbohydrate that the authors recommended that English walnuts be consumed, but not other types of nuts, for the reason that the English walnut has a lower carbohydrate content than other nuts do. This is certainly reducing the carbohydrate intake to the *n*th part of a hair. If it is startling to the reader to find the *Journal of the American Medical Association* publishing as a "new approach to obesity" a diet which, when published by Dr. Taller previously, was denominated as an evidence of food faddism, the reader is now face to face with the reality toward which this book has several times pointed. There are two bodies of truth in science today: the total truth, such as may be exemplified by a book of this type; and the partial truth, defined as the "authorities" decide to define it.

The secret of the more successful reduction of some individuals on a diet devoid of carbohydrate, compared with their lack of success on the same number of calories with some carbohydrate as the source, appears to lie in the action of carbohydrate in promoting the retention of salt. This in turn, of course, leads to the retention of liquid in some individuals. If water is retained in the tissues when food is burned, it is obvious that weight loss is not going to be very satisfactory.

A popular misconcept has it that the *addition* of polyunsaturated fat to an ordinary, adequate diet will somehow magically melt the pounds away. Calories added to an ordinary diet spell nothing but weight gain. The myth derives from a distortion of a fact: if a diet is held to 60 grams of carbohydrate daily, generous amounts of fat and protein, in six meals a day, taking 20 per cent of that fat in the form of polyunsaturated oils and margarine will actually help to burn body depot fat. Please note the qualifying phrases: the public has leaped into a broad generalization deriving from a very highly qualified and restricted proposition.

And now, the reducing diet we recommend, which will safely reduce a normal person at a rate of not over two pounds a week. Faster than this is dangerous; slower than this is frustrating. The individual in normal health who does not lose weight on the diet that follows may be a candidate for the low-carbohydrate, high-protein, high-fat diet under medical supervision.

It will be noted that vitamin supplements are stipulated as part of this diet.[3] The supplementing of the diet is necessary for two reasons: First, when food intake is drastically reduced, so is vitamin intake, and the supplements thereby act to prevent defi-

---

[3] Vitamins have no calorie value; can't contribute to weight gain. If they could, the millennium for "skinnies" would have arrived.

ciency. This may explain why this diet with its supplements is rarely guilty of causing nervousness, irritability, fatigue, and some of the other common consequences of reducing diets not protected with supplements. Second, in research by the senior author in association with a medical man, we were able to demonstrate

IDEAL WEIGHTS FOR WOMEN
(Ages twenty-five and over)

HEIGHT (in shoes with average heels)	WEIGHT IN POUNDS (as ordinarily dressed)		
FEET INCHES	SMALL FRAME	MEDIUM FRAME	LARGE FRAME
4 11 ...	104-11	110-18	117-27
5 0 ...	105-13	112-20	119-29
5 1 ...	107-15	114-22	121-35
5 2 ...	110-18	117-25	124-35
5 3 ...	113-21	120-28	127-38
5 4 ...	116-25	124-32	131-42
5 5 ...	119-28	127-35	133-45
5 6 ...	123-32	130-40	138-50
5 7 ...	126-36	134-44	142-54
5 8 ...	129-39	137-47	145-58
5 9 ...	133-43	141-51	149-62
5 10 ...	136-47	145-55	152-66
5 11 ...	139-50	148-58	155-69

IDEAL WEIGHTS FOR MEN
(Ages twenty-five and over)

HEIGHT (in shoes with average heels)	WEIGHT IN POUNDS (as ordinarily dressed)		
FEET INCHES	SMALL FRAME	MEDIUM FRAME	LARGE FRAME
5 2 ...	116-25	124-33	131-42
5 3 ...	119-28	127-36	133-44
5 4 ...	122-32	130-40	137-49
5 5 ...	126-36	134-44	141-53
5 6 ...	129-39	137-47	145-57
5 7 ...	133-43	141-51	149-62
5 8 ...	136-47	145-56	153-66
5 9 ...	140-51	149-60	157-70
5 10 ...	144-55	153-64	161-75
5 11 ...	148-59	157-68	165-80
6 0 ...	152-64	161-73	169-85
6 1 ...	157-69	166-78	174-90
6 2 ...	163-75	171-84	179-96
6 3 ...	168-80	176-89	184-202

that the vitamins, when properly used, help to direct the weight loss so that it is more likely to be uniform. This is a distinct help to those women[4] who complain that, when they lose weight, the loss shows up first on the face, making them cadaverous; and last or not at all in the areas that really need reduction.

DIET FOR REDUCING

This diet is balanced in protein intake, and contains enough fat and carbohydrate to keep body function unimpaired. By the code system employed, and the lists of foods, the need for set menus is eliminated, and there is no need for counting calories.

Every effort has been made to keep vitamin-mineral intake as high as possible. However, a diet below 2400 calories is very likely to be deficient in vitamins and minerals; that is a risk inherent in reducing the gross intake of food. It is recommended therefore that this diet be supplemented with multiple vitamins and minerals in capsules. These will not interfere with reduction, but will help to avoid deficiencies of the type that have made reduction hazardous in the past.

On this diet, which permits much more generous meals than most, a normal person should lose about 6 pounds a month. On it, some have lost as much as 150 pounds—safely, sanely, and without discomfort.

> *For breakfast you may eat . . .*
> One serving of fruit
> One egg or egg substitute
> ½ slice (thin) whole wheat toast with ½ level teaspoonful butter
>   or One glass of skimmed milk instead of whole wheat toast
> One cup of coffee or tea (optional) (no sugar; no cream or milk)

[4] The technique is effective for a smaller percentage of men.

Prepare your egg in one of the following ways:
  Plain omelet
  Poached
  Soft boiled
  Hard boiled
  Raw

Substitutes for one egg are:
  Buttermilk (one glass)
  Calf's liver (two ounces)
  Cottage Cheese (four tablespoons)
  Lamb chop (one small, lean)
  Lamb kidney (one)
  Mutton chop (one small, lean)
  Skimmed milk (one glass)

For lunch you may eat . . .
  One helping of lean meat, fish, fowl, or meat substitute
  One vegetable from vegetable list A
  One salad (from salad list)
  One serving of fruit or dessert
  One glass of skimmed milk or buttermilk
  One cup of coffee or tea (optional) (no sugar; no cream or milk)

For dinner you may eat . . .
  One cup of soup (optional)
  One helping of lean meat, fish, fowl, or meat substitute
  Two vegetables from vegetable list A; plus one from vegetable
    list B

          or

  One vegetable from vegetable list A; plus one from vegetable
    list B

          plus

  One helping of salad (salad list)
  One portion of fruit or dessert
  Coffee or tea (no sugar; no cream or milk)

Substitutes for meat helping are:
  Buttermilk (two cups)
  Cottage cheese (¾ cup)
  Eggs—poached or omelet (two eggs)
  Skimmed milk (two cups)
  Whole milk (one cup)

CHOOSE FOODS FROM THESE LISTS:

Soups:
   Beef broth
   Chicken, mutton broth
   Clear vegetable soup
   Consomme
   Other clear soups
   NOTE: No creamed soups, none with milk or content of vegetables, meat, or cereals.

Salads:
   Celery and cabbage
   Pimento and greens
   Radish and watercress
   Stuffed Tomato (cottage cheese, chopped celery)
   Tossed greens
   Watercress and lettuce
   NOTE: If butter is omitted from vegetables at lunch, one teaspoonful of salad dressing may be used. Divide between lunch and dinner, if salads are eaten twice daily; use vinegar or lemon juice to augment.

Fruits:
   Apple (one, small)
   Apricots (two, medium size)
   Berries (one half cup)
   Cantaloupe (one half, medium size)
   Cherries (ten)
   Grapefruit (half, medium size)
   Grapes (twelve)
   Melons (two-inch section of average size melon)
   Nectarines (three)
   Orange (small)
   Peach (one)
   Pear (one, medium size)
   Persimmon (one half, small)
   Pineapple (two average slices)
   Plums (two)
   Tangerines (one, large)

Fruit juices:
   Grapefruit, Orange (unsweetened): 6 ounces (¾ of water glass)

Vegetables:

List A
    Asparagus (fresh or canned: eight spears)
    Beans: String (½ cup)
           Wax (½ cup)
    Beet greens (two heaping tablespoonfuls)
    Broccoli (one five inch stalk)
    Brussels sprouts (½ cup)
    Cabbage, cooked (½ cup)
    Cabbage, raw (¾ cup, shredded)
    Cauliflower (½ cup)
    Celery (five stalks)
    Chard (½ cup)
    Chicory (½ cup)
    Eggplant (½ cup)
    Endive (ten medium stalks)
    Green pepper (one, medium size)
    Kohlrabi (two heaping tablespoonfuls)
    Leeks, chopped (⅓ cup)
    Lettuce (ten leaves)
    Radishes (five, medium size)
    Sauerkraut (½ cup)
    Spinach (½ cup)
    Tomatoes, fresh (one)
    Tomatoes, canned (½ cup)
    Tomato juice: four ounces (½ cup)
    Watercress (ten pieces)

List B
    Beets (two heaping tablespoons)
    Carrots (two heaping tablespoons)
    Dandelion greens (three heaping tablespoons)
    Kale (two heaping tablespoons)
    Onion (one, small size)
    Parsnips (two heaping tablespoons)
    Peas (two heaping tablespoons)
    Pumpkin (three heaping tablespoons)
    Rutabaga (two heaping tablespoons)
    Squash (two heaping tablespoons)
    Turnips (two heaping tablespoons)

Meats:

Beef kidney (¼ lb.)
Beef liver (one slice, three inches square, ½ inch thick)
Beef, roast (two slices, about three inches square, ¼ inch thick)
Beef tongue (two average slices)
Beefsteak, lean (¼ lb. about one inch thick, 2½ inches square)
Calf's liver (¼ lb.)
Hamburger (¼ lb.)
Lamb chop (one, about two inches square, ½ inch thick)
Lamb kidney (two, average size)
Lamb, roast (one slice, 3½ inches square, ¼ inch thick)
Mutton, boiled (one slice, four inches square, ½ inch thick)
Mutton chop (two, medium size)
Veal cutlet (one, average size)
Veal kidney (two, average size)
Veal, roast (one slice, three inches by two inches, ¼ inch thick)

Poultry:

Chicken, broiler (½ medium size)
Chicken, gizzards (two, average size)
Chicken, livers (two whole, medium size)
Chicken, white meat (two slices, four inches square-cut very thin)

Fish:

Bass, sea (¼ lb.)
Bluefish (¼ lb.)
Carp (¼ lb.)
Cod, fresh or salt (¼ lb. to ½ lb.)
Flounder (¼ lb. to ½ lb.)
Frog Legs (¼ lb.)
Haddock (¼ lb. to ½ lb.)
Halibut (¼ lb.)
Herring, lake (¼ lb.)
Kingfish (¼ lb.)
Perch (¼ lb.)
Pike (¼ lb.)
Porgy (¼ lb.)
Red Snapper (¼ lb.)
Salmon (¼ lb.)
Smelt (¼ lb.)
Trout (¼ lb.)
Weakfish (¼ lb.)

Shellfish:

Clams, round (10 to 12)
Crab meat (one crab or ¾ cup flakes)
Lobster (½ small lobster or one cup flakes)
Mussels (four large or eight small)
Oysters (twelve large)
Scallops (⅔ cup, raw measurement)
Shrimp (⅔ cup)

Desserts:

Fruit cocktail (fruits from fruit list; small portion)
Cantaloupe cocktail
Orangeade (one and one-half oranges; one-half lemon; egg white; saccharine for sweetening)
Milk and ginger ale (half and half)
NOTE: Low calorie desserts don't exist; will power is the best dessert.

Appetite cheaters:

If your appetite is hearty—and dieting annoying because of hunger pangs—do the following:
Avoid soups: they are optional, anyway; and they tend to stimulate appetite.
Choose salad instead of one vegetable, at meal.
Protein tablets or wafers are useful as appetite cheaters. These are a concentration of essential food values such as in meat and milk—concentrated to the point where several tablets are the equivalent of a fair portion of such protein foods. They have little calorie value, but they do help to check the appetite.

Special notes

Sugar substitute: Use saccharine if you must have beverages sweetened.
Water consumption: No more than four glasses daily for first four days; then as much as you please—provided that you do not drink more than one glass of water with each meal.
Extra butter allowance: At luncheon or dinner, one level teaspoonful of butter may be used on your vegetables. If you prefer, you may use a teaspoonful of salad oil as a dressing on salad (at lunch or dinner—not both). If you use the salad oil, it replaces the butter.
Broil, pan broil, bake or roast meat, fish or poultry—*DO NOT*

FRY. Remove all visible fat before eating—*DO NOT EAT GRAVIES OR SAUCES.*

Do not eat or drink of the following without advice from your doctor or nutritionist:

alcoholic beverages	jello
beer, wine, whiskey	ketchup
avocado	mayonnaise
bacon or bacon fat	muffins
cake, candy, chocolate	nuts
coconut, cookies, crackers	olives
cream, sweet or sour	pancakes, peanut butter
doughnuts	pies, popcorn, potato chips
french fries, fried foods	pretzels, puddings
gravy, honey, ice cream	soda, ginger ale, cola
ices	sugar, syrups
jam	waffles
jelly	

Diet supplementation

The purpose of a reducing diet is to cut your calorie intake so that you will be forced to burn your own body fat. However, in reducing the quantity of food, we must be careful not to reduce your protein intake since this would create a loss of your own protein reserves.

High vitamin and mineral intake is essential so as not to deplete your reserves and perhaps injure your health. Optimal supplementation of vitamins and minerals is recommended since it does not interfere with reducing, but guards against dry skin, weak finger nails, brittle hair, and more serious deficiency disorders.

Keeping the body efficient in burning calories is another function of vitamin and mineral supplementation. This helps to avoid the weakness some people experience when they restrict their food intake.

Practically every vitamin and mineral—with the possible exception of vitamin C—is limited in a reducing diet. We therefore supplement the diet with: multiple minerals, multiple vitamins, the entire B-complex, and vitamin E.

These can be used in either syrup or capsule form. Those reducers who complain of the "sinking in" of the face will find additional supplements of vitamin E and lecithin useful because they preserve the depth of fat beneath the skin of the cheeks.

What to do to stay where you are:

When you have lost as much weight as your physician tells you it is safe to lose, increase your milk intake to two full glasses (for an adult), and use as much of the leafy vegetables as you wish. If you do not gain—or if you continue to lose—you can then increase your intake of bread—whole grain, please! If you still do not gain, the root and starchy vegetables may now be added cautiously, and with them, a little more butter. The vitamin supplements may and should be continued.

11. Mental illness: Do you fear it?

It is estimated that one American out of every ten will at some point in his or her life become a patient at an institution that treats the mentally ill. Now, think of the millions more who are classified as suffering from acute neurosis, those who are sufficiently in touch with what is termed "reality" but who recognize their illness and seek private treatment. The total number of sufferers from mental illness is alarming.

Neurosis and psychosis (insanity) threaten all of us, no mistaking that, as man's life becomes ever more complicated and tension ridden. We are faintly doubtful about the "average" (that word again!) psychiatrist's efforts to readjust his patient to a manifestly mediocre world, a world in which it is demonstrated to the intelligent person a thousand times a day that he is living on the third planet from the sun, a planet on which social order has not advanced much beyond the primitive state, and a man, in order to "succeed," must be almost as ruthless as were his cave ancestors in establishing primacy among themselves and over the animals.

Add to this the frustrating disillusionment that many of us experience when confronted with the fact that there is really *no escape*, and it is not surprising that we find the vast numbers of psychotics and neurotics who have given up. They feel they have *no hope*. Yet it has been demonstrated repeatedly with animals and humans that when they are offered a way out of their various "maze" problems, a proper incentive, they tend to be rejuvenated psychically.

But what has nutrition to do with mental health? And how can a man, dispirited, disillusioned, cynical, yes, even psychotic, ever make a comeback to the world of what he considers mediocrity— and even not only improve that world but imbue the world within his brain-pan with renewed hope, courage, and vitality? In ortho- dox medical circles you will be told that nutrition has little or nothing to do with neurosis or psychosis. Doctors will then "prove" their point by electro-shocking a man's brain until he is only too happy to come back to even a mediocre, frustrating exist- ence. There is an old biological concept: Pleasure or happiness is merely a cessation of pain. In spite of the monumental and signifi- cant research that others have published, few orthodox mental healers know anything about nutrition's role in preventing or cur- ing mental illness.

Can *we* offer hope for neurotics and psychotics? Yes. You see, we, unlike some psychiatrists, do not wish you to adjust to the mediocre, or to the world as it now exists. We want to develop *true* revolutionaries in the ultimate sense, clear-eyed and healthy, who will overthrow the old concept of medicine that attempts to *cure* disease rather than *prevent it*. And we have excellent evi- dence that poor nutrition is responsible for many of the world's ills. Once you become an informed, zealous revolutionary, you will find the real reality is not mediocre and that the battle *is* worth fighting. For there *is* hope, far beyond any hope proffered by current orthodox medical theories.

We will offer the record, which clearly shows that malnutrition produces profound changes in the human mind, not just in the body, and we will show that these neurotic and psychotic changes can sometimes be *reversed* with proper nutrition. But our thesis is not easy to grasp in spite of our attempts to make it so. We must begin with our explanation of "mental" illnesses.

Modern medical spokesmen now talk glibly of psychosomatic ill- ness, of the power of the mind over matter, and consider not at all that the scales may also tip in the other direction: that we should also be concerned with the influence of body on mind. Part of the difficulty lies in our continued separation of the concepts of emotional illness and physical illness. As one of the senior author's students remarked: "Is it not remarkable that an emotion can cause a change in the acid-alkaline balance of the saliva, and thereby contribute to tooth decay?" The author noted in reply that the change in the pH of the saliva *is part of the emotion.* Perhaps the best way to illustrate this point is to suggest that you try, with the cooperation of your doctor, an injection of epinephrine (adrenaline). The administration of this hormone, one of the factors released by the adrenal glands when the body is under stress, physical or emotional, is followed by all the emotional stigmata of fright; and so you will come to realize that being terrified, with all the symptoms that come with it, is neither an emotional or a physical manifestation, but a dynamic interplay between the two. It becomes futile, then, to talk about the influence of mind over matter. It is likewise unprofitable to deny that, among the factors contributing to abnormal reactions in the emotional area, there are physical contributions. Freud himself thought neurosis to have a physical basis.

Some somatic (body) factors such as adrenaline (and there are many others) not only can alter behavior, but can result in changes of perception and behavior that would undoubtedly be labeled as neurotic or even psychotic by many a psychiatrist.

The classic example of such a physically based altering of the personality occurs in vitamin-B deficiency. We must, however, appreciate the esoteric nature of the type of deficiency with which we are about to deal. Let us consider two levels of deficiency in thiamine (B_1). At the first level, one-third of a milligram or less per day, the body is totally unable to adapt to the interferences with metabolism that it suffers for want of an adequate supply of this nutrient. The "burning" of carbohydrates (starch and sugar) is interrupted midway; just as a fire for want of oxygen will yield a smoky flame, so does the combustion of carbohydrates with inadequate thiamine intake yield half-burned products of interrupted combustion. Some of these by-products are highly toxic; the nursing mother with an intake of thiamine as low as half a milligram a day will produce toxic breast milk and kill her baby. Pyruvic acid accumulates in the body; apathy overtakes the sufferer. Multiple neuritis develops and ultimately the patient will die—by drowning in internal fluid in the "wet" type of beriberi, or perhaps by heart failure in the "dry" type. Beriberi, incidentally, means "I cannot." Semantically, it is a happy choice, for lack of a "will to do" is a principal symptom of this disease.

Turning to an adequate thiamine intake, we can say that an individual who has at least a milligram of thiamine a day is not likely to develop any clear-cut symptoms of a deficiency, although one milligram may be far below the optimal intake for many individuals.

Between these two extremes is a kind of twilight zone of thiamine deficiency, which we may frivolously liken to social security: too much money to license one to starve to death; not enough for a full life. At this level of intake of the vitamin, the body has enough of the nutrient to make an attempt to carry on its activities, but too little to permit it to function properly. In a sense, this is a more devastating type of dietary deficiency than the level which, by inducing complete collapse, gives a quick warning.

Perhaps the best way to illustrate the insidious effects of such a twilight-zone deficiency is to trace the history of a group of volunteers who agreed to subsist for an extended period on a diet that pushed them down to this level. The experiment was conducted under the direction of the late Dr. Russell Wilder, Senior Physician of the Mayo Clinic.[1] His subjects were women. For the duration of the experiment, they agreed to be confined in a psychiatric hospital. Their diet was an interesting one. It consisted of reasonably lean beef, skim milk, fruit, vegetables, cheese, and desserts: in other words, one of the typical reducing diets on which count-

[1] *Symposium on Nutrition in Nervous and Emotional Disorders.* Williams and Wilkins, 1943.

less American women develop nervousness and irritability. (If this is the diet you are now following, *please* add more vitamins and minerals to it.) One element of the diet needs emphasis: the desserts. These were typical American desserts, marked by a high sugar content. Thiamine requirement is related to sugar intake; sugar raises the vitamin B_1 requirement but does not supply the vitamin. Since there was no restriction on dessert portions, the amount of vitamin B_1 provided in Dr. Wilder's experimental diet, which at first glance would seem to be adequate, became inadequate, swamped by the torrent of sugar that the subjects permitted themselves.

Let us follow a typical volunteer. She entered the experiment as a psychologically normal, well-adjusted, congenial person. Her physical examination was entirely negative. After three months of the diet, she complaimed of loss of manual dexterity. Her fingers felt like five thumbs. She broke the laboratory glassware she had been washing as part of the work assigned to keep her busy. Her attention span and her memory span were shortened. She suffered from nightmares, and awakened dripping with perspiration and apprehensive about a sensation of constriction—as though an iron band on her chest were interfering with her breathing.

Interpersonal relationships in the group broke down by the end of three months, and our volunteer complained that she couldn't get along with the others. She described unprovoked feelings of apprehension ("as if something terrible was about to happen").

Any psychologist or psychiatrist watching her, and aware of these strong sensations of unprovoked anxiety, would unhesitatingly have labeled her a neurotic. How many patients horizontal on a psychiatric couch should be vertical at a lunch counter is a moot question: for as yet there are no laboratory procedures that will let us clearly identify the twilight zone of thiamine deficiency; and the subtle symptoms are certainly not listed in the textbooks dealing with beriberi and pellagra.

The physical examination of the typical patient at this point showed a drop in the basal metabolism, which had been in the normal range, to a minus 33. Iodine deficiency is listed in the textbooks as the only deficiency in a nutrient that contributes to an underactive thyroid gland. If you find it surprising that thiamine deficiency will also cause hypo-thyroidism, you are referred to studies in Swiss veterinary medicine, in which you will learn that goiter in cows is reduced as satisfactorily with thiamine as it is by iodine. Here, we may note that today's senior Americans, having eaten unenriched bread and flour products for a majority of their years, are undoubtedly suffering with some mild degree of thiamine deficiency. As attempts are made to indict cholesterol for the responsibility for cardiovascular disease in this group, let it be remembered that subacute thiamine deficiency will cause hypothyroidism, and that hypothyroidism will permit cholesterol to rise even in the absence of a high cholesterol diet. The underactive thyroid, Cheraskin[2] has shown, occurs with striking frequency.

Another deficiency that affects the human brain and nervous system is inadequate intake of niacin. Pellagra, formerly a foremost killer, particularly in the Deep South, was found to be due to a deficiency in the vitamin-B complex. Tom Spies, M.D., at the Hillman Clinic in Alabama, had the curiosity to investigate the previous histories of patients under treatment for pellagra. He found many in which, with easily recognizable symptoms of pellagra evident, the patients had come to the clinic earlier, complaining of nervousness, "swimmy-headedness," a sense of confusion, hypersensitivity to noise, vague feelings of unprovoked anxiety, and difficulty with memory and attention spans. Indeed, Dr. Spies managed to set up a diagnostic procedure that would identify which deficiency was dominant in a patient suffering from mixed symptoms. He would tell the patient a funny story. If the patient did not laugh, the deficiency was predominantly in niacin, for loss of sense of humor is one of the very early symptoms of niacin deficiency.

[2] Emanuel Cheraskin, M.D., D.M.D., Department of Oral Medicine, The University of Alabama Medical Center. Personal communication (C.F.).

Yet arguments on nutrition rage on. When you have two scientists in one room you can depend on debate or argument, and lacking an opponent, a scientist will develop a "schizo-split" and argue with himself. The emergent field of nutrition intrinsically invites sharp difference of opinion, and no battle has been more bitter than that which has been fought over the prevalence of dietary deficiency. Food manufacturers are, logically, sure that the American diet is the best of all possible diets.

No one really educated in nutrition—and this would include familiarity with the entire literature—would uphold the concept that the American public is well fed. Yet there are those—medical men, primarily—who insist that vitamin deficiency to all intents and purposes does not exist in this country, except possibly among alcoholics and the poor whites of the Deep South. Yet other scientists will declare that vitamin deficiency is almost universal. This is not only a case of the blind scientists examining the nutritious elephant; they are not even dealing with the same animal, because basic to the formation of such diverging opinions are differing systems of semantics and concepts. What do these men mean by deficiency?

The physician who says that one must go to Skid Row or the alcoholic wards to see deficiency is concerned with outright scurvy, pellagra, or beriberi. Those who see deficiency as a national condition are thinking in terms of the patients Dr. Spies commented on, or the women of Dr. Wilder's Mayo Clinic experiment. You must understand that the physician who defines deficiency in terms of full-blown beriberi and pellagra will necessarily dismiss as vague and lacking in significance the tenuous preceding symptoms described by Dr. Spies. He would call such symptoms subclinical. If the term means anything, it means the symptoms are unrecognizable. Not only should the term be erased from our scientific vocabulary; we must realize that this school of thought relegates to the area of the subclinical any symptoms that it has not learned to recognize and classify.

To translate the philosophy of these medical men into plain

English: they are saying that the human being who eats a diet deficient in protein and B vitamins will over a period of years develop a purple tongue, cracks at the corners of the mouth, diarrhea, skin disturbances, and delirium. At this stage he can now be labeled as having pellagra; but, says the exponent of this school of thought, in the years preceding the emergence of this disease, deviations from the norm of physical and mental health do not occur or do not constitute clinical symptoms, and can therefore safely be ignored.

This is to say that a fire must burst through the roof before we grant that a disaster is in progress. Obviously, a fire begins somewhere—and so does a deficiency. When the diet is inadequate or the mechanics of digestion and absorption fail, the first tangible effect is the reduction of the level of the particular nutrient in the blood. At this point, the blood begins to draw on the tissue reserves, in what is apparently an attempt by the "wisdom of the body" to mete out the inadequate supply to the organs most critically affected by the deficiency, such as the nervous system and the brain. When the tissues are depleted, the organ reserves are called upon. Note that a deficiency is now definitely in progress and yet, at this stage *there are no symptoms whatsoever.* Should an unusual stress be placed on the person at this period, the deficiency will undoubtedly make its presence known, but even at this stage the discovery will be equivalent to the well-known locking of the stable door after the horse has departed.

The next stage involves changes in functioning. This may take the shape of nervousness, irritability, overactivity of the reflexes as the body tries to compensate; grinding of the teeth in sleep, perhaps stammering, constipation, indigestion, or easy fatigability. Psychometric testing at this stage will reveal undue susceptibility to suggestion and reduction of the ability to make value judgments. The personality trends at this stage will be toward the neurotic. Even so, in the average diagnostic clinic or physician's office the patient will still unhesitatingly be labeled "well nourished." The symptoms? Psychosomatic.

Following this as yet unrecognized stage, miscroscopic changes in the tissues develop. Because of their nature, sections of tissues would have to be cut out for laboratory examination, and understandably both patient and physician are averse to the procedure. Finally, there comes the stage at which even the ultraconservative doctor is willing to acknowledge that the patient is the victim of a bad diet. Changes in the tissues are now visible to the naked eye. Now, and only now will the doctor prescribe the vitamins, the lack of which caused the illness! The vitamins that, prescribed earlier, could have prevented it.

Another type of nutritional disturbance can cause symptoms very likely to be labeled psychosomatic that needs a reverse label, somatopsychic. This is *idiopathic functional hypoglycemia,* which is translated as "low blood sugar, of unknown origin."

The disorder is either appallingly common or relatively infrequent, depending on the authority you consult, for the same division of opinion exists here as is exhibited in the debate concerning the prevalence of subclinical vitamin deficiency. Low blood sugar is a condition first recognized in 1923 by Dr. Seale Harris, but now, forty years later, it is still not a significant element in the physician's thinking in differential diagnosis. He is not only not watching for low blood sugar, ordinarily, but may be understandably myopic when confronted with it. For low blood sugar, like subclinical vitamin deficiency, often exhibits its presence by symptoms that seem perfectly to fit the picture of neurosis. To add to this difficulty, the ordinary diagnostic testing procedure for low blood sugar involves considerable time and expense and the taking of frequent blood samples. Moreover, the prime treatment is dietetic, and however dramatic the response may ultimately be, it is slow in appearing. Both diagnosis and treatment of the disorder are therefore unlikely to make it a "popular" disease. To make the situation even more difficult, low blood sugar can be a disorder of physical origin that causes emotional as well as physical symptoms, or a disorder of emotional origin that intensifies the original emotional disturbance.

The symptoms produced by low blood sugar can be found in any textbook under the heading "neurosis," or sometimes under "psychosis." Anxiety, clear-cut, omnipresent, and imperative—is almost an invariable concomitant of the disorder. Irritability, fatigability, hypersensitivity to noises, difficulty with the attention and memory spans, slurring of speech, migrainelike headaches, epilepticlike attacks, pains resembling those of gastric ucler—they are all typical. A feeling of detachment from reality is also a common symptom.

The disorder begins with, understandably, a craving for sweets. Yet if the craving is indulged, the condition is always made worse. It may seem paradoxical that eating sugar will not remedy low blood sugar, but it is not. Let us see why.

Probably the most apt synonym for this type of low blood sugar is hyperinsulinism. This describes the sufferer as paying the price for a condition opposite that of the diabetic. The diabetic, theoretically (but not probably in fact, as we have seen in Chapter 8), does not produce enough insulin and so suffers from an excess of sugar in the blood. The hypoglycemia patient, again theoretically, produces too much insulin and thereby suffers with too little sugar in the blood.[3] If, however, he eats sugar, the pancreas promptly responds by producing still more insulin, which promptly "burns" the sugar. The end of the process inevitably drops the blood sugar, sometimes below the level before sugar was consumed. Despite the fact that this phenomenon was pointed out by Harris when low blood sugar was first discovered, to this very day we meet individuals who have been fortunate in that their hypoglycemia was recognized but unfortunate in that the pat orthodox prescription of "carry candy in your pocket" has been the suggested remedy. (Our suggested low blood-sugar diet is given at the end of this chapter.)

A determination of the amount of sugar in the blood at a given moment serves no useful purpose for the hypoglycemic patient.

[3] Another cause—prime or contributing—may be failure to *absorb* carbohydrates properly.

Such a test might reveal the opposite condition, diabetes, but identification of low blood sugar necessarily involves a study of the *dynamics* of the body's management of sugar. By the common testing method, the blood sugar of the fasting patient is determined. If it falls within "normal range" the test is usually stopped at this point. This represents a grave error. If the initial sugar value proves to be low, sugar is then administered to the sufferer, and the blood sugar levels are determined over a period of from two to six or even eight hours, depending on the philosophy of the practitioner. Out of such a study, three possible interpretations could arise: namely, normal sugar levels; flat glucose (sugar) tolerance curve; or outright hypoglycemia.

The normal blood reaction to the eating of sugar, if graphed, would show the "normal bell-shaped curve." The eating of sugar is followed by a rise in blood sugar to a "normal" height, and then the action of the blood's insulin brings the level down until, in a time period differing from person to person, the original level is regained. A flat glucose tolerance curve, which, incidentally, is often the hallmark of the neurotic, the jaded, the frustrated, and those without a sense of achievement, simply represents a milder variety of insulin overactivity, which allows the sugar levels to rise but not to normal height. The third result, low blood sugar, would parallel the flat curve but at a lower level. Here the insulin overactivity is so great that the initial sugar level is much too low and the curve never gets a chance to rise appreciably. Of course these statements are oversimplifications, and human beings display innumerable variations in these responses.

Recently, Dr. Herman Goodman of New York City devised a new test for low blood sugar that takes little time, is inexpensive, and is more efficient than the older test. In Dr. Goodman's test, the fasting level of blood sugar is determined preceding breakfast; the person is then instructed to eat his accustomed breakfast. If the blood sugar level 45 minutes after the meal does not rise 50 per cent, he is suffering with low blood sugar even though his fasting level is within "normal range." Undoubtedly there are individuals with low blood sugar who may elude this test, but as a screening procedure it is likely to identify the great majority of sufferers.

At this point the discussion may seem somewhat academic, so let us translate it into the experience of a real person. Take the case of Gloria, a young woman so vivacious that her friends nick-named her "Peppi." She retained her vivacity and zest for life until she bore her first child at the age of twenty. (Low blood sugar often develops after a period of a stress such as pregnancy.) She now found herself weeping without provocation, melancholy without cause, tortured with claustrophobia. Her strength had ebbed away. She could not continue her housework, she could not care for her child, and the task of preparing a meal became insuperable. As her ability to concentrate faded, and as she was gripped by an alarming degree of anxiety, she was taken to several diagnosticians. The diagnosis was "post-partum melancholia" (depression after childbrith), which is ordinarily a self-limited disorder. This diagnosis was proved wrong by the duration and continued worsening of her symptoms.

A year later, she was under psychiatric care; after a few months of analysis she had an appointment for shock therapy, that ultimate and atavistic torture of modern civilization.

Driving his wife to the psychiatrist's office for her first shock treatment, the husband turned on the radio and by chance heard the senior author discussing the picture of low blood sugar. The husband changed their destination, arriving at the family doctor's office with a *demand* rather than a request for a blood sugar determination. Fortunately for her, the initial value was below 50; had it been within "normal range" the tests probably would not have continued. The significance of this finding will be clear only if you realize that if you were given an injection of insulin that quickly dropped your blood sugar to such a level, you would undoubtedly be unable to function, if not unconscious. Somehow, persons with low blood sugar learn to live and to seem to half-function with the blood sugar thus depressed, and the process represents a testament to the magnificent capacity of the body to accept punishment.

There is a happy ending to our story. It took two years to convert the girl into a normal human being: two years of applied dietetics and vitamin therapy. And it was most difficult for her to accept the realization that the sweets she craved and in which she had lavishly indulged could not be used to correct low blood sugar, but would make it worse.

Her later history gives us an indication of the complexity of this nutritional problem, for while she is perfectly well as long as she refrains from eating sugar or quickly absorbed starches, her blood sugar levels persistently are below the "normal range." Elsewhere in this book, her later history is described: for the dietary habits that initiated or aggravated her low blood sugar caused other disturbances, which ultimately caused cystic mastitis and, later, uterine fibroid tumors. Both conditions were brought under control as they appeared, by progressively stricter supervision of her nutrition, and intensification of the vitamin therapy.

This patient was fortunate in having a cooperative physician. She was hospitalized at the time that she developed hemorrhages, which revealed the uterine tumors. A gregarious person, while she was convalescing she visited with other patients on the same floor of the hospital. In the next room was a woman about fifty years of age, who had been hospitalized in preparation for shock treatment: her third course, to be administered because of her periods of semipsychotic mood and behavior. As Gloria listened to this woman's story, for obvious reasons she speculated on the possibility that the older woman's "psychotic" symptoms might, like her own original behavior, be traceable to low blood sugar. When the woman confessed to an unusual craving for sweets, Gloria urged her to seek a sugar tolerance test. This the woman did, though not without a battle with the physician who had hospitalized her.

She too, it developed, had low blood sugar—a rather tragic finding when one realizes that she will wear a brace for the rest of her life because of the fracture induced by the convulsions she suffered in her first bout of shock therapy for her "psychosis." (We learn by fractures; shock so violent is now not medically fashionable.)

We must remember that while the causes of low blood sugar of the functional type are not definitely known, we know this as a disorder that can create a vicious circle. Emotional disturbances—a sense of frustration, monotony, or lack of achievement—can initiate low blood sugar; anxiety can also cause it; and low blood sugar itself can cause these very symptoms or reinforce them when they pre-exist. The purported "wisdom of the body" translates into foolishness, which leads the sufferer into the deadly peril of a craving for sweets. Yet we must admit the body is in desperate need of sugar and its urgency is for sugar of *any* type: not just the type obtained from substances that the body utilizes more slowly and therefore does not call upon the drastic action of the pancreas to burn quickly.

Why it is that frustration or boredom or anxiety or lack of achievement can initiate low blood sugar is not difficult to understand, once we have obtained a clear picture of the condition. To give an oversimplified explanation: man's skull houses two brains. One, the cortex, is the thinking brain. Housed within it is man's earlier and more primitive brain, the thalamus, in which the emotions originate and are controlled. Or are often not controlled.

The maturation of a child from an asocial little animal, his behavior largely impelled by the emotional brain, to the civilized human being, is a process in which some degree of control is achieved by the cortex or the thinking brain over the thalamic or emotional brain. At best the relationship is an uneasy armistice. The intellectual, calculating cortex would dictate, for instance, continuing to work in a job with no goal, no room for pride of achievement. The emotional brain rebels like a small child, but the cortex controls the communication system, which impels voluntary activity. Unable, therefore, to achieve a break in the monotonous activities by bickering with the thinking brain, the thalamic brain in its own devious way turns its attention to the mechanism in the blood, which it can influence. One of the thalamic ploys is stimulation of the nervous system and the glands that largely control sugar metabolism. It is as if the emotional brain says: "I cannot induce the thinker to pay any attention to the fact that this job is monotonous and unrewarding. He insists that we must stay with it to earn a living. I don't care. Therefore I shall lower the blood sugar until the cortex gets so little that he must stop what he's doing!" In carrying out this fantastic biochemical war, the thalamic brain drives the organism to the point where not only the cortex suffers as a result of the low blood sugar: the thalamic brain itself becomes irritable. In its blind frustration, the emotional brain has created the seeds of its *own* anarchy as well as that of its hated rival. This mental process may be somewhat analogous with cancer, in which the rebellious cells grow beautifully for a time at the body's expense, but later, of course, are destroyed themselves when the body dies as a result of their actions.

The anxiety arising from the conflict is not difficult to comprehend. It is obviously a protective mechanism of the human organism—because a lack of sugar in the brain is the equivalent of lack of oxygen, and serious, even irreversible brain damage can take place if the condition is too long ignored. If the postulated wisdom of the body exists in this instance, it is lacking in the rest of the behavior induced by hypoglycemia, for indulgence in the craving for sweets simply perpetuates the vicious circle.

So it is that low blood sugar becomes an excellent example not only of the influence of mind on body, but of the reverse equation often neglected: the influence of body on mind.

We could offer many other examples. Some twenty years ago, German nutritionists published the observation that individuals suffering from a toxic thyroid—usually overactive—were quieted by dosages of vitamin E. This vitamin the Germans administered because it was known to affect the diencephalon, an area of the emotional brain. They reasoned that the patient's nervousness and anxiety were curbed when the vitamin dampened the transmission of the nervous impulses from the diencephalon to the cortex.

It was probably as a result of this reasoning that vitamin E was administered to nervous and anxious menopausal women. Unsurprisingly, it acted for them, too, as a physiological tranquilizer—one sometimes as effective, by the way, as the artificial tranquilizers widely used in the United States today.

The pathway of action of the vitamin undoubtedly involves more than the diencephalon. It probably includes stimulation of pituitary function. Not only is this gland closely related anatomically to the emotional brain, but we know from research that vitamin E is involved in the formation of the pituitary gland in the embryo. When a pregnant rat is partially deprived of vitamin E, its young are born with pituitary glands half formed. A commonsense axiom in the field of nutrition indicates that a nutrient needed for the formation of an organ or tissue is usually required for its maintenance. Since it is undoubtedly the pituitary gland that "decides" when the menopause is to take place, it is logical that a nutrient that the gland requires might have profound effects on processes in which the pituitary is involved.

Here it should be noted that Dr. Roger Williams, a former president of the American Chemical Society, has protested against the tendency of the medical profession to force the nutritionist to equate his suggestions for physiological therapy with the unphysiological, and frequently dangerous methods used in medicine.[4] Specifically, Dr. Williams asked why pantothenic acid (one of the vitamin-B complex), which is useful in at least one type of constipation (among many other uses) is measured by the medical man against laxatives. Now, following Dr. Williams' reasoning, why should vitamin E treatment be forced into a comparison with shock therapy, which is at least unphysiological and at worst dangerous?

The United States Food and Drug Administration has repeatedly assured Americans that deficiency in vitamin E is not possi-

[4] The reader should become familiar with Dr. Williams' *Free and Unequal, Biochemical Basis of Individuality,* and other texts and papers.

ble. This propaganda gambit collided with the fact of vitamin-E deficiency in sizable segments of the American population, as disclosed in recent papers delivered before the American Public Health Association. Whether vitamin-E deficiency can cause mental disease is not the issue, although it is possible that in subtle ways, which our present testing instruments are not sensitive enough to detect, vitamin-E deficiency has an impact upon brain function and total personality. But the fact is indisputable that administration of the vitamin[5] has been helpful to neurotic and psychotic individuals. It matters little whether such results are obtained by correction of deficiency or as an exhibition of a pharmaceutical effect of the vitamin, unrelated to the presence or absence of deficiency.

Still another example of the body's influence over the mind is shown in the area of "subclinical" calcium deficiency. Ordinarily, calcium levels in the blood fluctuate within a very narrow range. Here the "wisdom of the body" is well illustrated, for a small drop in body calcium levels will bring on tetany—convulsions. The body, via the parathyroid hormone, maintains a system of blood calcium replenishment that operates *independently* of the dietary supply of the mineral. If this were not so, the very first day of a menu low in calcium, as consumed by millions of Americans, would result in drastic changes in neuromuscular function and in personality. To maintain a constant supply in the blood, the body draws on calcium in the tissues and the bones. Yet it obviously cannot continue this process forever. The calcium must eventually be replenished or the body suffers.[6] At every level of medical practice, from pediatrics to geriatrics, persons are seen whose behavior has been altered by calcium inadequacy.

The pediatrician sees the colic-prone baby and the spasm-prone child, the preschool child given to holding his breath when frus-

[5] And other vitamins and minerals, as demonstrated by Watson. Consult files of *Journal of Psychology* for his papers, in mid-1950s.
[6] The brittleness of the bones mistakenly attributed to old age may result from a lifetime of inadequate intake of calcium, often the result of a diet low in milk and cheese.

trated, to the point of unconsciousness (which his mother seldom sees because she faints first!). The typical mother's reaction to "breath-holding" is spanking or dousing the child with cold water. Actually, the child is sometimes being punished for a deficiency in ionized (usable) calcium in the blood. A determination of the gross amount of calcium in his blood would undoubtedly show it to be within normal range, but our ordinary testing methods are hard put to maintain a reasonable level of accuracy when dealing with quantities as minute as ten milligrams of a nutrient in one hundred cubic centimeters of blood.

The pediatrician competent in biochemistry treats the breath-holding child with dosages of calcium bromide. The sedative (bromide) quiets the nervous system until the added supply of calcium has at least in part raised the blood content of the usable form of the mineral. The mother then watches the mystifying spectacle of a problem child being "cured" with doses of a physiological substance. In other words, the "bad boy" thought to be a psychological problem is cured by a physical medicine—not by psychoanalysis or psychotherapy. Yet heaven knows how many children are treated by the latter methods when no attention is paid to the underlying physical cause of their difficulties.

The rationale for the physical treatment will be obvious if you understand that spasm of the muscle is a direct consequence of a deficiency of calcium in the only form in which the muscle will accept it: the ionized form. While a gross deficiency in calcium will cause involuntary convulsions, a qualitative deficiency can, in the breath-holding child, cause a spasm that will prevent the child from venting his breath and resuming a normal breathing cycle. Since calcium deficiency will cause cramping of muscles, which is a form of spasm, it is obvious that the petulant or angry child who would ordinarily hold his breath for only a few seconds may, if he is deficient in ionized calcium, suffer a spasm that will not permit him to release his breath. In this sense, the breath-holding becomes completely involuntary.

Some years ago, Dr. E. V. McCollum remarked that with a

small drop in blood serum calcium, there is a tendency to muscle spasm; a still larger drop and an unwholesome personality develops, with manical outbursts of uncontrollable temper. How many "neurotics" and "psychotics" are primarily or secondarily suffering from nutritional deficiency no one knows, but their number must be legion. Yet they might be helped if present-day medicine were not prejudiced.

You may be wondering, if the wisdom of the body controls blood serum calcium, how these "psychotic" symptoms can develop. It happens that there is a *qualitative* type of calcium deficiency as well as a *quantitative* one. And as we have seen in the example of the breath-holding children, it is the usable form of calcium that makes all the differences in behavior.

Apropos of the ability of certain nutrients to affect the mind, the senior author some years ago conducted an experiment with several hundred subjects in which an attempt was made biochemically to change the *contour* of the body *without changing body weight*. In the course of this experiment it was demonstrated that it is possible to reduce or add to the dimensions of an area of the body without general weight gain or reduction.

During the experiment, which involved a change in the distribution of body fat, dosages were given of the nutrients important in fat metabolism. These included lecithin, a substance found in brain and nerve tissue. But the lecithin did more than help redistribute the fat, amazing though that may be. Circumstances made it possible to distinguish between the effects of this and other nutrients administered. The reaction of one woman is perhaps typical. She said: "The vitamins you have given us, I have taken before. The lecithin was the only supplement I have never used. It descended upon me like a blanket of peace." Compare this action of lecithin with the comparable effects of vitamin E.

A question arises out of "twilight zone" deficiency and mental illness. These borderline deficiencies are obviously mild ones, but how long would it take for them to exhibit their effects? Fortunately, though the average physician is not even aware the problem exists, there is a clear-cut answer to this question. It has been established, for instance, that the first symptoms of deficiency in vitamin-B complex are exhibited in subtle changes in personality and brain functions, and can appear after just *five days* of such a diet.[7] However, their subtlety is such that delicate psychometric testing is needed to establish their nature. The earliest changes appear to be difficulty in making decisions and value judgments. This is accompanied by undue susceptibility to suggestion. Hypochondria also appears early in the sequence.

Anatomically, such vitamin deficiency appears to attack brain function in a phylogenetic sequence, man's newest brain faculties first becoming disturbed. The attack then proceeds backward from the cortex until it reaches man's original, primitive brain, the thalamus. It is interesting, as we have seen, that sensitivity to low blood sugar is also directly related to the embryological age of the brain structure, so that man's thinking brain is the first to be affected. The vital functions of the brain stem seem more resistant, and thus the older brain structure holds out much longer.

While this chapter does not pretend to be a definitive examination of all the nutritional deficiencies that influence brain and personality, it must be clear to you by now that our nervous, tense, and neurotic culture deserves something more than tranquilizers, psychotherapy, and shock treatments. Although we do not allege that nutritional deficiences are a major, demonstrated cause of psychosis except in conditions such as advanced pellagra, certainly the *presumptive* evidence indicates a vastly more important role than has heretofore been admitted by the "authorities." [8] It is our belief that nutritional treatment of neurotics and psychotics should take place in four areas:

1. Correction of dietary error and deficiency, frequently a byproduct of the bizarre selection of foods encountered in many mentally and emotionally ill persons.
2. Correction of the nutritional deficiencies of the diet in the in-

[7] In some individuals. Responses differ to bad and good diet.
[8] How many patients in psychotherapy eat a good diet?

stitutions and agencies that care for the mentally sick. (The diet in many of these institutions, as in most institutions, including our best hospitals, is less nutritious than anyone has a right to expect.)

3. Compensation, by increased intake of nutrients, for the poor utilization and absorption that seem to characterize digestive function in certain mental disorders.

4. Experimental usage of vitamins and other nutrients that may hold therapeutic promise.

The fourth proposal includes massive dosage of certain nutrients. Thus, the disoriented old person need not be the victim of a deficiency of glutamic acid to receive help from doses of the substance. It may even be unlikely, since this material is synthesized in the body, that outright deficiency is possible. The favorable response to doses of the acid may be explained on the basis that it is given alone, unaccompanied by the carbohydrate that would be present in the diets that are natural sources of glutamic acid. Or it may be that in high doses this acid, like many other nutritional substances, begins to exhibit beneficial actions not related to its nutritional effect, and not achieved at lower dosage. An analogy would be high dosage of vitamin C, which yields an antihistamine effect completely unrelated to the presence or absence of vitamin C deficiency.

Here is an example that touches on all four of our proposals. Years ago, the senior author was asked to improve the diet of a group of schizophrenics who refused to eat, and were being tube-fed. The thin gruel used for the forced feeding was not difficult to improve upon. Surprisingly, as their nutrition was reinforced with protein and vitamin-mineral supplements, not only did the patients show a heightened well-being, with needed weight gain, but they also came closer to the world of reality, and began to respond more to the psychiatrists' efforts to communicate with them. The significance of this *mental* response to nutrition, however, was lost upon the psychiatric thinking of the early 1930s.

In the years that followed, as new nutrients were isolated, identified, and synthesized, they were used experimentally in the treatment of the emotionally disturbed and mentally sick. Among these nutrients was glutamic acid.

Originally, experiments with glutamic acid were based upon a happy accident of the kind that was responsible for such other scientific discoveries as penicillin, X-ray therapy, ether anesthesia, and aspirin. Let us use the discovery of aspirin to illustrate our point. The usefulness of the salicylates in the treatment of rheumatic disorders was first hinted in the folklore notion that plants and trees indigenous to an area must surely be useful in the treatment of that area's disorders and diseases. The willow was common where rheumatic disease was rife, and the willow's bark contained salicylates—and thus we obtained modern aspirin and the allied drugs helpful in rheumatic disease.

The same type of thinking led to the trial of glutamic acid in epilepsy. An osteopathic physician had found that starvation seemed helpful in reducing the frequency of epileptic convulsions. The pathway of action of this treatment was determined to be the acidosis caused by starvation, as fat is burned in the absence of a carbohydrate "flame." This led to a deliberate attempt to create a more controlled type of acidosis by the feeding of large amounts of fat in the absence of carbohydrate intake. This in turn was followed by the trial of glutamic acid, in the mistaken belief that this harmless amino acid might cause the desired acidosis without the risk, expense, and inconvenience of fasting or high fat intake. Had the experimenters reviewed their biochemistry they would have realized that glutamic acid could not possibly produce such an acidosis.

Proceeding on a faulty hypothesis, they discovered a completely unexpected benefit for the epileptic. True, the glutamic acid did not affect the major convulsions of epilepsy in the form and dosage employed, but it profoundly altered toward the normal the mental functioning and personalities of some of the sufferers. Asocial, indifferent, hostile patients became more agreeable and cooperative. In mentally retarded epileptics, the IQ rose, alertness increased, and there were improvements in memory and in attention span. Moreover, some of these results were obtained in persons who were not epileptics and in those who were not mentally retarded.[9]

Encouraged by this research and by some of the responses obtained in children with cerebral palsy, the senior author applied the nutritional treatment of massive dosage to the seriously mentally ill, such as paranoids. Although delusions of persecution have appeared in individuals suffering from outright starvation, there is no significant scientific evidence to prove that nutritional deficiency has ever been a contributing factor in a paranoid psychosis. Yet here is the suggestive history of one of the patients:

Beginning treatment, the woman suffered from the typical paranoid symptom of an elaborate structure of delusion of persecution. Shopping for groceries, she could accept only factory-sealed packages: otherwise she would run the risk, so she thought, of being poisoned through the machinations of men who were following her for the specific purpose of destroying her.

After three months of improved nutrition and large doses of vitamins, the patient no longer saw the men who were said to be following her, but expressed the fear that they were still following her. Two months later, a total of five months of treatment, she was asked about the men who were pursuing her. Her response was: "What men?"

This massive dosage technique has also been applied to manic-depressives, victims of dementia praecox, and individuals with compulsive behavior of an order approaching psychosis. In many cases there were significant benefits.

We must emphasize that we are dealing here with the *pharmacodynamic* effects of high dosages of nutrients. We must differentiate between this response and that obtained, for instance, in the case of the schoolteacher who found herself weeping in the classroom, without the provocation normal to educating a group of

[9] Apropos of conspiracy of silence: any advertiser citing these reports on glutamic acid can find himself threatened by the FDA with injunction, fine, and jail sentence.

rowdy youngsters. Frequently she herself was unaware of the tears. The symptom disappeared, never to return, when her intake of vitamin B_1 was raised to a level approximately three times that established as the normal requirement. In her case we are dealing with a deficiency, and the only unanswered question concerns the nature of that deficiency. Were we rectifying a vitamin B_1 deficit in the diet, as related to the alleged minimum daily requirement; or were we meeting the needs of an individual whose requirement for a nutrient far exceeded the average, and which was difficult of fulfillment even from a well-balanced diet? In the case of the teacher there was a definite demonstrated deficiency; with the psychotics, while there may have been deficiencies, the massive doses were used for their *pharmacodynamic* effect.

In recent years there has been further confirmation that nutritional treatment of neurotics and psychotics will produce amazing results. Undoubtedly the most significant and conclusive experiment was that performed at the University of Minnesota's School of Physiological Hygiene. It was first extensively reported in a national magazine by the junior author. Healthy young men were placed on a semistarvation diet for six months, and the deterioration of their minds and personalities was carefully followed. Let us quote one significant finding here: "Amazingly, however, the significance of the study, which in six months turned thirty-six young, healthy, idealistic, fun-loving men into old, cynical, suspicious neurotics, *has escaped the attention of all except a comparatively few scientists.*"

Now, do you see what we mean by prejudiced thinking on the part of those in control of "organized" medicine? Why did the Minnesota experiment escape the attention of all but a few? Whatever the answer to this, there is clearly something *you* can do about it. There is a valid nutritional approach to the prevention and alleviation of many emotional and mental disorders, and it is one that you can employ.

There is, first, the correction of any deficiencies in your diet. Here, as in other chapters, we must refer you to details in Chapter

19; in Chapter 15 we discuss the supplements that should be added to guarantee that deficiencies do not contribute to initiating or worsening emotional and mental disorders.

The second area of nutritional therapy in these disturbances takes us into the problems of individuals, possibly those of the weeping schoolteacher, who may require a larger intake of certain nutrients than the standards of the authorities would lead us to expect. This problem, too, can be managed by the housewife, and it, as well as the previous one (deficiency related to normal requirement and a poor diet) simultaneously overcome. The suggested supplements should take care of a vast majority of those falling in these first two areas.

The third area is that of the pharmacodynamic. Here the nutrients are used in very high dosages to yield actions unrelated to the overcoming of deficiency or the satisfaction of high requirements; the nutritional substance, because of the dosage, functions as a medication. This area is clearly the prerogative of the physician. An example would be the administration of vitamin E in dosages far beyond those required to satisfy even a high need; acting medicinally on the emotional brain and the pituitary gland, it may yield a beneficial effect approximating that of shock therapy.

This procedure compensates for dietary inadequacy, whether related to normal or abnormally high requirements:

1. Supplementing of the diet with a high-potency therapeutic vitamin capsule, a multiple mineral supplement (including trace minerals); a vitamin-B complex supplement, preferably in liquid form so that it can supply a generous amount of a source of the natural unknown factors of the B-complex group; and a vitamin-E supplement, providing 100 milligrams of the vitamin measured in terms of alpha tocopherol potency.

2. Vitamin B_{12}, 100 micrograms, daily by mouth, accompanied by desiccated stomach tissue. B_{12} is more efficiently utilized if the physician administers it by intramuscular injections; hence our attempt at improving the oral dosage utilization with the stomach tissue, which helps the body to assimilate B_{12} when it is taken orally.

3. Wheat germ oil, 1½ teaspoons daily, best taken in divided amounts, between meals.

4. A palatable protein concentrate[10] of high biological efficiency, supplying at least 50 per cent complete protein, to be used as a beverage or in wafer form between meals.

5. The preceding regimen, which can be instituted by anyone, should be utilized by the physician *as a basis* for added individual doses of nutrients that he may choose to give *therapeutically* in much higher dosage.

SUGGESTED DIET FOR LOW BLOOD SUGAR (ALSO A GOOD DIET FOR THE EMOTIONALLY DISTURBED)

The most important feature of the diet is a substantial breakfast. This will not produce unwanted weight gain, for there is automatic compensation for a large breakfast in the reduction of the amount of food taken in later meals.

Self-diagnosis of low blood sugar should not be attempted, although the diet and the vitamin supplements are harmless and would represent good nutrition for anyone. Inasmuch as certain physical disorders may cause hyperinsulinism, the physician should be consulted.

Professional readers are advised that the vitamin supplements suggested here are an integral part of the dietetic attack. While the diet alone may control a persistent hypoglycemia, the response will be more adequate and more enduring if the concentrates are used as an adjunct. Likewise, protein foods may be used in place of the protein concentrates suggested for between-meal feedings, but the protein powders and tablets are often convenient for many individuals who do not have access to food between meals. The diet is based on the premise that a high-protein, medium-fat, low-carbohydrate diet, free of sugar, is the diet of choice; that frequent feedings are indispensable for such individ-

10 Nonfat milk suffices.

uals, and that carbohydrate chemistry and liver function must be normalized if the condition is to be stabilized.

ON ARISING:

One glassful of warm or tepid milk, with one teaspoon of nonfat dried milk added.

BREAKFAST:

Fruit, or four ounces of juice. Two eggs, with or without two slices of ham or bacon. Only one slice of bread, whole wheat, or reinforced with wheat germ. Use plenty of butter as a spread. Beverage. Immediately after breakfast, take: one multiple vitamin capsule; one multiple mineral capsule; one teaspoon vitamin-B complex syrup in a natural base of rice bran, and especially potent in choline, inositol, pyridoxine, thiamine, para-amino-benzoic acid, and niacinamide; 100 milligram vitamin E capsule daily, prior to 4 P.M.

Two hours after breakfast:

Protein concentrates in powder or tablet form (as much as desired.)

LUNCH:

Meat, fish, cheese, or eggs. Mixed green salad with mayonnaise or French dressing. Vegetables. Only one slice of bread, plenty of butter. Dessert. Beverage.

Three hours after lunch:

Eight ounces of milk, plus one teaspoon nonfat dried milk, or protein concentrate or tablets (as much as desired).

One hour before dinner:

Four ounces of juice.

DINNER:

Soup if desired (not thickened with flour). Vegetables. Liberal portion of meat, fish, or poultry. Only one slice of bread, if desired. Dessert. Beverage.

Two or three hours after dinner:
Eight ounces of milk.

Every two hours until bedtime:
Four ounces of milk or a small handful of nuts.

Allowable vegetables

Asparagus, avocado, beets, broccoli, brussels sprouts, cabbage, cauliflower, carrots, celery, corn, cucumbers, eggplant, lima beans, onions, peas, radishes, sauerkraut, squash, string beans, tomatoes, turnips.

Allowable fruits

Apples, apricots, berries, grapefruit, melons, oranges, peaches, pears, pineapple, tangerines. May be cooked or raw, with or without cream, but without sugar. Canned fruit should be brands packed in water, not syrup.

Lettuce, mushrooms, and nuts may be taken as freely as desired.

Juices

Any unsweetened fruit or vegetable juice, except grape juice or prune juice.

Beverages

Weak tea (tea ball, not brewed). Decaffeinated coffee. Coffee substitutes. May be sweetened with saccharin.

Desserts

Fruit, unsweetened gelatin, custard, junket (made from tablets).

Alcoholic and soft drinks

Club soda, dry ginger ale, whiskies and other distilled liquors in moderation.

Avoid absolutely

Sugar, candy and other sweets such as cake, pie, pastries, sweet custards, puddings and ice cream. Caffeine: ordinary coffee, strong brewed tea, beverages containing caffeine (your doctor will tell you what these are). Potatoes, rice, grapes, raisins, plums, figs, dates, and bananas. Ordinary spaghetti, macaroni and noodles. (Gluten spaghetti and macaroni with wheat germ may occasionally be used.) Wines, cordials, cocktails, and beer.

12. Alcoholism: You may not think this problem affects you—but it does!

Dr. Roger Williams, in his research on the subject of nutrition vs. alcoholism,[1] has shown that unsatisfied nutritional needs will, if alcohol is available, pervert an animal into alcoholism. He has also demonstrated the converse: that satisfaction of the nutritional needs of the animal will cause the appetite for the alcohol to diminish or disappear. Further, he was able to demonstrate that these unsatisfied nutritional needs sometimes originate with inborn nutritional requirements so high that satisfaction of them with the ordinary good animal diet becomes improbable if not impossible. He did not, however, attempt to ascertain why certain animals come into the world with such high requirements for certain nutrients as to make satisfaction of them most difficult.

We are interested in Dr. Williams' work for several reasons. The problem of alcoholism seems to be growing rather than diminishing in spite of all efforts to overcome it. Practically all theories that attempt to explain its cause have not apparently made much of an inroad into the realm of practicality: we see around us a steadily increasing army of several million "confirmed" alcoholics and many more millions who are "problem" drinkers. In one way or another the problem touches the lives of most of us.

The attack on alcoholism has largely been monopolized by psychiatrists and psychologists, who have explained that alcohol is

[1] Roger Williams, *Nutrition and Alcoholism.*

the device by which the drinker escapes unpleasant realities that he does not feel equipped to endure. This, when we examine it, is revealed as another of the pat explanations with which, alas, the field of psychology is filled. It does not, for instance, explain why the subject chooses liquor as his pathway to a more pleasant dream world. Some people escape reality with a movie, a novel, television, food, a blonde, or a dose of heroin. Excepting the latter method, which of course carries severe physical, mental, and societal penalties, escapism is indulged in by practically all of us, with few disastrous effects for most. There are some who would argue that such escapes are really not escapes from reality at all but efforts to achieve total or full reality. Their reasoning goes like this: The reality experienced by most men and women in our present-day existence is so shallow, banal, and boring that man's mind, being filled with the curious thirst for knowledge that made him a man, seeks something better, seizes on any promising departure from the norm, the average, the typical. The view is presented here only to show there is another possibility in "psychological" explorations of alcoholism.

But, then, why does alcohol specifically become the addiction of so many? Why are we, as nutritionists, interested in the problem? Alcoholism is a disorder which, by the substitution of liquor for food, creates nutritional deficiencies. These deficiencies produce effects that go beyond the delirium and beyond the brain and the nervous system disturbances that threaten the confirmed alcoholic. For instance, it is perhaps not coincidence that along with the development of an alcoholic liver, the male alcoholic tends (as we noted in Chapter 7) to retain a full head of hair and lose his interest in the opposite sex. Since these phenomena mark a change in the *gynic* index, from male characteristics toward female characteristics, we should remember that liver disturbances will allow female hormone to accumulate in the male body, and that retention of a full head of hair and loss of sexual interest in women are the predictable results of a process of femininization.

The nutritionist is also interested in another part of the picture:

those drinkers who, between bouts, have a tremendous appetite for sweets. This is a possible sign of low blood sugar; and we have also observed that known hypoglycemics will often stop drinking liquor when their low blood sugar has been competently treated.

Another premise for the nutritionist's interest in the possible role of nutritional deficiencies in creating the appetite for alcohol lies in the possibility upon which Dr. Williams speculates: the alcoholic human being, like certain individual animals, comes into the world with extraordinarily high requirements for a specific nutrient or nutrients.

This leads us to speculate upon the mechanism by which the newborn come into the world with an exaggerated need for a nutritional factor or factors. One possibility is logical. We are aware that long-continued nutritional deficiency changes tissues in a way that ultimately makes them inefficient in utilizing a missing nutrient, so that massive doses become necessary if the process of degeneration is to be interrupted before it reaches the point of no return. Several nutritional deficiencies are common in the diet of the American expectant mother, among them folic acid and vitamin B_6 (pyridoxine). In an earlier chapter we spoke of the tendency to convulsions which can be interrupted only by administration of relatively large amounts of vitamin B_6. After reading Dr. Williams' papers and book, we are inclined to wonder whether there are not some babies who escape the convulsions, but *later* arrive at alcoholism because of the "inherited" deficiency. Significantly, the delirium of alcoholics has often successfully been treated with vitamin B_6.

Williams comments on the fact that all agencies dealing with the alcoholic, whatever their philosophies, whatever their mode of therapy, begin with food. This is true, whether it is the intravenous glucose administered at the sanitarium (and here heaven help the alcoholic who has low blood sugar, as sugar is put into his veins!) or the Salvation Army, with its bowl of soup.

Of course, the best test of a theory lies in application. Was Williams able to stop the appetite for alcohol with nutritional therapy? He was. He tells the story of a confirmed alcoholic who, after good diet and vitamin therapy, was able for the first time in his life to take two drinks and *stop*. We ourselves have seen the same response in a significant number of alcoholics. And must not Alcoholics Anonymous evaluate its own fine work in terms of the possibility that the alcoholic is not only receiving moral support and psychiatric help, but is being persuaded once again to eat regularly?

We may say, then, that all real alcoholics need nutritional therapy, since by definition they are substituting alcohol for food. In addition, some who are consistently given good nutrition at the heroic level may very well emerge cured of their appetite for liquor. And let us remember that the alcoholic who eats large quantities of candy and sweets between binges deserves the kindness of a test for low blood sugar. Should this dysfunction be found and competently treated, the senior author's experience indicates that this individual's liquor problem may disappear.

Nutritional factors requiring emphasis for the alcoholic are protein and the vitamin-B complex. All other vitamins, of course, and the essential minerals, must be supplied. The unknown factors of the B complex are administered most profitably by injection of crude liver and by dosage of "40-degree" liver concentrate by mouth.

Now then, if you happen to be reading this chapter simply to see what we say—if you have never had a personal problem with liquor—we suggest you *reread* it, substituting the word *sugar* wherever the word *alcohol* or *liquor* appears. For if you are an average American, it is almost certain you have a sugar problem, and the excessive consumption of sugar, substituted for needed foods, will have *nutritional* effects not easily distinguishable from those of alcohol.

The preceding statement may startle some of our readers. Actually, it is completely justified. There are individuals whose compulsive drive toward sugar has about it the hallmarks of the obsession of the alcoholic with his favorite beverage. There is also an interlocking of the two compulsions, for there are alcoholics—of the type who go on periodic binges—who in periods of sobriety intervening will evidence a marked craving for sweets. In such individuals, there is the possibility that the craving for sweets derives from the same source which dictates the appetite for alcohol: low blood sugar. Specific diet therapy of the type recommended in Chapter 11, accompanied by the recommended vitamin supplements, has in some instances completely eliminated the desire for liquor.

The alcoholic substitutes alcohol for food; the sugarholic substitutes sugar for food. The effects overlap and both go into nutritional deficiency. Both show an exaggerated need for the B vitamins. Both show disturbances of glandular function which may interfere with libido. Both show constipation. And both will give you a rationalization which completely explains away the undesirability of the particular pattern of diet.

13. Your Glands: They control you—can you control them?

Do you know that your glands—pituitary, thyroid, adrenals, and others—control your functions almost entirely? By *functions*, we mean many functions of both body and what we call mind.

This is saying that on this earth, at least, and in your present body-mind state, your glandular activity controls *what* you are. Your glandular condition is a determining factor in how and why you will react at any given time to any situation. It will determine what your reaction toward life itself will be: whether one of jubilance, controlled optimism, "neutrality," or deepest pessimism. Although these moods can and do fluctuate within you almost every day, nevertheless the basic pattern of your personality is fairly constant if you are "normal," if you live under fairly regular circumstances and receive a fairly regular nutritional allowance each day.

There are no gland specialists who would disagree with what we have stated thus far. In fact, the endocrinologists have pinpointed many of our actions in our glandular behavior. For example, whether we will fight (be aggressive as the hungry lion) or flee in terror (as the hunted gazelle) depends in part upon the amount of epinephrine (adrenaline) released by our adrenal glands. But whether we fight or flee depends on an even more subtle action of the adrenal glands than the gland specialists at first thought.

Adrenaline (we stick to the name everybody knows) is now known to be manufactured by the body in two forms. The two forms do not have the same effect on the body, even though they are closely allied in chemical structure and manufactured by the same gland. The first is now dubbed *nor*-adrenaline. This type gives the lion (and the human being) his courage and aggressiveness, while the "regular" adrenaline produces the flight reaction in gazelles, rabbits, and human beings. It also appears in lions and elephants as well, so they will know when properly to be frightened and run away in the face of unknown or overwhelming disasters.

All these intricacies concerning the animal and human body and mind our friends the endocrinologists are only too willing to admit. In fact they are only too proud to admit them because it gives them (they think) added proof of a mechanistic universe in which one has only to push the correct buttons in order to get the desired results. Yet, as if to prove their inconsistencies, few if any of these specialists will acknowledge the role of nutrition in the functioning of the glands. They think logically in one area. That is, they understand the function of the glands in the behavior of the body and "mind." But they will not go further and admit that nutrition governs the function of the glands themselves. In other words, they will not agree that what the glands manufacture and release is dependent upon what the glands receive in the form of nutrition.

The senior author was lunching one day with an endocrinologist in the physicians' dining room of a large New York City hospital. We had eaten a poorly balanced meal, improperly cooked, and plainly revealing the oxidizing influence of the steam table. The endocrinologist, finishing a piece of cake calculated to destroy his few remaining teeth, turned to the author and said: *"You broadcast on nutrition five hours a week?"* When this was confirmed, he said unbelievingly: "Why, I could tell the world all I know about nutrition in three minutes!"

The comment is a reflection of our culture in which specialization has proceeded to the point where a gland specialist, for instance, considers most of his patient's anatomy to be merely an appendage to a set of glands. The fact that this remark came from a physician may be surprising to some. You might suppose that a profession that freely recommends diets and freely prescribes vitamin concentrates would not plead guilty to inadequacy in an area so intimately a part of the healing art. The glands are not only directly affected by the diet (remember what happens to the thyroid when iodine is lacking) but in turn are directly concerned with the utilization of food. A poor diet will almost certainly disturb the glands; and disturbed glands may make it difficult for the eater to profit by what he is eating. And so it was that, in response to the doctor's remark, the author commented: "You have just disqualified yourself for the practice of endocrinology."

"Dietary insufficiency equals endocrine imbalance" is axiomatic to the nutritionist, and it should be to the endocrinologist. But specialization in gland function to the medical man is a matter of dispensing small but potent dosages of this hormone or that, and of dealing with the diseases that visit the body when one or more of these glands is overtly over- or underfunctioning. Actually, endocrinology is merely an aspect of biochemistry; and biochemistry is merely nutrition at work; and the relationship, therefore, between nutrition and the functioning of the glands is so intimate and so complex that it is literally impossible to be competent as a "gland specialist" unless one is also a competent nutritionist. Yet such incompetent "specialists" exist—and treat patients. Is this ignorance their fault? Most medical schools do not offer more than a few hours' instruction in nutrition. Nutrition is not yet a medical fad, which means it is not yet popular with the hierarchical cliques that control medicine. However, we are not examining here the current medical curricula, the penalties for overspecialization, or the failings of the endocrinologists. Let us proceed by going back for a moment to the fateful lunch from which this chapter was born. The endocrinologist demanded an explanation for the "insult." The author's reply was a quotation from a German textbook on vitamins: "Among vitamins and hormones there exists a state of co-play and counter-play, with the actions so intermixed that a deficiency of one of these factors may appear only as the effects of a deficiency of the other."

The statement appeared in the early 1930s. We are writing more than a quarter of a century later. This is an example of cultural lag: the time lapse intervening between research that has a potential impact on, for instance, our fight against disease, and the ultimate acceptance and application of such principles in public health and medical practices. As we have already said in a number of ways, we want to shorten, happily eliminate, the cultural lag.

The endocrinologist of today is in the unhappy position of knowing more and more about less and less, since it is an unfortunate aspect of his conventional medicine that it largely investigates the sick organism. Indeed, medicine studies health from the negative aspect, attempting to appraise well-being by assaying the symptoms of illness.

The gland specialist, particularly, occupies this unhappy position. Studies of the effects of the glands are, like those of the effects of the vitamins, carried on with the subject in a state of deficiency. Thus we achieve some understanding of the often dramatic results when the body is deprived of a hormone, just as we have knowledge of the catastrophic effects that follow deprivation of a vitamin. We can well define the effects of deficiency in hormones and vitamins, but we are somewhat hard pressed in absolutely defining the results of an optimal supply.

The term "optimal" is the root of the evil. Dietitians have warred themselves into two-and-seventy sects in an effort to define optimum nutrition. Endocrinologists have been too specialized to fall into the trap: Your glands are sick or they are not, and if they are not, they say in effect, you are of no conceivable interest to the world of science.

Between the maintenance diet that keeps body and spirit together and the optimal diet that confers buoyant health, there is a gap. There are speculations concerning the nature of that gap, but nothing definitive has been established except its recognition. But between optimal and marginal functioning and outright failure of the glands there are also gaps. Present-day science can determine only that your glands are grossly overactive or underactive. Between these two classifications are millions of people, presumably well if not optimally fed, ably possessed of functioning glands adequate to meet the needs of the organism. This is what the specialists tell us.

There is another concept that you must grasp before we propound a thesis that equates glandular function and diet. There are investigators who do not recognize that a diet need not produce symptoms of deficiency, and yet may fail to support ideal function of mind and body. These workers, trained in an older school, insist that a diet is not deficient in vitamin C unless symptoms of scurvy appear in the eater. They hold that beriberi is the price for a diet deficient in B_1 and, lacking the emergency of a full-fledged set of symptoms adding up to beriberi, the eater need have no concern about the vitamin B_1 worth of his diet. (As might be expected, orthodox medicine, for the most part, accepts this narrow viewpoint. And therefore very likely your doctor does too.)

In short, such a school of thought does not recognize the twilight zone of nutrition, in which the diet is neither truly good nor truly bad, and produces an individual who, similarly, is neither truly sick nor truly well. We think there is a similar order of deficiency in glandular function: a netherland in which the glands are neither functioning badly enough to cause the manifest symptoms of excessive or insufficient activity of these organs, nor functioning well enough to allow the individual to reach his full potential for a healthy and productive life. Let the reader remember that no gland misfunctions without repercussion on the function of other glands; the symptoms of a vitamin deficiency must reflect its impact on the actions of other vitamins and other nutrients.

Still another concept deals with heredity. Judging from the literature of genetics and from personal communications the senior author has received, specialists in heredity seem to be convinced that observations on heredity should be their unique province—presumably on a hereditary basis. However, let us offer here our thought on heredity as it relates to the functioning of the glands. It has been said that each of us comes into the world with an omnibus of ancestors riding on his shoulders. This is another surrender to the concept of the immutable nature of the "dictates of heredity," which are supposed to limit our potentials and determine our destinies. A woman, for example, inherits a tendency to underactivity of the thyroid gland. Also her ovaries are weak—but so were her mother's. This is "bad heredity," the phrase goes.

Now, let us deal with a new approach in which the term "bad heredity" is discarded in favor of a more helpful one: "interrupted heredity." It is a more realistic even though a more optimistic term, as we shall see. It denominates heredity as a force for good. When it does not operate for the benefit of the person, we maintain the force for good has merely been interrupted; and interruptions, unlike the concept of "bad heredity," may not pose insoluble problems.[1]

With these ideas in mind, let us look at a "well" woman who inhabits the shadowland of glandular function where failure or overactivity of the glands is not present in sufficient degree to produce the classical symptoms succinctly described in the textbooks of pathology. Now, she has a few physical complaints—but who does not? For instance, the soles of her feet are calloused. Her skin is sensitive to friction—the rubbing of a girdle, of tight hose or shoes, of a garter belt or brassiere. She occasionally suffers from headaches. In the premenstrual week, she is likely to be tense, irritable, weak, and afflicted by an unprovoked craving for sweets, drawing sensations in the thighs and breast, and a feeling

[1] Dr. Helen Mitchell in the *J.A.M.A.* (Vol. 30, 9, Sept., 1954), has suggested that supraoptimal doses of nutrients may compensate for hereditary inability of the body efficiently to complete essential enzyme reactions.

of being bloated. The menstrual period itself is a stormy episode, marked by pain and backaches. And she may have some allergies —as, again, who does not?

All these are such minor and common complaints, so characteristic of millions of women, that they certainly do not constitute a license to use hospital facilities. Nor is there any basis on which to expect consolation, advice, or treatment from a physician. Indeed, the patient may be wary of the physician, for the reason that she is likely to find herself called neurotic—not alone on the basis of the symptoms described, but because of her own description of herself when asked: "Psychologically speaking, how do you feel?" To this, her answer is: "Inadequate."

Women suffering with the organic failure we are describing not only consider themselves inadequate, but are so labeled in medical literature, where the term is embellished as "constitutionally inadequate." These are presumably, then, the weak reeds who are cursed with a constitution not capable of bearing the stresses normal to everyday living.

The typical sufferer rises in the morning unrefreshed by her night's sleep. Either she has slept so soundly as to feel, on awakening, more or less drugged or she has slept so lightly that the slightest sound awakens her. In any case she awakens, as she says, more tired than she was when she went to bed. She finds it difficult to gather momentum during the mornings. She cannot function at all without her morning cup of coffee. Addiction to coffee and cola drinks—leaning on the beverages in the therapeutic sense, craving them as needed stimulants—is another persistent characteristic.

In medical literature she is often sketched like this: "By the time that she has the children off to school and her husband off to work, she has barely enough energy to reach for another coffee and a cigarette. Planning the day's activities, the shopping list, and the menu for the evening meal—these activities exhaust the remainder of her slender stock of energy, and now she must lie down to recover."

Little wonder this woman characterizes herself as "inadequate."

It should be made clear that in her own mind this characterization is not based on easy fatigability. It is a capsulated description of her whole personality. When she rises, she looks forward to the day's activities with dread, desiring to avoid all but the unavoidable in tasks and responsibilities. Asked why, she says, "I don't feel adequate—to cope with my husband, to mother my children, to run this household, or, for that matter, to manage myself."

If she presented this complaint to a psychologist, the practitioner might well reply: "You are entitled to an inferiority complex, because you are inferior." If she goes to a clinic or a medical office, will she be received seriously as a patient suffering from calloused feet, premenstrual pain, fatigability, and a sense of inadequacy? Or will she be hastily brushed over in favor of persons "genuinely" ill? Or, if she is well to do, will she be put through a series of expensive tests that prove little, and then given any one of a number of "pep" pills?

There is a specific physical aspect of this woman that deserves our attention. If you want to play the role of scientific investigator, ask her to open her mouth so you may see the entire "horseshoe" of her upper teeth. Look at the distance across the dental arch—from the rear molars on one side to those on the other. In such a woman it is almost invariably a narrow arch, high and Gothic.

How many individuals have this narrow dental arch? Ask a group of dentists, as the senior author did, and the response will be: "Ten to 15 per cent of our practices." If, however, you display pictures of dental arches of primitive peoples, and ask the dentists to use these arches as their yardstick, they will say 90 per cent of their patients have narrow arches.

Question: Who is abnormal: the primitive or you?

Part of the answer to this question was sought by Dr. Weston Price, an internationally known dental researcher who traveled all over the world in an effort to ascertain why primitives have beautiful teeth in their mouths while ours are on the night table. He encountered this disparity in the width of dental arches, and he noted with interest that the nutrition of the white man's grocery stores in the primitive community brings with it, in the second generation, a narrowing of the arches of the primitive children in a degree so marked that the youngsters do not physically resemble their parents or their forebears.

The upper dental arch is, of course, the palate. The palate is formed in the embryo simultaneously with the formation of the pituitary gland. Both are formed from the same basic tissue. If a narrow dental arch represents a genetic abnormality—one which we shall call "interrupted" heredity—what is the possibility that the pituitary gland, formed from the same tissue at the same time, has likewise encountered interruption of heredity? And if the pituitary gland in some way, if not structurally, is functionally altered in this process, what might the impact on the individual be?

We must remember that the pituitary[2] epitomizes our ignorance of the functioning of the glands. For years, chemists have speculated upon the chemical identities and the exact functions of the appallingly large number of hormones attributed to this small gland. Growth factors, factors affecting the utilization of food, factors stimulating other glands, the hormone affecting the production of breast milk, an anti-insulin factor—these and innumerable other functions were identified or speculated upon as being present among the many hormones believed to be produced by the pituitary. Endocrinologists considered the pituitary to be the ruler of the glands. Recently, however, there have been surgical removals of the pituitary in cases of cancer that pointed in a new direction. The patients were kept alive, surprisingly, by doses of a single hormone (cortisone) or perhaps two. None lived very long, and all eventually died of cancer. Nonetheless, several mutually exclusive conclusions might be drawn from this remarkable operation. Perhaps the seemingly innumerable principles supposedly produced by the pituitary are not all necessary. Perhaps, which is likely, with the removal of the gland the body induces compensa-

[2] This chapter concentrates largely on the pituitary because it controls and interlocks functionally with all other glands.

tory activities by the remaining glands. The third possibility—and there may be others—is the chance that the pituitary is not the source of the hormones it has long been credited with producing; and thereby the removal of the gland deprives us only of a depot that awaits but the command of the body to release the trains of the necessary hormones.

The fascinating possibility that the pituitary gland functions like a catch basin rather than a chemical factory is a concept which, if accepted, would throw the neurologists into a tizzy from which the psychiatrists, themselves already confused, could not rescue them. It would also place the endocrinologists in the interesting position of having their domain extended to include the brain itself,[8] for such a theory would make it mandatory that the brain itself produce the hormones now credited to the pituitary gland. (For specialists accustomed only to thinking in their usual narrow confines, such an idea might easily prove too shocking, and we would have the amusing spectacle of endocrinologists seeking solace on psychiatrists' couches only to have psychiatrists disclaiming the responsibility and forthwith demanding treatment from the endocrinologists. Neither, of course, would seek the logical source of adjunct treatment—from the enlightened nutritionist!)

Anatomically speaking, such a hypothesis is easily supported. The palate is the floor of the brain; above it is the pituitary gland, directly beneath the "emotional brain" (the thalamus), which in turn is encased in the "thinking brain" (the cortex) like the meat in a walnut. If emotional disturbances are transmitted from the feeling brain to the glands via the pituitary gland, as has been supposed, perhaps it is not surprising that we have been unsuccessful in demonstrating intimate and plentiful nerve interconnections between emotional brain and pituitary. Such voluminous neural connections would not be demanded if the message trans-

[8] There is an ancient theory that all organs produce their own unique hormones.

mitted from the emotional brain to the pituitary is partially endocrinal—chemical—rather than neural.

If this is the machinery, it is easy indeed to understand that an emotionally disturbed brain might transmit to the pituitary "abnormal balance" or "abnormal" types of hormones. This, in turn, would result in a pattern of "abnormal" repercussion in other glands. The process would lead ultimately to the familiar "psychosomatic" diseases.

To understand even partially the influence of the pituitary gland on the personality requires an examination of the anatomy of personality. Let us proceed with an oversimplified view of the functioning of our brain, of which we have really *two*, and our nervous systems, of which we have *three*. Surely such a perspective should be of value beyond understanding of the immediate premises, which are developed in this chapter.

Our children at birth are controlled by the emotional brain, strongly bent on survival of the organism, functioning crudely and yet efficiently in terms of the needs of the organism, at whatever cost to other organisms. Babies' needs are imperative and of first concern to baby. This emotional brain is *not* left behind as baby grows up. Instead, housed and protected by the developing thinking brain, the emotional brain continues to function throughout life. Oddly enough, this is fortunate, for although this brain may be a center of greed and hate and belligerence, it is likewise true that the emotional brain gives us—and lets us enjoy—music, dancing, and poetry. It is barely possible that if amputation of adult man's emotional brain were possibly without threat to life, it would rid the world of man's most undesirable traits, but it simultaneously would banish *feeling* and leave behind it the cold, the gray, the disproportionate, and the objective. A little of this is seen in inverse in the operation called lobotomy, which is used only on persons who are completely out of touch with "reality" and are often violent. Here some of the association bands linking the thinking brain with the emotional brain are severed. The individual no longer worries—or worry at least does not rise to confuse thinking; but he likewise loses the capacity to feel responsibility, of which worry is the progeny. He returns to society, but no longer feels the necessity for accomplishing anything.

So the child grows up and becomes, instead of a little animal, a civilized human being. That is, the insatiable, ruthless, egocentric, selfish, and imperious demands of the emotional brain are brought into an uneasy equilibrium by counteracting controls exerted by the cortex, or thinking brain. The angry child throws a rock at a hated teacher; the college student murmurs to the hated professor: "No other authority I've read quite agrees with you." Between the two statements is a network of association bands, maturing as the child matures, and establishing an armed truce between the two brains. For there is no victory: the intellect never reigns alone.

The anatomy of the brain is such that it is highly doubtful that any stimulus, any sensation, reaches the thinking brain without traversing the emotional. For example: you stroke some velvet, you stroke some sandpaper. Without the emotional brain, one would be merely soft, the other merely rough. Because the emotional brain has, by a fraction of a second, priority in appraising the sensation, recognition of "softness" is instantaneously associated with recognition of "pleasant softness," and the roughness of the sandpaper is instantaneously linked with "harsh and unpleasant." This seemingly innocuous observation carries within it the grain of a singular truth: it is physically impossible for man to have a completely objective, dispassionate, emotion-free thought. Perhaps the ideal judicial temperament may be defined in these terms: while his thalamus continues to function, it never rules his head.

Those who may have wondered about the cofunctioning of Siamese twins might wonder even more about "normal" man, who has two brains and frequently gives the impression of using neither, perhaps because one brain impulse cancels out the other, so that he is left in a state of frustration.

The emotional brain, we have noted, cannot be amputated. It

happens to have within its province the management of those body activities that we may term "uncontrollable," meaning that we cannot exercise voluntary control, hence no emotional control. These would include the beating of the heart, the breathing reflex, the mechanisms that dilate and contract our capillaries, and, among others, the undulation of the digestive tract as it moves food through the body. It is very fortunate that we do not have to concentrate on these activities, for they would leave us little time for abstract thinking. Therefore, the nervous systems that are involuntary are closely linked with the emotional brain.

Yet it is the emotional brain that deprives you of your poise, however desperately you try to maintain it when you are applying for that all-important job. It is the same autonomous machinery of the body that leaves you trembling with rage after an insult. And, before you wonder whether the machinery is worth the price, remember that the same mechanism gives you the flash of added strength—the instantaneous and unthinking reaction that allows you to leap out of the path of a speeding car. The first man's primitive brain functioned in a way that meant survival in the day of the ferocious cave bear and mastodon. The caveman cursed with a dominant cortex tended not to survive: one cannot pause very long to think about courses of procedure when in the darkness of the primeval jungle an earth-shaking roar suddenly calls for instant action. Scientists have speculated that the Cro-Magnons, the earliest true men, who produced the first great art in the caves of France and Spain about thirty thousand years ago, did not survive because their cortexes were too highly developed. Their brain capacity was indeed much greater than ours—we, the "modern" Homo sapiens. It is likely they were too thoughtful and too sensitive for their parlous times, odd as it may seem.

However, the autonomic nervous system has great disadvantages, now that man has become "civilized." Among the difficulties that beset us, we can include one that nature did not create, except indirectly. The machinery of fight or flight is like an electric light switch. It knows only yes or no, which means that you may turn the light on or off. In our generally Judeo-Christian culture, however, we are frequently confronted with situations in which neither fight nor flight is seemly or proper. This is inherent in the doctrine of "turn the other cheek." Unfortunately, the autonomic mechanisms of the body cannot prepare for this inaction; faced with a situation where the thalamus is screaming for the privilege of running or giving battle and the cortex is suppressing any such desires, the autonomic machinery still diverts the blood circulation to the muscles. The muscles are prepared; they are geared to the thalamus. Here, possibly, is the beginning of essential hypertension, high blood pressure, another of the prices we pay for the split in purpose and function between the thinking and the emotional brains.

In returning to our main discussion, the relationship of pituitary function, function of the brain, the personality, and the body, let us briefly examine the now discredited Lombroso theory, which once made phrenology popular. This was the attempt to appraise personality primarily by the bumps on one's noggin, and it resulted in alleged identification of a "criminal type." The anthropologists and the psychologists have long since buried Lombroso and his bumps, but his ghost still haunts the scientific battlefield, for serious research is in progress at Harvard University and in the constitutional clinics of several hospitals in an effort to appraise the extent to which characteristics of body structure *can* be linked to aspects of personality and susceptibilities to disease.

If a malfunctioning of the pituitary gland, reflected in a narrowing of the dental arch,[4] has definite impact upon personality, we should be able to establish some association between this type of facial structure and the individual's attitude toward society. Certainly the woman we have described, the victim of the "anterior pituitary syndrome," cannot be accused of being asocial because she feels inadequate. It is equally possible that the vagaries of a malfunctioning pituitary gland may be reflected in symptoms

---

[4] Only of late are papers appearing on narrowing of the palate as one of the stigmata of certain heritable diseases.

other than those described. Among these is inexplicable, unprovoked asocial behavior. Without attempting to connect mental retardation and abnormal and/or criminal behavior, let us realize that the hallmark of mental retardation very frequently is malformation of the mouth. We picture the Mongolian idiot with his tongue lolling out of his mouth. Yet it is not that his tongue is too large; it may be normal in size. Rather, the *mouth* is too small. On at least one occasion, the dentist mentioned earlier, Dr. Weston Price, experimented with surgical widening of the dental arch, wondering whether the procedure would stimulate the pituitary gland. The retarded child who was the subject of the experiment showed a remarkable improvement in mental function. More notable was his gradual retreat to previous retardation when the surgical appliance, which held his teeth in position as his gums healed, fell out of place. The child resumed his "interrupted" progress when the dentist restored the appliance to its proper position. We consider this last response highly significant and almost in the nature of a controlled experiment.

Dr. Price became interested in the narrow palate from his observations among primitives as he conducted research aimed at isolating the causes of tooth decay. Identifying our overprocessed foods as being responsible for the decay, he studied the effects of these foods on his primitive subjects into the second generation. He observed a narrowing of the palate in the children. With it, Dr. Price observed other impacts on mind and body: asocial behavior and congenital deformities of the feet. The observation was made that the children with narrowed palates did not resemble their parents, but began to look like us.

To link the "primitive" behavior with our own: we have had, in the United States, almost continuous "sporadic" outbursts of asocial behavior or actual crime by some of our children, particularly teenagers. For these seemingly "inexplicable" acts our psychiatrists have had glib explanations: some of them, interestingly, offered without personal contact with the youths involved. A classic example, a few years ago, was a group of teenagers who beat girls, tortured old men, and wound up with a senseless, unprovoked assault on an innocent father of two children, who drowned in the East River of New York City after a brutal beating.

Said the psychiatrists (we are paraphrasing) "This boy was overprotected; this one received inadequate affection; that one was insecure." While these pundits were holding forth in the daily press, no one rose to ask the pertinent question: "Why have we not been decimated with murders committed by overprotected children? Why have not the insecure teenagers blistered, tortured, and murdered most of the adult population?" In short, although we acknowledge fundamental need for security accompanying all of us into the world, how do the psychiatrists dare give a single explanation for the widely different responses of children (and, for that matter, adults) to emotional environments which, in the psychiatrist's own terms, appear to be similar?

Although many psychiatrists will reject this fact as representing an attempt to trace psychic disturbances to a purely somatic source, it is a fact that there is a high incidence of narrow mouths (reflecting narrow dental arches) in individuals convicted of crimes of senseless violence. Of course, we recognize that Wide Palates also commit crimes and that Narrow Palates are often upright pillars of the community, but it should be remembered by the "doctrinaire" psychiatrists that Freud himself indicated that certain common emotional disorders probably have a physical basis. Freud also stated that all so-called mental and emotional diseases would probably be cured by "chemical" means: a statement that his closest followers of today choose to ignore. (The authors of this book, it becomes necessary to note, certainly believe in psychotherapy but not when it is practiced as offering the *only* road to the truth.)

Remembering the control that the cortex must exercise on the emotional brain to produce the pattern of behavior we call "social"; remembering the linkages between the emotional brain and the glands involved in "behavior"; mindful of the dominant role of the pituitary gland in mediating between the emotional brain and the other glands; and remembering, finally, that the medication of choice for certain types of mental dysfunction is the administration of pituitary extract, the thesis developed here does not originate from pure speculation.

Perhaps the best test of such a thesis is observation of the results when remedial steps are taken predicated upon the theory. What happens to personality when our typical female victim of the anterior pituitary syndrome is treated on this basis? And—an unanswerable question, because the test has not been made—what happens when the "juvenile delinquent" is medicated on the supposition of faulty pituitary function?

There is a difference between the nutritional approach to support of the glands in an individual who is reasonably healthy, and nutritional therapies aimed at stimulation of the glands in an individual woman who is in the twilight zone of being neither truly sick nor truly well because her glands are neither functioning properly nor failing totally. For the "constitutionally inadequate" woman, small, almost homeopathic doses of pituitary-supporting nutrients—paba, pantothenic acid, vitamin E, copper, cobalt, and manganese—have been found to work subtle changes in the personality, as the first response.[5] Under such therapy, the author has seen such women after about six weeks of treatment suddenly announce that they feel more "adequate"—this, although they did not know that a feeling of inadequacy is a distinguishing feature of the group of symptoms that we look for in such women. Interestingly, if the doses of the nutrients are too high for the limited capacity of the pituitary to respond in such women, the symptoms worsen instead of improving. Quite apart from the fact, then, that this book is not intended to promote self-medication, we aim this chapter at nutritional support of glands not too seriously in trouble because the management of the therapeutic approach requires expertise—the supervision of a competent medical nutritionist-endocrinologist.

[5] Personal communication to the senior author from John Myers, M.D.

Our discussion of several related theses suggest that we now, for clarification, summarize what we have been saying:

1. In the field of nutrition, there is a strongly entrenched school of thought that still does not recognize the twilight zone of health caused by diet neither truly bad nor truly good, resulting in people who are neither truly sick nor truly well.

2. In the field of endocrinology, there is a similar failure to recognize the malfunctioning of glands neither overactive nor underactive enough to produce classical symptoms of glandular disturbance, and yet not functioning well enough to support buoyant health and balanced personality.

3. Between the twilight zone of dietary failure and the similar zone in glandular failure, there is a relationship.

4. This relationship is exhibited in certain effects of twilight diet on the pregnant woman and the unborn baby.

5. One of these effects is a narrowing of the palate, which indicates possible interference with the proper development and the function of the pituitary gland.

6. The disturbances produced by such failure of the pituitary are very much in the twilight zone, and the effects, singly or accumulatively, may be ignored as nonpathological, accepted as "average health," or labeled "constitutional inadequacy" or "juvenile delinquency."

7. The kind of "average health" thus tolerated wrecks the functioning of the individual, and its impact on personality may be such as to bring the individual to the psychiatric couch.

8. Among the forces operating on the diet that may interfere with proper nutrition of the unborn baby are consistent heating of protein foods and overconsumption of overprocessed carbohydrates, the consumption of both of which represents a dietary experiment on man's part.[6]

It has long been recognized that minute amounts of the chemicals produced by our glands are essential to life. Examination of

[6] In this chapter will be found part of the data supporting an inimical influence of cooked proteins, as we eat them, on the pituitary glands of the unborn.

the chemical structure of these glandular products showed, as might have been expected, that the hormones manufactured by the glands are primarily fatty in nature or constructed of protein materials. The implication was immediately accepted that the diet was obviously the source of the building materials. A crucial point, however, was glossed over: the endocrinologists were so hypnotized by the indefatigability of these organs that it was somehow assumed that, come hell, high water, or bad diet, the glands would go on extracting the needed building materials— virtually out of the blue—and manufacturing their hormones. Thus, one would not expect to find an endocrinologist examining a patient and reporting "glandular disturbance causing, caused, or aggravated by vitamin deficiency." Yet this *is* the concept that burst upon the minds of investigators exploring the intricate network of the relationship between diet and glandular function. As far back as 1936, German researchers made a proposal that tended to break down the distinction between vitamin and hormone. They proposed a definition in which the vitamin is an "exogenous" hormone, a hormone an "endogenous" vitamin—in other words, that vitamins and hormones are chemical substances, both vital to cellular processes, both needed in minute amounts, both essential to life, the chief distinction being that the body manufactures one and must ingest the other. This appears to be pure caprice on the part of nature: vitamin B_1 is so essential to life that it has seriously been proposed that the requirement of the organism for this substance be made part of the definition that will distinguish between the living and the dead.

The attempt of the Germans to break down the artificial distinction between vitamins and hormones became more logical as research progressed, and it was found that the hormones themselves are manufactured in the plant world. Testosterone, or male hormone, is manufactured from a basic substance found in the sarsaparilla root; both male and female hormone activity have been found in wheat germ oil.

The Germans had pried a small toehold in a tenuous area that has received little further exploration. Here and there, enlightened endocrinologists in personal correspondence with the senior author (thus escaping cries of "crackpot" from their colleagues) have recognized the deeper truths within the German's statements. In a letter, one such practitioner explicitly acknowledged the principle:

> I have this morning examined Mrs. ———. She shows clear-cut signs of a mixed vitamin deficiency-endocrine disturbance.

Fleeting notes in the literature fortify the impression that these men are pioneers in science. A Swiss doctor remarks that he can cure colloid goiter in a cow as quickly with vitamin B_1 as he can with iodine. A Boston endocrinologist found that the administration of para-amino-benzoic acid (a vitamin that is removed from most of our carbohydrate foods) restored fertility in 55 per cent of a group of women who had, for five years or more, been unable to conceive and deliver living babies.

Another investigator found that doses of cortisone, a highly dangerous hormone drug, can be lowered if para-amino-benzoic acid is given simultaneously. Still another endocrinologist, in a personal communication, remarked: "This vitamin (para-amino-benzoic acid) not only stimulates the pituitary gland; it likewise stimulates the adrenal." A biochemist reported that deficiency in vitamin E (also removed from our daily bread) resulted in young rats being born with the pituitary gland half completed. Vitamin C has been reported in dozens of papers to be essential to the adrenal gland. Deficiency of vitamin B_1 has been noted to cause a severe drop in thyroid activity, a condition which, in the human being, becomes irreversible after a few months of such diet.

In the senior author's own research, the administration of folic acid has been noted to increase the response to female hormone in tissue sensitive to that hormone, with the result that enlargement of the bust sometimes follows doses of this vitamin. To prove that the female is always feminine, a similar response is found in the young chick: given female hormone, with an adequate diet, the young chick responds with a fortyfold increase in the size of the oviduct, or egg-laying channel. If folic acid is removed from the diet, the oviduct growth response is only fourfold. Graying of the hair, traced to a disturbance in the adrenal gland, is known to follow the feeding to animals of diets deficient in pantothenic acid; and the human beings as well as animals fed substantial doses of this and other vitamins sometimes respond with the re-coloring of gray hair. Although para-amino-benzoic acid is often referred to as "the anti-gray hair factor," there are other nutrients which have an effect on adrenal or pituitary function, and thereby on the synthesis of hormones by these glands, with resulting impact on hair color. These include pantothenic acid, choline, iodine (indirectly), and possibly copper.

There are many similar reports to be found in the medical literature, from which we make our point that the function of the glands, and therefore all the body functions, mental and physical, are dependent on the intake of dietary factors. While we recognize that such a statement is beyond the pale of orthodox medical thinking at the present time, we would refer both our professional and non-professional readers to the experiments we have cited. But even a careful review of such research does not give us a revealing perspective on all the forces which alter the glandular structure and function of man. Any attempt to "explain" modern man's health, or lack of it, and the role of his glands in this state of twilight ill-being, must take cognizance of the impact of man's environment, practices, and diet on these organs. For it is not only that man's foods are divorced from the composition dictated for primitives by inherited wisdom. He has also altered his environment, specifically to escape from the atmosphere of unremitting stress which in eons of evolution guaranteed the survival of the fittest.

Let us therefore inspect three important—and largely unrecognized—forces that affect man's glands.

The first, already cited, is the diet—with particular stress on the cooking of protein, and the overconsumption of highly processed carbohydrates.

The second is the shift from breast to bottle in feeding of infants.

The third is man's persistent and successful effort to create for himself womb-to-tomb shielding from environmental stress.

Mention has been made of the effect of modern diet in causing in the unborn a narrowing of the palate. It has been produced in animals experimentally by the simple process of feeding them protein foods cooked as most of us eat them. The protein foods in our diet comprise eggs, milk, and dairy products, meat, fish, and fowl, and the less significant contribution of protein from cereals, vegetables, and fruits. The dominant protein intake comes from foods of animal origin.

A moment of reflection will remind you that 99 per cent of our protein foods are cooked. With the exception of raw eggs, clams or oysters, and a possibly dangerous (because of the presence of parasites) "cannibal" or "tartar steak" sandwich, the average person in this culture rarely encounters a protein that has not been heat-treated in some degree. The pasteurization of milk represents the application of heat to a high-quality animal protein. Most of our cereals are roasted; our bread, of course, is baked. Our canned protein foods are actually overcooked in an effort to protect the public against contamination. How early in his history man encountered Charles Lamb's device for making pork more succulent we do not know, but certainly the application of fire to food came comparatively late in man's history.

What is the effect of heat upon protein food? Answer: We do not yet fully know. Authorities in nutrition have written much about destruction of vitamins in cooking, and loss of minerals by certain cooking techniques; we are aware that burned fat may be irritating (even cancer-causing), if not actually indigestible, but we know little about the effect of heat on our always heated protein foods. Evidently acting on the theory that the best defense is an offense, the "authorities" assure us that heat does nothing to protein foods, thereby declaring the pasteurization of milk an innocuous procedure that produces a great health benefit. Although pasteurization was originally proposed as only a temporary measure intended to give us safe, clean milk, you may be sure that any move to appraise the effects of heat on milk classifies the nutrition researcher as a "faddist." However, pasteurization, and the cooking of all protein foods, must be evaluated, for the evidence leans toward indicting heated proteins consumed in pregnancy as being responsible for the narrowing of the palate in the offspring, and thus—as we have seen—with possible repercussions on the pituitary gland.

In addition to Dr. Weston Price's observations of primitives, numerous references in the scientific literature explicitly or implicitly point a finger of suspicion at cooked proteins as failing to shoulder their metabolic responsibilties in maintaining the health of the organism. These appear in papers reporting the feeding of animals and children with various types of milk. Respected medical journals such as the British publication, *Lancet,* have carried many reports indicating that the growth of children, like that of young animals, is more satisfactory on raw milk than on pasteurized. Dr. Albert Sobel, chemist then of the Brooklyn Jewish Hospital in New York, had noticed that the blood chemistry of the newborn baby on raw cow's milk is similar to that of the baby on breast milk, but different fron the chemistry of infants fed formulas comprising the conventionally twice-cooked milk.[7]

Probably the experiment of Dr. Francis Pottenger[8] is the classic in this area. Involving cats fed various types of milk, the experiment produced anatomical changes in the animals closely resembling those observed in primitive people by Dr. Price. Dr. Pot-

[7] Personal communication.
[8] "The Effect Of Heat-Processed Foods And Metabolized Vitamin D Milk On The Dentofacial Structures Of Experimental Animals," by Francis M. Pottenger, Jr., M.D., F.A.C.P., which appeared in the *American Journal of Orthodontics and Oral Surgery,* Vol. 32, No. 8, Oral Surgery Pages 467-485, August, 1946.

tenger fed several generations of his animals on a diet one third of which was derived from foods known to support good health in cats and the other two thirds of their intake representing the type of milk being tested; raw, pasteurized, evaporated, and condensed. The cats were run-of-the-pen mongrels, in good health at the beginning of the experiment.

The adults of the first generation, on raw milk, continued to exhibit good health. Skin and fur were in good condition; shedding the hair was minimal; neuromuscular coordination, normal; mouths in good condition. The first generation of the pasteurized milk group showed less satisfactory condition of skin and hair, with a marked tendency to shed, and some inclination toward abscesses of the gums. The cats on evaporated and condensed milk were in still less satisfactory condition.

These results differ from those reported by some other investigators, but it is noteworthy that the investigations that have resulted in complete vindication of pasteurized milk have invariably stopped with the *first generation*. In the Pottenger research, it was revealed that this omission in other investigations is a critical one, for in the second generation of cats, sharp and significant differences appeared among the groups. The cats on raw milk remained healthy. Reproduction was normal; the kittens were normal. Cats on *all* the other types of milk encountered difficulty in reproduction, including stillbirth, miscarriage, spontaneous abortion, or resorption of the young in the uterus. In addition, the young cats showed eczema, neuromuscular disorders, calcification of the soft tissues, allergies of the nose and eyes. Could one of the cat mothers have spoken, it is probably she might have said: "I don't understand it—nobody in our family was ever allergic."

Some of the kittens in the second generation were so sick—so ridden with degenerative disease—that they were barely able to crawl. Some cats ostensibly in normal health showed abnormalities in neuromuscular coordination. Homosexuality also appeared in this group; it was missing from the raw milk group. Merely allowing the kittens to support themselves by clawing a wire mesh fence quickly separated the lucky raw milk feeders from the others. The former lowered themselves quickly; the others remained in place, crying feebly, and lacking strength to descend.

The mention of homosexuality leads to another observation made by Dr. Pottenger. Anatomical distinctions between the sexes in the cats fed the various types of cooked milk became less apparent in succeeding generations. This phenomenon is not confined to cats, as Pottenger demonstrated. He photographed from the rear groups of nude male and female teenagers, then tested the pictures at a medical convention. Attempting to guess the sexes of the individuals, the visiting physicians were wrong a majority of the time.

But what is of prime significance to our discussion is the narrowing of the dental arch that appeared in the second generation of cats fed the cooked milks. Profiles of these cats were sharply different from those of the raw milk group. Temperaments were different, too. The raw milk cats were playful, spirited, and mischievous. The others were querulous, irritable, and, when strong enough, belligerent. Notable, too, was the tendency of the cats on milk other than raw to pace their cages restlessly. This phenomenon, familiar to those who have visited zoos, did not appear in the raw milk group. And let us note that the nutritional differences in the milk influenced even the excreta of the cats. Bean crops were deliberately planted in the pens after the animals had been removed. This had been suggested by the noticeable difference in the growth of weeds in the idle pens. The growth of the beans paralleled the growth of the weeds. In the raw milk pen both were luxuriant. There were fewer weeds and bean plants in the pasteurized milk pen. There was scarcely any crop in the evaporated milk pen, and the plants did not survive when droppings of the cats consuming condensed milk were the only soil fertilizers.

Many enzymes in raw milk are destroyed in pasteurization. Their importance to the body is still largely problematical, though at least one, *phosphatase*, has been proved important in the nourishment of infants. In the early days of research with vitamin D, it became apparent that animal reactions, usually valuable as a guide to human needs in nutrition, could not be trusted for this particular vitamin. Estimates of the needs of a human baby for vitamin D were predicated on a per pound body weight basis established by research with young rats. However, the dosages of vitamin D that protected the rats against rickets did not protect a considerable percentage of human infants. This might have been attributed to a species difference, had it not been for the observation that the rats were being nursed and the human babies were not. This, in turn, might have been dismissed as another of the puzzling phenomena surrounding the values of breast milk, and, in fact, some nutritionists concluded that breastfed baby, for an unknown reason, required less vitamin D for antirachitic effect than the formula-fed baby.

Further study, however, showed that the nursing rat was receiving a protection that the baby consuming twice-cooked (formula) milk did not receive: a supply of phosphatase, which is present in raw milk and missing from pasteurized. The crowning irony resides in the test for pasteurization. When a health department wishes to determine whether milk has been pasteurized, a search is made for phosphatase, and if any phosphatase activity is found, the milk is condemned!

Among other enzymes present in raw milk and missing from pasteurized are those concerned with fat utilization. There is also one enzyme that has a germicidal effect. This natural protection in raw milk disappears spontaneously in twelve hours, but during that time raw milk remains *constant* in bacterial count, while pasteurized milk gains until the bacteria swamp the fluid.

Still more evidence tips the scales in favor of raw milk. Experiments with monkeys show that it possesses an antianemia effect missing in pasteurized. Tests on both animals and children demonstrate a growth-promoting effect in raw milk that is missing in pasteurized. The so-called antiulcer factor, discovered also in cabbage juice, is present in raw milk. It disappears both from cooked cabbage and pasteurized milk.

In experimenting with raw versus pasteurized milk, therefore, we are not dealing with a single variable, but with many. It is definitely known that heat tends to lower the digestibility and thereby the biological efficiency of protein. Technically we think that this effect is caused by a toughening of the bonds between the protein acids that are the building blocks of protein. You can actually see this when you heat egg white. This coagulation effect is believed to make it more difficult for the body to break down the protein, a necessary prerequisite to proper utilization. Protein in liquid form, such as milk, is reported (by some authorities) not to suffer significant alteration in this way, yet it is noteworthy that the experiments supposedly attesting to the innocuousness of the pasteurization procedure and its effects on protein have, as previously noted, usually been conducted with only one generation of animals. Dr. Pottenger's experiment, which went as far as it could be carried—since in the third generation he encountered reproductive disaster in the cats—appears to be the only such research that has thoroughly investigated the long-term effects of pasteurization of milk and cooking of meat. Reproductive disaster means what it says, but perhaps we should elucidate. There was no fourth generation of Pottenger's cats because the third generation (what there was of it) was such a miserable set of creatures that even copulation, much less reproduction, was out of the question.

Research on cooked meat versus raw meat was part of the Pottenger project, and similar results were obtained. Other experiments indicate that cooked meat and cooked eggs lose their ability to support the protein needs of the organism in an even greater degree than does heated milk, but most of this research has as yet been confined to one generation of animals. However, at this point we might well pause to think about the infant whose first eggs are hard-cooked and whose milk is cooked, not only in pasteurization but in the preparation of the formula.

John Dewey remarked that, thinking being painful, the average person prefers to know rather than to think. And, of course, every American mother "knows" that babies are healthier today, on their twice-cooked formulas, than babies of yesteryear, and they emerge from the uterus in glowing well-being, even though they are produced on a diet of heated protein and overprocessed starches. The mother—and the propagandists who keep her "informed"—ignore the fact that the mortality rate of babies in the first thirty days of life has shown nothing like the improvement in the mortality rate at other periods.[9] Since the newborn is a product of the genetic and the nutritional environment, we may well wonder why the first thirty days of life continue to be precarious in this day since, if heredity is no better, nutrition is, they tell us, remarkably so.

This theme reminds us of the advertising of evaporated milk for babies and of the fact that, some years ago, there was a report that young puppies maintained on evaporated milk tended to develop myocarditis, a form of heart disease. Interestingly, an abstract of the report first came to the senior author's attention via a bulletin published by an evaporated milk producer. The advertising of evaporated milk as a perfect and safe food for babies is largely predicated upon the robust health of small infants maintained on it. However, in nutrition research it is axiomatic that effects of a diet on animals cannot be evaluated by any trial involving only the period of infancy. For instance, short periods of certain dietary deficiencies produce no demonstrable effects until the animal reaches middle age. Then, at man's equivalent of fifty years, many animals develop hypertension. Might not one, with full propriety, ask the evaporated milk manufacturer to display his prize babies after fifty years of growth? And would he do so with the knowledge that, as insurance statistics clearly reveal, 36 per cent of the survivors at age sixty-five would be faced with a degenerative disease, ranging from diabetes to heart trouble, from hardening of the arteries to cancer, ulcer, or arthritis? To this, the manufacturer would naturally reply that the lifetime nutrition is not entirely based on evaporated milk. But this is an interesting

[9] And the United States improvement is far below that reported by many other nations.

rejoinder, for the cooked milk industry attacked the Pottenger experiment on the very grounds that the animals *were* fed milk as a lifetime diet. You really can't win. The heavily vested interests will cheerfully quote experiments that prove or seem to prove their point of view, but experiments that disprove it are ignored, if possible, or are attacked as "unscientific."

Time will tell to what extent the heating of protein may alter its ability to support health, reproductive efficiency, and normal longevity in man. And, if this area demonstrates itself to be another example of the cultural lag in which science marks time while the public and the vested interests catch up with it, you will at least have the consolation of knowing that you and your progeny are the victims not only of the heating of protein but of the reluctance of the public, the professions, and the great food industries to act promptly on the basis of verified information. That is, if you last long enough. Meantime, we recommend that certified raw milk be used by every person who can obtain it, adult as well as child, since it represents the only widely available food in which the "complete" uncooked protein can be obtained. We certainly do not advocate the use of ordinary raw milk, for the dangers in its use were what led to our pasteurization laws. But the average physician, when certified raw milk is proposed, almost always becomes indignant. For one thing, he probably does not hear the word *certified,* and if he did, he might not know what the term means, even though this milk that is produced under the supervision of the medical profession is highly recommended in his own trade journals. But like good news, truth takes a long time to spread. If the milk is not available in your community—in many places it still cannot legally be sold—we urge you to begin agitation for it.

A few pointers about this milk: Its producers claim that no disease has been traced to certified raw milk in a half century has been accepted in advertising in medical journals affiliated with the AMA. Against this record, some 70 per cent of milk-borne epidemics have been traced to pasteurized milk. Certified raw milk is produced by cows that receive *daily* veterinarian inspection. Cows producing ordinary milk may be inspected as infrequently as once every six months. The bacteriological examination of certified raw milk is both for *quantity* and *type* of organism. For pasteurized milk there is only a quantitative count. The policy of the certified raw milk industry is delivery of the product as soon as humanly possible after production. While pasteurized milk is dated on the label in many cities, the date refers only to the time of pasteurization and gives no hint of the real age of the milk. Thus, many a customer, after tasting pasteurized milk and certified raw milk in succession, awakens to the realization that most of his life he has been drinking partially sour milk.

The bacteria count of certified raw milk is actually lower than that of pasteurized milk. This is attributable not only to a natural germicide contained in raw milk but to the exquisite care exercised in the production of the milk. The cows are milked by machine with sterilization preceding its use, each cow is shampooed daily, and the workers themselves are required to undergo frequent medical inspection.

Certified cows are not turned out to pasture, for the variation thus caused in spring and fall milk makes the first laxative and the second constipating. In addition, the dry winter feed fed the average cow may or may not be stored properly. If not, the vitamin A value of the milk will drop in winter. The certified cow is fed a balanced diet all year round, scientifically calculated to support good health in the animal and maximum nutritional values in the milk.

It should be understood that we do not say pasteurized milk is a bad food. We are dealing here with relative differences. If certified raw milk is available in your community, we say it is worth buying. When clams and oysters are available, fresh, from uncontaminated waters, their uncooked protein is worth consuming. Other safe sources of uncooked protein are hard to come by. On the basis of Pottenger's work and other studies, we suggest it is highly probable that two glasses of certified raw milk daily may bring health dividends, not only to this generation, but to those as yet unconceived.

The heating of protein is of course not the only influence on the diet that has as yet received inadequate attention. There are dietary deficiencies not recognized as deficiencies, yet they have demonstrable effect on such organs as the pituitary. These center about the starch-sugar content of the diet. In Chapter 2 we sketched the long history of agriculture and food processing, showing how civilized man who evolved on a diet primarily comprising protein and fat, is today ingesting approximately half his calories in starches and sugars, with some of these carbohydrates deliberately overprocessed in an attempt to make them uninviting to the lower forms of life. Subjected to this type of diet, modern man is indubitably surviving, but surviving is not living healthfully. Ultimately, he will survive, much as bacteria adapt to penicillin or other antibiotics. Challenged with an antibiotic, the bacteria without resistance die. Ultimately, the survivors breed a strain that tolerates the antibiotic. Many generations later, they have learned to *feed* upon it. It is entirely probable, though a vantage point is difficult because of man's infinitely longer lifetime, that man—generic man—will survive his dietetic experiment of 250 centuries, but the process is hard on those who cannot adapt, and we are today no longer dedicated to survival of the fittest—not even the fittest to survive an unfit diet.

The hypotheses discussed here at so technical a level should not prevent the reader from remembering that we are not dealing with the purely theoretical and the abstract. We are presenting possible explanations of the actual responses of human beings to alteration in "average" diet—in the direction of less total carbohydrate, elimination of processed carbohydrate, and consumption of unheated protein. One has to see an asthmatic respond to such improved nutrition, or the response of a rheumatoid arthritic, or the change in personality of a hypoglycemic, or the tightening of loose teeth after only three days of such diet therapy to realize that there is something grossly—qualitatively—wrong with the food pattern of Americans, and something very much more right when these changes are made. We may be wrong in our interpretation of the pathways of action, though it is not likely that we are far from the truth. We are not in error in appraising the responses.

The preceding discussion brings into focus a totally neglected role of nutrition in shaping structure and function of master glands. But the processing of food and the cooking of proteins are not the only influences man has brought to bear upon his endocrine glands.

He struck hard at pituitary-adrenal function when he invented the bottle, as replacement for the breast.

He weakened these glands, which help us to resist stress, by creating a welfare state as free of stress as he could make it.

The superiority of breast feeding nutritionally is discussed elsewhere in this text. Its superiority in creating larger and more efficient pituitary-adrenal glands, better equipped to meet stress, is *not* based on better nutrition. It is an emotional phenomenon, difficult to appraise in the human being, easily assessed in the animal. For it is known that young animals which are petted and fondled by laboratory attendants do develop larger pituitary and adrenal glands than animals which are neglected. Substitute for the breast, a bottle propped up on a diaper, and you have more than a nutritional change!

The growth increment in the glands of the petted animal is a phenomenon running counter to the trend in the domesticated laboratory animal, for the effect of the welfare state of the stress-free laboratory on the rat is in the direction of smaller and less efficient stress-resisting glands. Since man is desperately trying to avoid or at least minimize stress upon himself, and has created a welfare state for that purpose, the parallel between man and the laboratory rat may be significant.

The domesticated animal is free from the stresses of searching for food, shelter, and a mate. He has so been free for many generations. His wild brothers, who refuse to mate with any but their own particular kind, are therefore useful controls. A comparison of the Norway rat in the wild with his domesticated counterpart in the laboratory should give us some idea of the effects of domestication; i.e., the effects of the laboratory welfare state on the animal—and thereby, perhaps, a new perspective on man in his own version of the welfare state.

The tamed laboratory animal is more docile than the Norway rat in the wild. This would seem to be a truism, but it is not—nor is it directly a product of the stress-free laboratory state. It is just that the more ferocious wild animals refuse to mate under laboratory conditions, and thereby a selection is made of the more docile types.

The tamed animal has smaller pituitary and adrenal glands, less able to resist stress. The difference is of great degree: where 1 milligram of a given poison kills the laboratory rat, 1200 milligrams may be required for the lethal dose for the untamed animal. (Speculate here on man: housed in a similar welfare state, seeking freedom from stress from womb to tomb, and exposed to foods seasoned with DDT and Sr^{90}, water spiced with insecticides and detergents, and air laden with tons of carcinogens!)

The domesticated animal has a smaller and presumably less efficient brain. Exposed to artificial stresses calculated to induce animal "neurosis," the tamed rat is much more susceptible than the wild, by a factor of about 9 to 1. It is also more susceptible to convulsions.

The wild animal does not operate under the dominance of the sex glands that is exhibited in the domesticated rat as other glands become smaller and less efficient. (And thereby, one assumes, we will not find in the wild Norway rat any counterpart of man's preoccupation with pornography.)

Finally, we obviously see in the laboratory the survival of many strains and types of animals which could not for an hour survive in the wild—toothless, bald, convulsive, otherwise unfit.

Now take a good look at man in his welfare state. His entire philosophy is based on avoidance of stress. He cushions himself with life and health and accident insurance, with pension plans, with air conditioning and heating systems, with pollen filters and vaccines. He has his unfit and keeps them alive—if only by dependence on the clinic, laboratory, and pharmacy; and lets them reproduce. "Take it easy" is his favorite farewell. Carlyle knew better: he said: "Produce—in God's name, produce!" Nature knows better: the laboratory rat can testify. But man does not muse upon this: he is too busy taking injections of ACTH and cortisone even to speculate on the obvious failure of his own pituitary and adrenal glands to produce enough of the stress-resisting hormones.

Please remember diet freed of processed carbohydrate, or reinforced with added vitamins and minerals, or supplemented with high quality protein has in *three days* tightened loose teeth; helped high blood sugar to fall, and low blood sugar to rise; improved irritated gums; helped to normalize both high and low blood cholesterols; aided oldsters in better toleration for new dentures; begun the process of reversing resorption of jaw bone. The authorities who belittle these responses can very often be shown to have a vested interest in the *status quo*, which in nutrition may be defined as the dietetic anarchy created by an endless tide of overprocessed starch and sugar, heated proteins, artificially saturated fats, and other artifacts of man which masquerade as health-supporting foods, presented under the slogan of: "Get your vitamins and good nutrition in well balanced meals."1

An earthy reminder: before executives of the television industry, Paul Willis, President of the Grocery Manufacturers' Association, pointed out that his organization had been successful in teaching magazines "the interdependence of their editorial and advertising departments." This pressure, he announced triumphantly, had resulted in the publication by these magazines of a long series of articles condemning food faddism. What is food faddism to Mr. Willis? Any credo which does not involve complete endorsement of the many highly processed products made by the companies associated with his organization. And the purpose of the speech? Mr. Willis was explicit. "It is time," he declared, "that you [the television industry] learned the same lesson [the interdependence of your editorial and advertising departments]"!

Has the reader come to realize that with his overprocessed, overheated diet, he has also swallowed a large dose of propaganda?

14. Arthritis: Do you believe what you are told?

Arthritis may not kill you, but it can be so painful and crippling that you will "wish you were dead." This is the grim, pathetic comment of many who are seriously afflicted with one of mankind's most prevalent ailments. Regarding the prevalence of arthritis, we should include *all* vertebrate life, not just man, for the records show that even some dinosaurs—a few that reached old age—were afflicted with the disease. Some of their bones afford definite evidence that before their uneasy lives were completed, they were subjected to the miseries of a progressively crippling disease. And likewise with all the bony inhabitants of this planet we call Earth—a goodly portion of them, that is, that achieve old age. This form of old-age arthritis is termed osteoarthritis, or bone arthritis, and it is claimed that it represents "normal wear and tear" of the bone and joints.

From eight to eleven million citizens of the United States, it is estimated, suffer from one or another form of arthritis, a number vastly greater than those afflicted with the so-called "killers" such as heart disease and cancer.

In spite of the universality of the disease among the animal species, is there any hope that it can be successfully treated or helped or *prevented* by dietary processes of which the dinosaurs and other animals—and until very recently, man—were unaware? The answer is a qualified *yes*. The evidence certainly indicates that diet abetted with the proper supplements may provide distinct help and a degree of possible prevention.

Almost needless to say, you will not receive this answer from official medical circles, and although our facts come from orthodox medical research, it should not be surprising to you at this point in our book that you find striking contradictions between orthodox research on the one hand and official pronouncements on the other.

As you are probably aware, the Arthritis Research Foundation has issued statements to indicate that diet has nothing to do with arthritis.[1] Now, the Arthritis Foundation is an organization, similar to the American Cancer Society, which raises funds and presumably speaks for the medical world on its particular subject. But there is nothing in its pronouncements about diet to indicate that the foundation is voicing bias, rather than facts—nothing to show that many medical specialists in arthritic disorders would flatly disagree, nothing that would lead you to realize that even the *Journal of the American Medical Association* has on occasion carried papers which indicated that the diet is very much a part of the picture in arthritis (bad diet as a predisposing cause and good diet as a necessary component of recovery), nothing to indicate why arthritis alone of the degenerative diseases should be exempt from dietetic influence.

The senior author, in protesting the statements of the Arthritis Foundation, is aware that it may be reacting to the extravagant claims of various food faddists. A typical example of the misinformation against which the foundation may be overreacting is contained in the book called *Arthritis and Common Sense*. Any emerging science seems to attract the self-appointed authority, and nutrition has had its share, but *Arthritis and Common Sense* really abused the opportunity to take advantage of common scientific knowledge when it informed the arthritic public that taking water with meals "makes the joints rusty."

[1] As we go to press, this organization, after many years of "debunking" diet in arthritis, issued a handbook on it.

Life published a review of the book. Exactly why *Life* paid this tribute to the death of common sense, only its editors could reveal. The book also advises the arthritic that citrus fruits create acidity and are therefore harmful for the sufferer. A glance at any standard text on physiology and biochemistry should have let the author know that citrus fruits actually contribute to our alkaline reserves, but he was not a man to let beautiful theories come to disaster on the shoals of fact. Since this book sold nearly a million copies it may be granted that the Arthritis Foundation felt it necessary to counteract its author's attempt to exploit desperation. However, some objections to the foundation's statements are in order:

1. Their effect will delay still longer the acceptance by the public of the realization that poor diet is as bad for an arthritic as it is for anyone else and must therefore worsen the effect of the disease; and that good nutrition, if only by its general contribution to the body's welfare, must be helpful. *All* disease does not originate with poor nutrition, but there is *no* disease that does not ultimately involve nutrition, and arthritis is no exception.

2. The foundation's statements are not calculated to encourage the medical man, treating arthritis, to pay more attention to his patient's diet.

3. The statements completely ignore the fact that poor diet *has* been listed by many authorities as being on occasion a major contribution to arthritis.

There is a fourth aspect of nutrition in arthritis. Where this disease is a stress-caused disorder, poor nutrition becomes an added stress, and it seems to be axiomatic that the body can cope with but one major stress at a time. Second, if the dietary deficiency by evil coincidence should involve those factors which are needed by our stress-resisting glands, the deficiency then becomes an arrow striking a vital target, directly contributing to the worsening of the disease.

The foregoing academic phrases will not come to life until you examine the first few paragraphs of a letter we received from a retired physician, an emeritus professor of cancer research at Columbia University College of Medicine. He heard broadcasts in which we discussed the relationship between certain nutrients and the functioning of the pituitary and adrenal glands—this in the context of the employment of good nutrition in helping to weather stress diseases. The medical man's letter began thus:

> Dear Dr. Fredericks: If I were a religious man, I should say God bless you. Not being religious, I shall merely send my deep thanks —for last night I walked upstairs, using both good legs like an adult. (Prior to this I had dragged one leg and ascended with the other, because my arthritic knee gave me so much pain.)
>
> When I heard your discussion of the support which can be given the adrenal gland by paba, pantothenic acid, etc., I decided that it would be a lot cheaper to manufacture my own cortisone than to buy it at a drug store—not to mention the side reactions which accompany this drug. I decided to change my diet, emphasizing the foods you described as being rich in these factors, rather than using doses of the concentrated vitamins. Their result was my dramatic walk upstairs last night. It took about three months to arrive at my recovery.

The letter is fascinating for many reasons. Certainly the physician was entitled to his caution in using doses of cortisone: the literature is rife with side effects after prolonged dosage of this drug even in the form supposed to present less risk of "side reactions." He was perhaps overcautious in not employing the vitamin concentrates that we recommend, but one cannot quarrel with his response. Actually, as his letter indicated in a subsequent paragraph, he used large quantities of wheat germ to achieve the therapeutic effect.

We queried him and found that he had eaten white flour products all his life. Is it not ironic that a by-product of the processing of his food relieved him of the pain of a degenerative disease?

Before we examine the interrelationship of nutrition with the stress-resisting hormones, and thereby with certain types of arthritis, let us recognize that arthritis is not a single disease, or at least, that it has many faces. An examination of the medical texts will reveal that our rheumatic specialists are struggling with rheumatic arthritis, osteoarthritis, menopausal arthritis, gonorrhoid arthritis, palindromic arthritis, traumatic arthritis, and a host of associated conditions: bursitis, fibrositis, myositis, and so on.

The relationship of nutrition to these disorders has been challenged by other than the Arthritis Foundation, and affirmed by many others. In World War I troops in wet trenches were afflicted with trench fever, which, in retrospect, appears to have been rheumatic. American troops were peculiarly more subject than British. This was ultimately traced to a difference in dietary habits. The British Tommy ate and cursed bully beef, while the Doughboy was plied with doughnuts by the American Red Cross. This hint that a high carbohydrate diet increases susceptibility to rheumatic fever was at least partially confirmed by many other similar observations. For instance, rheumatic fever has been identified with poverty, poverty has been equated with inadequate diet, and starches are always cheaper than protein. A significant observation that confirmed this interrelationship in our mind was that made by a physician who noticed that failure to eat eggs is almost invariably a part of the history of a child with rheumatic fever. Often eggs are too costly for the budget, or allergy, not infrequent in children afflicted with rheumatic fever, forbids them, or the children just don't like eggs.

To test his observations, the physician assembled two groups of children suffering from rheumatic fever. The first, with light cases, were given the orthodox antibiotic treatment. The second, with severe cases, were given two eggs daily or two eggs above their accustomed intake. He reported that in one year the improvement in the severe cases given the eggs was so great—so much greater than the progress in the other group—that the "severe" group had now changed places with the other.[2]

Yet the orthodox treatment of rheumatic fever continues: pri-

[2] The senior author saw this response in a twelve-year-old boy, who recovered so completely that he was, seven years later, drafted by the army.

marily injections of penicillin. From what we know of the disorder, the treatment is obviously symptomatic, and symptomatic
treatment in preference to genuine therapy is certainly not recommended in any medical school curriculum.

If we are all supposed to get osteoarthritis finally, as some medical authorities tell us, are we then to assume that those who do
not develop osteoarthritis in old age are somehow abnormal? Are
we to consider young people with osteoarthritis as having encom-
passed in forty years the "normal wear and tear" of sixty or seventy? It will interest you to know that some specialists in arthritis—Dr. Esther Tuttle for one—do not consider osteoarthritis to
be produced primarily by wear and tear. Dr. Tuttle has labeled
this disease as a pathological process, a metabolic derangement
susceptible to a constructive therapeutic approach that would
capitalize on our modern knowledge of nutritional as well as
glandular and medicinal therapies.

The Nelson Clinic in California has made some interesting comments on the nutritional therapy which they employ in osteoarthritis. Their thinking is analogous to that of Dr. Tuttle. Dr.
Nelson remarked that the deposition of calcium in osteoarthritis
—which he recognizes as being denominated commonly as a wear-
and-tear disease—is actually an attempt of the body to bring
support to areas where calcium deficiency is paving the way for
erosion of bone. Therefore, though it may seem to be paradoxical,
Nelson treats osteoarthritis and its deposition of calcium by the
use of calcium. He regards the problem as being analogous to that
which the orthopedist faces in a person who has a fracture which
is not uniting properly. He uses vitamins and balanced diet and
medication, of course; but the important point is that in a disease
that is commonly dismissed as wear and tear, thereby relegating
the individual to years of unnecessary discomfort, Nelson and Tuttle both approach the patient on the basis that the disorder is a
disturbance of metabolism which can be treated successfully, like
so many others.

Rheumatoid arthritis is considerd by many qualified workers to be a stress disease. Stress is multifaceted. It can be emotional, it can be physical. The physical can range from a chronic infection to surgery, to exposure, to a violently shifting climate. After the loud hosannas that greeted the discovery of cortisone had ceased to echo, the disquieting realization grew that the drug was not a panacea, that its use is accompanied by many dangers, and that cortisone injections tend to discourage the body's normal production of this hormone. Result: those who receive cortisone dosage become more susceptible to subsequent stresses.

The British tossed a monkey wrench into the machinery grinding out cortisone when they discovered [3] that controlled groups treated with aspirin recovered from their arthritis, or at least found increased mobility and relief from pain, quite as quickly and completely as those dosed with the hormone. Moreover, the physician who performed much of the original research with cortisone has stated flatly that he believes the difficulty in rheumatic arthritis is not a continued deficiency in internal production of the hormone, but rather a peculiarity of the constitution of the sufferer, in that he has "tides" of cortisone production, and when the tide is low his disease flares. What a wonderful opportunity to explore the usefulness of the nutritional support of the adrenal gland, which is charged with the responsibility of cortisone production! Moreover, there is evidence to show that this can be done. But is the respectable physician likely to embark on nutritional research when the Arthritis Foundation for years announced that diet has *nothing to do with* arthritis?

It is in a sense unfortunate that a discussion of diet and arthritis cannot confine itself to that narrow area, because we are faced with the need for grappling with the more general concept of diet *vs.* glandular functions. This becomes obvious from what has already been said. Perhaps a clearer view will be more readily obtained if we consider vitamins as hormones originating from outside the body. (We discussed this concept more fully in Chapter 13.) A good deal of evidence exists to justify this view. For instance, let us

[3] As reported to the British Medical Council.

consider a staid and very conservative medical text, *Goodman and Gillman,* which remarks that dietary deficiency may cause underactivity of the pituitary gland. The authors did not proceed to the next logical point: when the pituitary gland is underactive, utilization of food is interfered with, and there now may be poor absorption and utilization of a diet already deficient. The possibility of a degenerative disease orignating in such a process has been confirmed by fifty years of nutritional experiments.

In Chapter 13 we reported that a cortisone-sparing action on the part of para-amino-benzoic acid makes it possible in some cases to reduce the dose of cortisone in the treatment of arthritis. Consider that para-amino-benzoic acid is part of the molecule of folic acid,[4] and that deficiency of folic acid reduces the responsivity of tissues to female hormone. Para-amino-benzoic acid has in fact been used successfully to treat infertility in the female. We cannot here deal with all such interrelationships between dietary factors and human glands, but once the concept has been established that our glands do not manufacture hormones from air and blue sky, but depend on factors from the diet, we then can approach the problem of diet in arthritis with a rationale.

One other concept must be understood before we indicate the use of therapeutic nutrition in arthritis disorders: Arthritis is not a disease of the joints. Yet this widely held misconception has been responsible for behavior reflecting superstition on the part of both professional men and arthritic patients. Many doctors tell patients they are depositing calcium at their joints; therefore, they must stop drinking milk and eating cheese. If they heed this negative advice they will continue to deposit calcium, but they will use calcium withdrawn from their own bones, thus adding porosity of the skeleton to their other conditions. *It is possible to halt calcifying of the joints with treatment aimed not at the joints but at the glands,* and it is possible to mitigate or to reverse collection of fluid at the joints with therapy not directly aimed at those areas.

The last point is easier to illustrate than some others. For in-

[4] Folic acid deficiency has been identified in many rheumatoid arthritics.

stance, when there is pain at the joints, with collection of fluid, the problem may originate with glandular dysfunction, but the target of the dysfunction is the blood vessels. The blood vessel wall must be permeable, for it is by virtue of this phenomenon that the blood in a closed circulatory system can feed the tissues and remove the waste materials. But if the walls become permeable to an abnormal degree, fluid may collect where it should not and in excessive quantities. The nutritional attack on this problem is aimed at the glandular disturbance as the primary goal and at the excessively permeable blood vessels as a secondary goal. You will note that the joints as such are ignored.

These observations are based upon clinical results of therapeutic diet and doses of vitamin and mineral concentrates. Now there are spontaneous recoveries in rheumatoid arthritis, just as there appear to be in other diseases we have discussed, and the skeptic may assume that a period of good nutrition happened to coincide with one of these spontaneous remissions. However, there is too much solid statistical evidence and too many actual case records of sustained benefit to accept the natural remission thesis. In addition, there is a vast correspondence from radio listeners of the senior author, covering almost a quarter of a century. One cannot ignore reports such as that from the retired physician already quoted, or the one-line report by a physician who was forced into retirement by Dupuytren's contracture (the hand permanently contracted like a claw), and who later wrote: "I am playing golf again—bless the vitamin E!"

The factors that specifically stimulate adrenal-pituitary function include: copper, cobalt, manganese, vitamin A, vitamin-B complex, vitamin D, vitamin E, and possibly vitamin C. In the vitamin-B complex, of the many vitamins that comprise it, those with the most specific interrelationship with pituitary-adrenal function are: pantothenic acid,[5] choline, paba, B_{12}, folic acid.

---

[5] Doses of pantothenic acid and "royal jelly" are known to benefit rheumatoid arthritics. Deficiency in vitamin B_{12} and in folic acid is common in this disease.

Unsaturated fats of the type obtained from wheat-germ oil appear also to stimulate pituitary function. Here it will be recalled that vitamin D in large doses was once treatment of arthritis, and with some success. Obviously, this treatment had nothing to do with the function of vitamin D as a preventive for rickets.

Generalizing about diet in arthritis is as difficult as generalizing about diet for healthy people: idiosyncrasy, intolerance, allergy, and constitutional factors enter to make a broad generalization risky. However, it can be said that a high protein, low carbohydrate diet appears to benefit the majority of sufferers. The diet can often be made more effective if it is fed in frequent, small meals, rather than the usual three larger ones. In other words, the dietetic pattern is very much like the one used for gastric ulcer and low blood sugar.

The vitamins and minerals should be supplied in the form of a multiple vitamin concentrate, a multiple mineral concentrate, and a separate source of vitamin E. A vitamin-B complex concentrate supplying a natural source of B vitamins as well as the crystalline factors should also be used. Added quantities of paba, pantothenic acid, vitamin C, and the bio-flavonoids would be needed when the basic supplements previously listed would not be likely to supply therapeutic amounts of these factors. It must be understood that this procedure is not intended as a substitute for needed medication and physiotherapy. The nutritional approach is an adjunct, but itself a helpful one. The physiotherapist likewise borrows from the field of nutrition, for wheat-germ oil ointment has been found very helpful for the fibrositis, muscle spasm, and pain that often are part of the difficulties of the arthritic.

Except for those with gout, the arthritic's diet should stress the usually recommended and nutritious organ meats such as liver, kidney, brain, sweetbreads.

The fact that we have labeled nutritional therapy for arthritis as an *adjunct* treatment should not obscure the compelling fact that nutritional therapy has often effected improvement where the primary treatments of medication and physiotherapy have totally failed.[6] It should be instituted routinely in all forms of arthritis except one, gout. There are misconceptions about this form of the disease at both professional and lay levels. While gout is not an allergic process in the ordinary sense of the term, it does represent an idiosyncrasy of reaction to a component of common foods. Moreover, it must be obvious that not all patients react to the disease or to the foods that aggravate it in the same way or in the same degree. This should preclude the prescription by the physician of any standard "diet for gout," which implies that the disease strikes all patients in the same degree, that all patients have the same effect of the disease processes, and that the dietary requirements of all such patients therefore can be formulated in a broad common denominator. A diet for gout would be about as rational as a standard diet for allergy. But while the field of nutrition does not hold positive therapeutic benefit for the sufferer with gout, the field of negative dietetics can hold harm. Arbitrary restrictions on the food intake, when unnecessary and when not warranted by the individual patient's sensitivity, constitute a pathway to dietary deficiency, which helps nobody. It is true that most patients with gout cannot stand concentrated doses of foods rich in purine such as liver and other organ meats, but some can stand a little of these foods, and they *are* good foods. Some gout patients cannot take vitamin B_1, but many others can.

In the senior author's professional experience, one woman could not partake of one teaspoonful of beef gravy without touching off unbearable pain in her big toe, while many other patients were happily able to eat quarter-pound portions of steak. Frequently, too, the fact is ignored that restrictions on the diet in gout that are necessary at the time of attacks may become unnecessary during periods of quiet. The patient may thus be kept on the severely restricted diet for long periods, or even permanently, without need. Finally, from the nutritionist's point of view it seems that the medical man should persuade his gout patients to realize that

[6] Dr. Tom Spies used hormone or drug therapies for arthritis only when nutritional treatment proved inadequate.

"high living" is not the necessary prerequisite for gout. A medical man is often unaware of the suspicion raised in a spouse's mind by this supposed association.

Climate in arthritis therapy has been grossly misunderstood. While New Yorkers leave for Arizona and Miami in search of climatic relief, one is struck by the Miamians and Arizonians who come to New York for treatment. The role of climate in arthritis needs reappraising in terms of stress. When arthritis has been initiated by stress of whatever nature, great variations in climate become an added stress, and as we have stated, the body seems able to cope with only one major stress at a time. A climate consistently hot or consistently cold seems better borne than a variable climate.

We must refer also to the novocaine treatment for arthritis. This therapy, sometimes referred to as H-3, has been the subject of violent and often ignorant medical attack in the United States. Yet it has produced unequivocal results. How little H-3 is understood by those who attack it most violently is exemplified in the comment of *Time* on the subject. Sarcastically attacking the Rumanian discoverer, Dr. Anna Aslan, who has spent more than a decade in research with this treatment, the magazine remarked that obviously the doctor was claiming for novocaine what it could not have: a vitamin-like action.[7] One medical firebrand arose at a medical convention and denounced Dr. Aslan as a faker on the grounds that her research would promise rejuvenation for anyone who receives an injection of novocaine from a dentist.

The senior author suggested that *Time* consult a reference text to learn the formula of novocaine: It is a compound of a solvent with para-amino-benzoic acid,[8] which has already been designated in this chapter as a vitamin with a profound effect on the internal production of cortisone, a hormone extensively used in the treatment of arthritis. With regard to the dentist's dose of no-

[7] Our knowledge of Dr. Aslan's work is first hand: a medical man, a consultant to our staff, visited her in Rumania, four times.
[8] A vitamin found helpful in fibrositis, arthritis, and scleroderma.

vocaine, we shall note that while the dentist administers only a few drops of the material once or twice, Dr. Aslan gives one sixth of an ounce by deep injection, three times a week for months, years, or even permanently. Further, Dr. Aslan maintains that the type of novocaine employed in H-3 therapy is in an acid medium quite different from that commonly used by dentists. There are many patients who do not efficiently utilize paba when it is given by mouth; for such, the novocaine treatment—which is inexpensive, can be given by any physician, and only rarely has side reactions—appears to be a way of administration in which the vitamin is better utilized. The potassium salt of paba is sometimes successfully administered by mouth.

Incidentally, Dr. Aslan reports therapeutic benefits not only in arthritis, but in so-called senile palsy. An American group, treating individuals with novocaine in a home for the aged, confirmed Dr. Aslan's finding that their resistance to viruses was increased. They also reported that a difficult patient in "second childhood" became more active and socially more cooperative. A patient with multiple sclerosis improved enough so that she was willing for the first time in years to try to help herself.[9]

It is instructive, too, to examine the death rate among the aged under Dr. Aslan's care. In a series of 875 cases treated with novocaine, the death rate over a period of four years was 2.7 per cent. She treated 495 patients of the same age distribution with other medicine over the same period, and found the death rate to be 10.3. The possibility of this difference occurring by chance is one in a thousand.

[9] Apropos of pressure by the authorities, the paper that reported these results wound up by categorically denouncing Aslan's claims for novocaine! The denunciation appeared in the summary, which is read by a far larger number of professionals than is the paper itself; the confirmation of many of Aslan's claims appeared within the paper, read by the minority. Most pertinently, the paper reported a sharp reduction in the death rate among aged people treated with novocaine who were exposed to an influenza epidemic, as compared with the death rate in the control group which did not receive the novocaine treatment. By the longest of possible and astronomical chances, the reduction in the death rate was identical with that reported by Aslan, whose conclusions are violently rejected in the summary of the paper!

We should also mention here a hitherto little-known but promising treatment for most forms of arthritis: bee extract, made from bee venom. For centuries, it has been observed that some beekeepers, stung occasionally, did not develop arthritis, even though living to old age. Some medical researchers, pursuing these empirical findings and meeting with outstanding success, ran into the usual stone-wall resistance from medical authorities who "knew" such an outrageous, barbaric treatment wouldn't work. However, it does work, very likely by inducing the body to produce its own cortisone. There are no side effects from bee extract, and it has now been refined, standardized (in Europe, not the United States), and even been formulated in tablets to be taken by mouth. The junior author has seen scores of undeniable "sustained miracles" on hitherto "hopeless" or far-advanced arthritis sufferers who have undergone treatment with bee extract. In fact, the results achieved are strikingly similar to those reported for H-3. There are undoubtedly other, as yet unknown, reasons for bee venom's remarkable results, and since the effects are sometimes far superior to those achieved by aspirin and cortisone, it seems unlikely that the action is only one of shocking the body into producing its own cortisone.[10]

Of course the nutritional therapy advanced in this chapter should be followed while the arthritic patient is under treatment of *any* sort.

[10] A physician, Dr. Joseph Broadman, called a quack by the Arthritis Foundation for espousing bee venom therapy for arthritis sued—and *won*.

15. Vitamins: You need them, but how many?

As these lines are written, before the senior author rests a printed statement from the American Medical Association. It reads: "Only in a deficiency state or an anticipated deficiency state are vitamin supplements necessary."

Vitamin supplements have been likened to an insurance policy. You may build a "fireproof" house; you still take out fire insurance. Some people would have you build the house, but wait until you anticipate a fire before you call your insurance broker. In the case of fire insurance, such behavior may invite a jail sentence. In diet, such behavior will earn for you second-grade health, the tragedy of a deformed baby, or impaired response to medication.

The outright cruelty of the suggestion that vitamin supplements should be used only in actual deficiency or *anticipated* deficiency marks many routine pronouncements in medical treatment of this area of nutrition. For instance, an article in a reputable medical journal suggests forcefully that the "balanced" pregnancy diet does not require vitamin supplements. Entirely apart from the fact that pregnant women often are not able to eat properly for the first four months, which is the period when the matrices for all the baby's organs are created, there is also the fact that biochemical disturbances are known to occur in all pregnant women, one of which interferes with the utilization of a vitamin (B_6). The article we mention grants that vitamin deficiency can cause the birth of a deformed baby, and concedes that after the birth of a baby with a harelip, cleft palate, club foot, or deformed spine, it would then (in subsequent pregnancies) be advisable for the mother to use vitamin supplements. Obviously, we have entered upon an era of *un*preventive medical nutrition!

The campaign against vitamin supplements is a strange one indeed. The opponents grant that supplements are desirable for the treatment of deficiency or even *anticipated* deficiency, but the important point seems to be that vitamin supplements are wonderful when prescribed by the physician, but useless or even dangerous when purchased in the very same form, over the counter, by the user.[1]

In a word, the campaign against vitamin supplements is pure propaganda. It is part of the same philosophy which in the state of Connecticut motivated the proposal of a law that would make a prescription necessary for the purchase of cough drops, on the grounds that a cough may represent tuberculosis! (Has your physician ever insisted on X-raying you or your child before prescribing a cough syrup?) If one took such statements seriously, it would be necessary to assume that physicians:

1. Are universally competent in nutrition;

2. Subject all patients to diet histories as a part of case histories;

3. Carefully evaluate vitamin-mineral intake (on the basis of diet histories and food assays, which are usually at least 40 per cent erroneous);

4. Have access to and employ competent comprehensive tests for nutritional status (which tests in the main do not exist);

5. Consider vitamins as nutrients with specific functions, none replacing another, in symptoms of deficiency that can and must be carefully distinguished from those arising from other conditions.

Most physicians actually make no distinction between vitamin supplements of one manufacturer and the other, thereby considering the content of the capsule to be immaterial. They consider

---

[1] But quite all right when purchased as a fortified cereal, enriched bread, or restored flour!

vitamins to be placebos, and therefore regard responses to supplements largely as reactions of hypochondriacs and those unusually susceptible to "ceremonial therapy."

The medical propagandists have had a field day with the supposed toxicity of vitamin supplements. Newspaper editors have found the toxicity pronouncements to be fine editorial material, but no newspaper or magazine, to our knowledge, has ever traced the background for these statements. None has ever searched the medical literature to learn that no one has ever been "poisoned" by the use of a vitamin supplement in the dosages recommended on the label. Where, then, do these reports of toxicity originate?

First, from the response of a group of infants to massive overdosage of fish liver oil concentrates. The mothers had been instructed to give the babies 10 or 15 drops a day of these preparations, rich in vitamins A and D. On the philosophy that, a little being good, more is better, these mothers gave the children teaspoonful doses, thus far exceeding the quantity recommended on the labels and the amount prescribed by the physicians. After a number of months of such overdosage, the babies began to show toxic reactions. This constituted no indictment of the vitamins as potential poisons. Anything is toxic at some point. As a matter of fact, there is a case in the Australian medical records of an idiot who succeeded in calcifying his tissues by drinking two gallons of milk a day. Shall we now have screaming headlines to indicate that babies should not be nursed? That adults should not drink two glasses of milk a day?

Second, there were some instances of Vitamin A poisoning in adults who took hundreds of thousands of units, whereas for most persons 25,000 units represents an optimal intake in supplementary form. These cases furnished grist for the AMA's propaganda mill. The average practicing physician was overwhelmed, and we recall one internist who said triumphantly that he had saved a patient from what—by his tone—was a fate worse than death. She had been taking a multiple vitamin capsule supplying 33,000 units of vitamin A in each daily dose! We pointed out that the internist's next meal including spinach, carrots, butter, chopped chicken liver, or broiled beef liver should be preceded by his making out his will. Look up the assays of these foods, and you will discover it is quite possible for the housewife innocently to "poison" her family with preformed vitamin A by serving 85,000 units of the vitamin in a single meal.

A few other cases of vitamin A toxicity were exhibited in patients whose physicians had prescribed hundreds of thousands of units of vitamin A for periods of many months. You may be sure that neither the headlines or the newspaper articles placed the responsibility on the proper shoulders, and that nowhere in any of these articles was there recognition of the fact that such toxicity is transient, the effects not permanent, and the condition completely reversible by a simple reduction of dosage. To this, the technician in the vitamin A field would add another note: vitamins interact, and these reports of toxicity should also be interpreted in terms of the irrational way in which many doctors prescribe vitamin supplements: large doses of one or two vitamins and no others. Actually, effects of huge vitamin A dosage suggest the impact of excessive amounts of fatty substance on the liver in the absence of similar dosage of those vitamins that help both liver function and the utilization of fats. It is quite possible that very large dosage of vitamin A would be better tolerated if the vitamin-B complex were simultaneously given in the same heroic dosage.[2] All the vitamins, minerals, and other known beneficial substances should be taken *together*, almost never alone, since vitamins, minerals, and natural body substances such as amino acids (protein's basic components), lecithin (the fat solvent and the cell guardian), and cholesterol (the fat), constantly act with and against each other every second of our existence. The cell, and therefore the whole body, exists in a continual and continuous state of dynamic equilibrium, and the "normal" equilibrium or "optional" balance is possible only when we have optimal supplies of each needed factor. The cell, itself, if well nourished and provided with proper

[2] There *is* a paper reporting this effect. (*Nature*, 1958, 182, 924.)

means of waste disposal, is potentially immortal, as the late Dr. Alexis Carrel dramatically demonstrated by keeping the tissues of a chicken heart alive for many years. It could easily have been a million or a billion years, had Dr. Carrel had the time. But he proved the point nevertheless.

With this propaganda campaign understood as another of the many attempts to maintain control of the public's efforts to improve its health, let us now consider the need for vitamin supplements and the manner in which they should be used. The regrettable part about the propaganda that has been unleashed is the allegation, explicit and implicit, that we are a well-fed people, that very few of us have any need for vitamin supplements, and that money spent on these preparations is therefore wasted. For remember this: if we accept the vitamin content of foods at the face values given in the food charts, a large segment of the American public is vitamin deficient. The authority for this statement is the United States Department of Agriculture.

But of course we have no scientific right to accept food chart assays of vitamin values. In the senior author's doctorate thesis there is a citation from one of the papers dealing with this elusive quantity: the actual vitamin value of the menus served by the American housewife. Two sets of figures are given: (1) the calculated value of a menu derived from the food charts; (2) the actual value as determined from samples of the foods, taken from the dining table as served. Some of the actual values were determined to be 40 per cent *below* the calculated values. In twenty-five years of analyzing diets the senior author has not seen a half dozen in which a 40 per cent correction factor would not have rendered the diet deficient in many essential vitamins. Moreover, frequently the 40 per cent correction factor served to explain symptoms otherwise inexplicable if the diet's calculated values were accepted.

We discussed these symptoms earlier, but to repeat, they are designated "subclinical" and most doctors do not recognize them as being caused by dietary deficiencies. To name a few: nervousness, irritability, apathy, hypochondriosis, sensitivity to noises, inability to work, fatigue, grinding of the teeth in sleep, lowered resistance to virus infections, undue susceptibility to suggestion, insomnia, crying without provocation.

Now these are actual symptoms, not subclinical as the average doctor has been taught. In many cases, they had been obliterated with institution of a proper diet with adequate vitamin-mineral supplementation. Proof that the nutritional therapy was responsible for the sustained improvement lies in the fact that placebos were methodically given in place of the supplementation (of course without the patients' knowledge); the symptoms returned, only to disappear again when nutritional therapy was resumed. Yet the typical medical therapy today for these "subclinical" symptoms still consists of superficial psychological "counseling," possibly some iron tablets (if anemia[3] is evident), tranquilizers for the nervous symptoms, and sleeping pills for insomnia.

The American Medical Association has long had a split personality on the subject of the vitamin concentrates. Scientifically, it fully recognizes the existence and the prevalence of subclinical deficiency. Officially, in terms of information to the public, it closes its eyes to both—indeed, as we have noted, has released the remarkable statement that vitamin concentrates should be used, even for nontherapeutic purposes, only under the direction of the physician, the pronouncement not explaining what criteria the physician will use to define the patient's need for such augmented intake. Factually, this "scientific" control of vitamin supplementing by the medical man, as the reader well knows, usually takes shape in handing out whatever vitamin samples are handy, with some such remark as, "These can't hurt you, if they don't do you any good."

We prefer the premise of Professor Alonso Taylor of Princeton University who, among others, has said the use of vitamin supplements is a sensible precaution in the absence of definite informa-

[3] It is possible for fatigue to accrue from iron deficiency, with no warning of an anemia displayed in the blood. This may also cause breath-holding in children.

tion concerning the composition of the diet. We know that the 50 per cent of the American diet derived from starches and sugars fails to contribute many of the vitamins and minerals normal to these foods, because more than 90 per cent of them are overprocessed, and what we earnestly call "enrichment" represents only a partial restoration of values that have been removed. And we know that foods are subjected to other influences that deplete vitamin value and sometimes mineral value too. Forces operating in cultivation, fertilization, storage, processing, and cooking can easily make the major contribution to the previously cited 40 per cent difference between the calculated and the chemically determined vitamin value of the diet. Moreover, it should be noted that the United States Department of Agriculture, when it declared a substantial number of Americans to be vitamin deficient, was measuring their diets without the 40 per cent correction factor, and against a set of modest and arbitrary dietary standards.

Here are two observations likely to be useful before we outline the procedure in vitamin supplementation that the senior author, in a quarter of a century of observation, has found to be most effective:

1. The inadequacy of the accepted tests for determining minimum requirements of vitamins is well illustrated by a recent paper on the subject of vitamin C requirements. The paper rejects the basic plateau of minimum excretion as a valid test of requirements for vitamin C, and offers a much more sensitive index: the condition of the experimental animal's jawbone. On the basis of this observation, the paper makes it possible that our human vitamin C requirement, instead of being in the neighborhood of 100 milligrams a day, may mount as high as 2,000 milligrams.

2. Dr. H. C. Sherman long ago learned that a multiple of the minimum daily requirement of calcium and riboflavin serves to lengthen the life span of animals by 10 per cent, and kept them in better health throughout their whole lives.

The intelligent use of vitamin concentrates aims at insurance of an intake high enough to cover all the contingencies of the tremendous variations both in the supply of vitamins from the diet and in the levels of vitamin requirement. They should not be taken in arbitrary handfuls; the supplement should be complete. It should supply not only the known vitamins, which are available in crystalline form, but the *unknowns*.[4] No distinction should be made between synthetic and natural vitamins, because no such distinction exists. Some quarters of the health food industry persuade the public into the belief that the natural vitamin is in some esoteric way superior to the synthetic. To do so, they capitalize by exaggeration on a germ of truth. While there is no distinction between any natural individual vitamin and its synthetic counterpart, foods do contain vitamins not yet identified, for which, of course, there are no synthetic counterparts. But it is deception to tell the public that rose hips yield a more effective kind of vitamin C than do the tablets. The greater effectiveness of the vitamin C in rose hips is based on the simultaneous presence of the bio-flavonoids, but these are also available in concentrated form, accompanying synthetic vitamin C.

The supplementing procedure, therefore, begins with a good multiple vitamin capsule. While such a capsule may contain a natural source of the unknown B complex vitamins, it is obvious that sheer lack of space will keep the manufacturer from providing any significant amount of the natural source. The concentrated alfalfa, yeast, wheat germ, rice polishings, or liver in an "all-purpose" capsule is thus more likely to make the label look impressive than make any real contribution to the usefulness of the supplement. A truly effective all-purpose vitamin-mineral-supplement capsule would have to be about the size of a golf ball.

It is intelligent, therefore, to add to the usual multiple vitamin supplement a separate vitamin-B complex concentrate; and this, preferably, should be in the form of a liquid. Not only does the liquid permit the incorporation of significant amounts of the natural B complex source in the daily dose; but it also allows incor-

4 See appendix for detailed review of vitamin sources and actions.

poration of significant amounts of certain vitamins for which the requirement is very large. Here, for instance, we are attempting to guide the reader away from use solely of multiple vitamin or B complex capsules, which offer not only inadequate amounts of liver or yeast, but as little as 25 milligrams of choline. How irrational such a formula is will be realized when the supply of choline in a good diet is stated. At minimum, it appears to be over 2,000 milligrams a day. Again, the manufacturer creates an impressive label by including "lip service" amounts of yeast, liver, choline, inositol, etc. The value of such a supplement as dietary insurance is obviously negligible. However, in a B complex liquid it is possible, even in a teaspoonful, to incorporate genuinely useful amounts of the desired natural B complex unknown factors. Certainly it makes more sense to use such a liquid as an adjunct to the multiple vitamin capsule, and obtain a significant protective intake of, let us say, choline, than to wait twenty years for hardening of the arteries and coronary thrombosis, hoping to survive long enough to be able to take heroic doses of the vitamin in an effort to prolong life. (It has been used successfully for this purpose.)

A supplement of minerals should accompany the multiple supplement and the vitamin-B complex concentrate. The need for the added supplement is based on the fact that factors which lower vitamin content, reduce mineral value as well; for example, the processing that removes the vitamin-B complex from white flour also removes an equivalent percentage of the mineral values. There is also a complicated web of interrelations between minerals and vitamins. It has been said that the vitamins are useless without minerals, and any biochemist would agree that the converse is also true.

The authorities are divided on the effect of poor fertilization on the mineral content of foods, many of them maintaining that soil poor in mineral value will produce good food but less of it. The process seems a little obscure by which a plant is able to pick up from the soil the minerals essential to a human being, merely because there are fewer plants competing for the inadequate quantity present in poor soil.[5] Interestingly, authorities of equal standing deny the validity of this thesis and insist that poor fertilization and poor soil give us poor food. It *has* been demonstrated that the vitamin content of food is more affected by the nature of the seed and the climate than by the composition of the soil; but it has also been shown that the percentage and the efficiency of the protein in a food crop rests upon the quality of the soil and the techniques of fertilization. However, let us be reminded here that when the knowledgeable physician desires to capitalize upon the usefulness of copper in helping the body to utilize iron, he does not rely upon the indefinite amount of copper in food, but prescribes a copper and iron compound, so that the two minerals may be simultaneously available in the digestive tract. The interplay between vitamins and minerals being what it is, we prefer to have them simultaneously available, with the comforting thought that the well-formulated mineral supplement that makes this possible is inexpensive, nontoxic, and may also serve to protect us against deficiency. If, after all, there is no need for such a supplement, we have wasted only pennies. If there is a need, we have protected ourselves and made our vitamin supplements more effective.

Many of the arguments that adduce a plenitude of minerals in our diets are specious, anyway. The argument goes that even if poor soil does produce poor food, we are protected by the fact that our foods are derived from many different soils. One has only to look at iodized salt to realize that this is a beautiful theory confronted by an ugly fact: the iodine deficiencies that have caused endemic goiter in adolescent school girls were not corrected by iodine supplies in foods coming from areas outside the so-called goiter belts.

We now have the basic supplements: a multiple vitamin capsule, a vitamin-B complex supplement in liquid form supplying

[5] Any farmer knows that the root system of a plant in poor soil is *stunted*, not enlarged.

substantial amounts of a natural source of this group of vitamins, and a multiple-mineral supplement. Let us now turn to cost. There is no need to pay $20.00 a month for products meeting these specifications. All three supplements, properly formulated, can be purchased for not more than $3.00 for a month's supply. Unbelievably, there are companies grossing $30 million a year by selling their products at the ridiculously high price level, justifying the exorbitant cost to the consumer on the basis of a content in the capsule of concentrated alfalfa or other vegetables. Were such alfalfa concentrates the El Dorado of nutritional goodness, the amount offered in such supplements (which are usually in capsule form) could not possibly justify either the extravagant claims or the extravagant price.

The special-purpose foods that are extraordinarily rich in B complex and other values should be used, too. These include liver, wheat germ, rice polishings, brewer's yeast, and dry nonfat milk. Each of these foods makes a contribution to the diet that is helpful, and they are not mutually exclusive. The user must be resolute, because in taking these vitamins and eating these foods, he will doubtless find himself called a food faddist. The term means whatever the user chooses to make it mean. The situation is reminiscent of the belligerent Irishman who was called "laconic." He punched his critic in the nose; he didn't know what "laconic" meant, but he was taking no chances. To a medical propagandist the user of a special purpose food such as wheat germ is a food faddist.[6]

The senior author's cookbook and that of Adele Davis are two of a number in which detailed instruction for the use of special-purpose foods will be found. We will note here that the housewife will vastly benefit the health of her family if she purchases vacuum-packed wheat germ (it is subject to dangerous rancidity unless shielded from air) and serves it as a cereal to her family. She can also add it to the nondescript average cereals, to convert them into better food. She can add a teaspoon or a teaspoon and a half

6 Babies are faddists—there is wheat germ in pablum.

of wheat germ to each cup of flour used in baking and other recipes. What will she accomplish with this addition? In one study,
the growth in weight and height of schoolchildren, as well as their
general health records, improved significantly when the bread and
rolls in their diet were improved with the addition of 2 per cent of
wheat germ. The control group, on the same diet without the
added wheat germ, did not so improve.[7]

Brewer's yeast is available in many forms, and can be taken in
tablets or added to food. There is a variety that tastes like cheese
in flake form; another variety has been smoked over hickory, and
has thereby a pleasing bacon flavor that is palatable in appropriate recipes. Four ounces of brewer's yeast daily and up to eight
ounces of wheat germ daily have been used by Dr. Tom Spies in
the treatment of deficiency disease in human beings.[8] The upward limit on the intake of these factors as special-purpose foods
for the average person would therefore be consideration of calorie
value or possible intolerance, meaning excessive laxative action or
the like, which to some readers would be welcome. On the other
hand, the public is daily buying enormous quantities of noxious
drugs for laxative purposes, so this action of these rich sources of
the vitamin-B complex may be highly useful.

The wheat germ, like the brewer's yeast and rice polishings and
liver, is rich in vitamin E and vitamin-B complex, richer than any
other cereal food; and low in calorie value when it is considered
that 150 calories from wheat germ, in round numbers, supplies
much of the vitamin value of a loaf of bread, with its 1200 calories. Which food is better suited to the needs of a public that is
experimenting with the new liquid reducing "foods"? And why
has the bread industry been so remarkably deaf to the plea that
they refrain from removing the wheat germ from their product or
take steps to restore it?

Wheat germ is also our richest source of vitamin E, which other

---

[7] This was reported by Dr. Agnes Faye Morgan, a quarter of a century ago.
[8] Two tablespoonfuls of each daily are a fine, effective, inexpensive supplement.

special-purpose foods do not supply in significant amounts. It has been reported that this and other vitamin values of wheat germ help to protect the user against certain diseases of the heart and the blood vessels, a topic discussed in Chapter 4.

Supplementary intake of liver yields many benefits, the sources of which are not yet clearly understood. There is an antifatigue factor in liver of remarkable efficiency; a factor that helps protect the woman against excessive activity of the female hormone. All the known B complex factors are in liver, and probably all the unknown factors, too.

However, the liver concentrates on the market, usually sold in capsule form, are often fractionated, heated, and frequently over-processed. The fractionation represents a selective concentration of certain liver factors for the benefit of those with pernicious anemia and other anemias. The excessive processing involves drying at temperatures of 180 degrees or even more. This can result in the destruction of unknown factors and the denaturing of the protein. Unfortunately, it is necessary to remove the fat from liver concentrates, for otherwise it would cause rancidity, but the negative effects of fractionation and the excessive heating can be avoided by the use of "40-degree" liver. This, as the name implies, is dried under vacuum, where the drying temperature can be held low. The product represents all the nutritional benefits of defatted liver. One or two tablespoons of this material daily is an extremely beneficial supplement for all age groups, particularly for older people.

We now have the basic trio of supplements, with the addition of added amounts of natural B complex vitamins, vitamin E, and liver supplements from the special-purpose foods. What gaps have we not covered in this form of dietary insurance? Only the possibility that for *therapeutic* purposes, or to meet uniquely large vitamin needs, we may have to raise the intake of individual vitamins. Thus, a man with a history of allergy or regional ileitis might require amounts of pantothenic acid larger than this program would normally supply. A man with a constitutional tendency to coronary thrombosis, with a history of an attack, or with a familial tendency toward it, might well profit by more vitamin E than these supplements and special-purpose foods will supply. A woman with a tendency toward premenstrual disturbances or cystic mastitis might well profit by larger intake of vitamin-B complex, and if her bent is toward varicose veins or spontaneous abortion, by a rise in the intake of wheat germ, wheat-germ oil, vitamin C, and the bio-flavonoids in addition. This is the point, however, for a consultation with a competent medical nutritionist, for here we leave the areas of insurance of the diet and enter the area of self-medication.

Even so, let us take a moment to study the concept of nutrition as a therapeutic agent. First of all, on the authority of Dr. Tom Spies, whose work we have already mentioned, there is *no* disease, of whatever origin, that does not ultimately involve nutrition. Even the process of repair of tissues and bone after, say, an automobile accident involves the chemistry of nutrition. Reading the conventional statements that high vitamin dosage, except possibly in such conditions as beriberi and scurvy, is useless at best and toxic at worst, the average person will probably be unaware that many physicians treat patients with therapeutic doses of vitamins for disorders not caused by bad diet or deficiency. For example, a New York physician, Dr. Lobell, published a paper on the improvement in his patients following injections of large amounts of vitamin A in the treatment of otosclerosis. A bone disorder, otosclerosis is certainly not caused by vitamin A deficiency, and yet the condition is reported improved by massive doses of the vitamin. Moreover, lower dosages are ineffective. Why should this be? The medical propagandists responsible for the antivitamin campaign might well be reminded of the law of mass action, which one ordinarily learns in a high school chemistry course. Translated into terms of high vitamin dosage, it means that the ability of the body to profit by the content of vitamins in the blood is directly proportionate to the amount of vitamins present in the blood. The higher the concentration of a solution of a chemical on one side of a membrane, the quicker and more efficient the transfer through the membrane to the liquid on the other side. Substitute blood for liquid, blood vessel walls for membrane, and tissues for the second liquid, and you will have the picture.

A second phenomenon leads us to expect a new order of reactions in the human body from large doses of vitamins. This involves a point we mentioned earlier, that in very high concentrates certain nutrients act like medicines, and the actions will be completely apart from the way in which they function as vitamins. Thus, large doses of vitamin C—1000 milligrams a day or more—have a definite antihistamine effect.[9] This can be demonstrated in a test tube; histamine and vitamin C destroy each other. Interestingly, an allergic person may exhibit low vitamin C blood levels even when the diet is rich in the vitamin. This simply means the person is producing enough histamine to destroy a significant amount of vitamin C. It also means that if the vitamin C levels are raised high enough, the destruction may go in the other direction. For some persons this reaction is enough to spell relief from hay fever and certain other allergies.

But under this phenomenon there is another. Vitamin C is used by the adrenal gland, the tissue of which is richer in this vitamin than any other organ of the body. When the body is under stress, and the adrenal gland begins to manufacture its antistress hormones, the adrenal supply of vitamin C is depleted with unbelievable rapidity. Since it is believed that good adrenal function will protect against allergy, it is possible that the high dosage of vitamin C is not only destroying histamine but helping to support the one gland that secretes the most powerful antiallergy hormones known, the cortisone group.

Some physicians give their patients with facial neuralgia an injection of 1000 micrograms of vitamin B$_{12}$, which may bring relief from the terrible pain of affliction. Why 1000 micrograms, when the normal human requirement is estimated to be seven micrograms a day? Simply because the medical man has learned by

[9] Reported by Harry Holmes, a chemist, about 25 years ago.

experience that lesser amounts do not yield results. Another example of the law of mass action at work—and another proof of the point that vitamins can be used therapeutically.

Another example of nutrition becoming therapeutic in diseases not caused by poor nutrition or deficiency appears in the treatment of such a disorder as a stomach ulcer. Here, doses of calcium pantothenate will sometimes interrupt what has been an apparently deadly sequence of ulcer attacks. Why? Because the calcium pantothenate blocks the action of cortisone on the target organ. A person with ulcers may have a personality structure that reacts badly to stress. Under stress, he releases large amounts of cortisone. Since cortisone tablets must be given cautiously to avoid creating an ulcer of the stomach, we can understand that self-produced cortisone may also produce ulceration. If the calcium pantothenate intervenes to shield the stomach from the attack of the hormone, it is obviously performing a prophylactic service in a disease that is distinctly not caused by nutritional deficiency or, for that matter, deficiency in calcium pantothenate. One might theorize that here is a person with a level of cortisone activity and a type of reactive stomach for whom the ordinarily satisfactory intake of pantothenic acid is inadequate. This, however, is still a matter for speculation. While the fact remains that vitamins can be used profitably to treat diseases other than the deficiency diseases.

THE UNCOMMON COLD

Since the "last frontiers" are likely to be internal to man, it is possible that our first Moon expedition will infect the ancient satellite with the organisms associated with the common cold. But though one would never guess it from the platitudes of the authorities, there *are* effective preventives and treatments for several types of the disorder. But first we must define a cold, for there seems to be a whole group of discomforts summed up under the generic term, and a whole host of organisms, viral and bacterial, that initiate, follow, or aggravate the cold.

In the climate of negation surrounding vitamins, let it be remembered that administration of so simple a vitamin supplement as cod-liver oil has been known to cut the incidence, severity, and duration of colds. Eastman Kodak established that with their employees back in the early 1930s; the senior author established it with a group of truck drivers (nearly a thousand) for a commercial bakery, using the modern multiple vitamin supplement. Such experiments have been duplicated and reported by dozens of investigators.

Yet if a physician writes to the *Journal of the American Medical Association,* requesting comment on vitamin prophylaxis or therapy in colds, he will be told: (*a*) the public doesn't need supplements; and, the obvious corollary, (*b*) supplements have no influence on resistance to or recovery from colds. Indeed, the AMA also takes a dim view of cold vaccines, and flatly declares that no cure for the common cold is known. Both statements, as the reader will learn, are value judgments masquerading as fact, and, indeed, both are contradicted by the literature as well as by the experience of millions of Americans who have fewer colds, thanks to the allergist's use of autogenous vaccines; the nutritionist's knowledge of the cold-breaking properties of vitamin A and vitamin C; and the psychologist's realization that the nose is a sensitive barometer of emotional pressures.

Let us begin by observing that the nose is a sex organ. Women recognize this—physiologically, with nose-bleeds which seem to substitute occasionally for the menstrual—and psychologically, when they fan the male biological urge with perfume. Less apparent to many sufferers with colds is the fact that this disorder is sometimes an expression of frustration; of a strong sex drive which has been throttled; of anger which can not be released; of hostility better not otherwise expressed. The reader will undoubtedly recognize the process in some of his friends, but not in himself—salt water being the last thing a deep-sea fish is likely to discover.

The process may result in sinus trouble and postnasal drip. Indeed, on occasion of a psychological catharsis—perhaps on the analyst's couch—the patient often experiences unaccustomed free breathing. To use the mixed metaphor of the chapter, the nose is sometimes the Achilles heel, where in the next individual the same dynamics of personality will yield a stomach ulcer, colitis, or cardiac fluttering.

Hives, eczema, and asthma need not be the response to ingestion of something to which you are allergic. A cold may be the only result. That is why the allergist eyes suspiciously the boast that aside from a half dozen colds a year, the person has no ailments. Such a history, or one of sinusitis and postnasal drip, may be the sole symptoms of allergy to food, bacteria, or dust.

Allergies to dust and bacteria are frequent contributors to colds. Even colds which are not initiated allergically reflect, in inflammation of the tissue and increased permeability and fragility of blood vessels,[10] an allergic reaction to the foreign protein of the organisms involved. These facts explain the helpfulness of antihistamine drugs in colds, even in those not directly of allergic origin. They also explain the action of vitamin C in aborting some colds, and minimizing others—of which, more later.

So it is that hives, eczema, and asthma may not be the response to ingestion of an allergen: the common cold may be the only symptom. That is why the allergist eyes suspiciously the person who says he has no troubles, no allergies—just six heavy colds a year. (Sinus trouble and postnasal drip may also result from allergies; polyps, too.)

The unfortunate who is allergic to dust and bacteria, two common allergens, makes tissue manufacturers rich. The dust inflames the tissues; the cilia which keep cleansing mucus in motion will bog down in swollen tissues, and conditions are propitious then for bacteria to breed. At this point, allergy to bacteria is piled on allergy to dust. Since dust and bacteria are ubiquitous, the

[10] This explains the benefits of the bio-flavanoids in some colds and virus infections.

sufferer says that he alternates between sinus troubles and postnasal drip, with intervening "colds." Remedies here are long range, but logical. Removal of dust from the environment (See Air Pollution, Chapter 19), hyposensitization against unavoidable dust, by repeated injections in gradually rising concentration, and immunization against bacteria with an autogenous vaccine, made from the sufferer's "favorite" bacteria, preferably harvested at the peak of a "cold." Such a vaccine is in distinction to the stock vaccines available commercially, which may not supply the particular organisms to which the sufferer is exquisitely sensitive. The whole process in no way differs from the technique of vaccination, even though, apropos of veils of silence, immunologists use a vocabulary different from allergists', do not meet together, and yet deal with the same phenomena, in the context of the same philosophy!

Two types of colds can be aborted or mitigated with simple vitamin therapy. Vitamin A is effective for one type; vitamin C for the other—and never the twain meet, meaning that the simultaneous use of the two vitamins in the requisite high dosage is not only ineffective, but may prolong the cold. This is to say that a vitamin A responder gains no benefit from vitamin C; and the sufferer with a vitamin C-responsive cold profits not by vitamin A. There is no way to discern which type of cold one commonly gets, but logic dictates that vitamin A be tried first, for if it is ineffective, failure is the only penalty. If vitamin C is not effective, it may move the cold from the head to the chest.

Dosages used are high, for we are not dealing here with a vitamin effect, such as prophylactic use of vitamin supplements would entail, but a medicinal action. C. Ward Crampton found several hundred thousand units of vitamin A, in one dose, repeated for three or four days, to be quite effective. (His paper was published by a society affiliated with the AMA, which still says there is no evidence, etc.!) The work of Harry Holmes and H. Curtis Woods led to the use of two or three grams (2,000 to 3,000 milligrams) of vitamin C daily, for a similar period, for the other type of cold.

Optimally, if the dose is taken at the first sign of a cold, all symptoms will disappear in less than 24 hours. If one becomes reckless in expending energy, though, the cold may reappear—and the magic of the vitamin will not repeat the performance.

"The first sign of a cold" is a phrase which brings us back to individual differences. Some persons betray a coming cold by depression, some by vivaciousness. Some have tenderness of the scalp, others indigestion, or dimness of eyesight, or constipation. It *is* important to know thyself, and recognize your first symptom as early as possible, if the vitamin therapy is to be effective.

VITAMINS—NO SUBSTITUTE FOR PROPER NUTRITION

It must be remembered that as a fire insurance policy is not a license for sloppy construction, so the supplements and special-purpose foods are not permits for dietary indiscretion. One cannot adopt the attitude, with the use of these protective factors, that it doesn't matter now what one eats. The first objective is the achievement of well-balanced diet within one's caloric limitations. The supplements and special-purpose foods now raise the intake of the protective factors, both guarding against deficiency and tending toward the optimal without the penalties of overeating.

We can now deal with the logical question: why bother? The senior author's reply is based on a quarter of a century of observation of the responses of hundreds of thousands of average Americans of all ages and of both sexes to this plan of improved nutrition. There is heightened resistance to infection, minor and major. There are fewer colds and sore throats, and those which do occur are shorter in frequency, duration, and intensity. There is heightened response to medication when ill. There is attenuation of the aging process—there is even recoloring of grey hair, in some individuals. The complexion improves, and, sometimes, visual acuity too. Blood cholesterol is better controlled; fats are better utilized; digestion and elimination are generally bettered. The hair benefits by improved sheen and texture, and, sometimes, growth. Nails are healthier. The tendency toward tooth decay is reduced quite as much as has ever been claimed for fluoridation, if the program is accompanied by reduction of sugar intake. Adverse reactions to potent and toxic medication, such as antibiotics, are mitigated. Sleep is improved; energy reserves are increased; zest for living— perhaps imperceptibly lost—is perceptibly regained. Muscle tone is bettered, and enjoyment of eating restored. Freedom from irritability is perhaps the most frequent by-product of improved nutrition.

While every statement made in this chapter is truth, the pity of it is that not one word concerning these benefits can legally be passed on to you by a vitamin manufacturer. Any such statements would constitute false and misleading advertising in the eyes of the Food and Drug Administration. How arbitrary this attitude is may be judged by the experience of one vitamin manufacturer. He reprinted as an advertising booklet a pamphlet on vitamins issued by a local board of health. The board promptly seized the booklet as "false and misleading advertising."

If you decide to take the plunge for your family, remember that the benefits will first appear in your children, who will flower as only children can. Responses in adults take longer. Not only is higher intake needed to overcome the long-term effects of a lifetime of improper or suboptimal nutrition, but time is of the essence. For some adults, this sometimes spells years of slow progress—so slow that a long-term perspective is sometimes needed before you can realize how far down you were and to what extent you have improved. Let neither the slow progress nor the derision and social pressures of the community deter you. It is not fashionable to eat intelligently, but it *is* rewarding.

16. Does your child eat correctly?

As you sow, so shall you reap. An obstetrician once confessed to his patient that he was somewhat startled that she realized that breast feeding a baby constituted ideal nutrition. She responded sagely with, "I know it is the latest thing, but—" Consider what has happened in a country where a highly mammalian blonde, Miss Lead Pipe of 1965, is the jacket decoration for a textbook on plumbing. The female breast has become the target of a huge brassière industry: a sales bonanza for popular magazines, an incitement in the male to the biological urge with a thin veneer of sentimentality, and far down the line, the source of "the latest thing" for feeding babies.

But a long time ago, Oliver Wendell Holmes observed that all the cunning of the chemists had not yet devised a food as satisfactory for babies as the product of the female breast. Certainly, the libraries are groaning with research that demonstrates this, and it ought briefly to be reviewed here. Groups of thousands of babies, breastfed and formula-fed, have been observed all the way through the tenth year of life. Children fed the natural way have had a more satisfactory health record, through the entire period.

An even more striking comparison of the natural and the artificial way of feeding babies is demonstrated in the difficulties encountered when the initial research to fix the vitamin D requirement of babies was performed. It turned out that the dose of vitamin D that had been calculated on the basis of animal research to be sufficient to protect babies against rickets was not enough. It seems that there was a variable that had not been controlled; the babies, obviously, were being fed cow's milk fortified with vitamin D, whereas the animals were being breastfed, and receiving their vitamin D in another vehicle. Why should a breastfed animal (or baby) have more resistance to rickets, and require less vitamin D than a bottle-fed animal or baby, body weight for body weight? As we noted in Chapter 14, the researchers found that there is an enzyme (phosphatase) in breast milk that lowers vitamin D requirement. The animals obtained this; the babies did not, for the enzyme is destroyed in pasteurization.

The mother who wishes to nurse her baby is often discouraged by her friends as well as her pediatrician. Her obstetrician may not be enthusiastic, and if her initial milk production is not adequate, supplementary bottles are promptly given to the baby, thereby depriving the mother of the only real stimulant to milk production, which is nursing itself. The hospital sometimes actually resents the procedure, because the baby must be brought to the mother "off schedule" and the conveyor belt line procedure in the nursery is interrupted. The indoctrination of the professional against breast feeding has reached the point where the mother must fight off doses of the antilactation hormone medications, because they are offered to her on the automatic assumption that she will not wish to nurse. The husband deplores the "inconvenience" of breast feeding, particularly because he has not yet had the experience of stirring the formula at 3:00 in the morning. Also, his concept of the function of the breast lies so largely in the esthetic rather than the nutritional that he prefers to sacrifice the baby's welfare rather than "jeopardize" the mother's figure. Since breast feeding is a process intimately and miraculously affected by the emotions, it is scarcely surprising that this unending barrage of cynicism and discouragement makes a woman who is able to maintain milk production a stout soul indeed.

Pasteurization of milk destroys an important enzyme (as well as other significant factors) and the milk is cooked twice—once in pasteurization, and once again when the formula is prepared. What is the nutritional impact of the addition to the formula of carbohydrates such as dextrose, in a vitamin-free form in which they do not appear in nature? You should appreciate the reasoning that underlies these concoctions. Cow's milk contains too much protein and fat for a baby. Water dilutes these values, but it also dilutes the carbohydrates, which should be restored. The recipe now takes shape as cow's milk—overcooked, twice cooked, diluted with water, and then treated to be a "duplicate" of mother's milk by addition of a type of carbohydrate completely free of body-building substances. The pharmaceutical industry that produces such formulas in dried form (on the assumption that the mal-nourished mother will not have strength enough to concoct them) gave mothers and pediatricians a lesson in the hard way to indi-cate that this procedure certainly does not yield a fluid equivalent nutritionally to mother's milk. A few years ago, for example, in one issue of a medical journal, there appeared both an advertise-ment eulogizing a proprietary dried formula as "close to human breast milk," and a paper on convulsion in newborn babies—sometimes lethal—caused by a deficiency of vitamin B_6, induced by the very same prepared formula being eulogized in the adver-tising section. Mother's milk happens to be a good source of avail-able vitamin B_6, which, incidentally, is largely removed from white flour and not restored in enrichment. This becomes more perti-nent in the choice of crackers, cookies, and bread, as the baby grows.

Some years ago, a pediatrician rose at a medical meeting where the senior author had delivered this kind of critique on infant feeding, and indignantly remarked: "In 1913, I was a pediatrician at a baby clinic in New York City on the lower East Side, where the women were too poor to buy decent food for themselves, and we doctors used to give them money as well as free pediatric care. Their babies were raised on formulas and they were fat, sassy, healthy babies." The senior author replied: "That was more than forty years ago. Where are those babies now? How many of them are left? For what diseases are the surviving now being treated? Are you satisfied with the knowledge that 36 per cent of those babies are among those who survived to the age of fifty-five and now have arthritis, pernicious anemia, diabetes, arteriosclerosis, heart disease, and a sprinkling of multiple sclerosis, epilepsy, myasthenia gravis, and Parkinson's disease?" In other words, how do you judge the infant's diet if not in terms of the entire life history?

Do you suppose that the pediatrician in question would have permitted a radical alteration in the pediatric diets on the basis of animal experiments in which the subjects were observed for the human equivalent of only a few weeks?

Some pediatricians are aware of the mischief that the addition of processed carbohydrates to formulas can perform. They realize that some cases of colic and other digestive disturbances in babies can be attributed to the added carbohydrate in the form in which it is used. For this reason, there are pediatricians who, when possible, will add to a formula nothing but water and a little honey. However, discussion of these techniques for laymen is academic, since the pediatrician controls the infant's diet. Although he may outrage the dentists by passing out lollipops, and the nutritionist by discouraging breast feeding, the pediatrician still dictates the infant's diet and must accept the responsibility for the outcome. Nonetheless, the intelligent mother can do a great deal to give her baby the best possible nutritional start. For instance, she can refrain from trying to outdo the commercial baby food manufacturers, by going to the time and needless trouble of preparing "fresh" vegetables and fruits at home. This is unwarranted for some very good reasons:

1. The "fresh" vegetables and fruits may not be really fresh. However, the baby food processor, for purely economic if for no other reasons, will locate his processing plant adjacent to the sources of the food.

2. The fresh foods may be contaminated with excessive amounts

of insecticide.[1] The reputable baby food manufacturer, out of a sense of conscience or the probability that his product will be government inspected, rejects crops that are too heavily contaminated.

3. The cooking methods used by the reputable manufacturer are designed to protect vitamin and mineral values as much as possible. The housewife cannot easily exert such protection.

Many of the prepared baby foods are heavily laden with sugar. While the young baby has no teeth to be attacked, it must be remembered that sugar raises the vitamin requirement without satisfying any of it. Moreover, the sensitive taste buds of the baby do not need very much sweetening to satisfy them, and there appears to be no point in encouraging a child's appetite for sweets in these formative months.

The baby cereals and some of the baby foods contain wheat germ, and in fact did contain it years before the public knew of its existence or considered its use to be the mark of the food faddist. Extra wheat germ, in small amounts, can profitably be added to a baby's food. Thus, when an emasculated cereal such as farina is given to an infant, its body-building values can be brought to respectable level by the addition even of a fraction of a teaspoonful of wheat germ. To avoid mechanical irritation for the baby, whose digestive tract is still tender even at the age when solid foods are being fed, a rolling pin can be used to pulverize the wheat germ before it is added to the cereal.

Referring to the "age" for solid foods, mothers compete with each other, striving to bring their infants to the solid food stage earlier. Babies are individuals, and mature at different rates. This competition, which sometimes drives pediatricians into feeding solid foods earlier than they really wish to, should be stopped. If solid food feeding is instituted too soon, it is inflicted on a digestive tract that has not yet learned to be selective in what it transmits to the body, and this can be a pathway to the start of allergies. On the other hand, the baby who is ready for solid food profits by

[1] Less than 1 per cent of our fresh produce is inspected for insecticide residues.

certain additions to the diet that are often unnecessarily delayed. The addition of strained meat to formulas has produced more contented babies with better growth and with more resistance to infection. The addition of brewer's yeast to the infant's diet has been practiced profitably even for premature babies.

Since sugar raises the vitamin requirement of babies (as well as adults), we now bring up the question of vitamin supplements. There are pediatricians who prescribe only supplementary vitamins A and D. There are those who go beyond this, with prescription of a multiple vitamin preparation in drop form. Supplements of both types are inadequate. Vitamins should always be used together, and this would include not only the noncrystalline vitamins, but the unknowns of the vitamin-B complex. Likewise, vitamins without minerals are not fully efficient. There is also the question of making the supplement complete enough so that the mother does not feel the need, arising out of anxiety, to exert coercion at the table. When the child reaches the age where he has become convinced that the pantry is adequate and the mother's intentions good, he is likely to try the experiment of refusing food. This is very gratifying (to the child), turns the faces of adults purple, induces father to do calisthenics to entertain the rebellious noneater, and brings with it the reward of TV or storytelling as part of the dinner menu. Our prime problem in such cases is to persuade the mother into performing two sensible actions:

1. When the child is old enough to rebel, he is old enough to be left alone with his meal; and, when he finds that refusal to eat earns no attention, the rebellion, being nonproductive of that attention, fades out.

2. If the vitamin-mineral supplement is adequate, it will fully protect the child against deficiency in such factors.

Years ago, the senior author expressed his dissatisfaction with the infant supplements by concocting a complete one for his own children. It was subsequently marketed by a pharmaceutical company and copied by many others, and is available to the public.

The supplement consists of two vitamin syrups. The first combines all the known vitamins in crystalline form, accompanied by the unknown factors from yeast, or yeast and liver. The second group incorporates mineral factors, chiefly calcium, phosphorus, and iron, accompanied by the trace minerals. This supplement was so complete that it could be added to a diet of starch, protein, and fat completely free of vitamin-mineral value, and allow the child to maintain good health. Such a procedure of course relieves the mother of anxieties.

At the stage of rebellion, many children go on a milk "binge." To this the mother ultimately surrenders, with the doctrine of, "Well, he won't eat, but at least he takes his milk." She may even feed cookies to create thirst for milk. By way of demonstrating that no food is a perfect food, such a diet produces children who are deficient and who show it in being sallow, pale, listless, constipated, fatigued, and oversusceptible to colds and other infections. The remedy? *Stop the milk!* No child has ever voluntarily starved to death, and when he realizes that you are adamant, he will go back to normal eating. When milk is reintroduced, consumption will drop to a normal level. The continued intake of the multiple vitamin-B complex and mineral syrup during this period of rebellion will help to protect the child.

For infants, the complete vitamin-mineral supplement is added to the formula. It is added not in a single bottle, but in the entire day's ration, so that failure to consume the entire contents of a bottle does not deprive the child entirely of his supplementary protection. For breastfed babies, the supplement is given in water, fruit juice when that is fed, or directly from the spoon. One does not, of course, begin with the labeled dosage for very small babies for whom a teaspoonful is a gigantic amount; one begins with a few drops, working gradually upward. This helps to control such possible reactions as excessive laxative effect from the vitamin-B complex.

Cookies, crackers, and bread for young children should be selected on the basis of the same criteria previously given in this book for adults. Commercial candy should be taboo, and the desire for sweets should be satisfied with good home-baked pastries, low in sugar. When white flour is employed, it should be reinforced with wheat germ and nonfat milk. Homemade candies based on fruits are easy to make. Ice pops can be made from frozen juices, unsweetened.

When children go to whole milk, *certified raw milk,* if it is available in your community, should be the choice. This can also be used as the basis for formulas; at least it avoids twice-cooked milk. For babies who are sensitive or allergic to ordinary milk, the conscientious pediatrician will try goat's milk, or cow's milk that has been modified with predigestion with enzymes. (Such products are available commercially, with the milk already predigested. Incidentally, such predigested milk often allows the milk-intolerant adult to partake.) Others can tolerate cow's milk if it is modified by fermentation or by the addition of lemon juice; the use of buttermilk or yogurt sometimes solves the problem of milk in those who are intolerant, too. Since there is no true milk substitute for small children, and since soy is conducive to goiter in susceptible infants, every milk possibility should be tried before soy milk is employed.

Often the question is asked: "Is it all right for very young children to be given bits of food from the adult table?" If it isn't all right, the adults are eating improperly!

Finally, forget the prejudices that deprive young children of the enjoyment of good, palatable food. There are mothers who would be horrified to see the senior author's two-year-old enjoying lobster. But what difference is there between lobster and lamb chop, except that the chop is laden with animal fat difficult for a child to digest? The only problem is that of mincing the lobster so that an impatient little nonchewer will be able to masticate it, although we should know that the body manages to digest protein even without chewing.

The story of the little boy who wrote to his parents from camp and asked them to send some food—on the grounds that the camp only served three meals a day—should remind us that children require frequent refueling. The senior author recalls investigating strange noises from the kitchen at three in the morning, to discover his six-, ten-, and fourteen-year-old busy destroying a roast chicken! While children do require refueling with extra carbohydrates, these need not be bad food and need not be oversweetened. Whole grain crackers and cookies *are* available, as well as some made with white flour reinforced with wheat germ. Given the opportunity, though, children will eagerly consume protein snacks. These supply body-building material as well as fuel. A good practice is to supply a trayful of ham, cheese, and the like, from which hungry little ones too busy to sit down for organized meals or snacks will snatch as they pass by.

In the preschool years, this pattern of good nutrition is easy to establish and maintain, and its rewards of beautiful skin, nails, and hair, fewer infections and faster recovery, limitless energy and zest for living are self-apparent. When the child reaches school age, parents become worried because children are cruel in their treatment of those who, in appearance or conduct, differ from their peers. This is a specious argument. You do not hesitate to make your child feel different when you forbid him to ride a bicycle in heavy traffic, even though the little boy next door is permitted to do so. Why hesitate to make him different by protecting him with good nutrition? Actually, the only real difficulty will come with candy and desserts. The nutrition-minded mother who knows her psychology will make quite sure that she substitutes for the poor nutrition and tooth-destroying action of the commercial product her own good confections, baked products, and desserts. No child will feel deprived if he is offered whole gelatin dessert, flavored delightfully with fruit and topped with whipped cream, instead of the commercial gelatin product, which is 85 per cent sugar and 15 per cent gelatin. The Brown Betty made with whole wheat bread crumbs or with whole wheat flakes reinforced with wheat germ, apples, butter, and a little honey actually tastes better than the concoction of corn flakes, white sugar, and apple. Several cookbooks designed to keep readers alive and in good health are available, such as Adele Davis' *Let's Cook It Right* and the senior author's *Good Nutrition Cookbook*, and offer concrete instruction in making bread, cake, confections, and desserts that contribute to better nutrition.

17. Fluorides: A substitute for dietary education?

Plastics are now being made from by-products of the processing of sugar cane. Poetic justice will be served, if these plastics can be used to make false teeth. For where the white man's grocery stores go, and more particularly where his white sugar goes, tooth decay appears. In certain primitive cultures, where the sufferers had no folklore in medicine to help them, the abcessed teeth resulting from "civilized" eating became a prominent cause of suicide.

Although we know that tooth decay is caused primarily by a combination of susceptible teeth and intolerable diet, our current "answer" to the problem is carefully to refrain from educating the public to eat intelligently, even though a diet that rots the teeth is not good for the rest of the body, and to drop a powerful protoplasm-poison into our reservoirs. Moreover, the public health do-gooders are very surprised when scientists do not unanimously close ranks and enthusiastically endorse the substitution of fluoridation for education. In the modern technique of adulterating reason with emotion in the field of science, those who object to fluoridation on perfectly sound scientific bases are called "crackpots" and terms less kind. For example, Stare of Harvard, and also the mayor of Grand Rapids, Michigan, recently put this label on *all* opponents of fluoridation. In reply, it is worthy of note that the death rate in Grand Rapids rose after fluoridation, although it did not change in adjacent cities where this chemical was not added to the reservoir.

It is rather pointless to discuss the nutritional causes of tooth decay and oral disease if the reader has already accepted without critical examination the thesis that tooth decay is no longer a problem, thanks to fluoridation. Let us therefore examine the evidence which, for the senior author, made acceptance of fluoridation impossible, though on the basis of the official releases we were initially enthusiastic about the proposal.

The fluoridationists remind us that there are foods rich in fluoride. Then why, they ask, should anyone object to a small additional amount of the chemical in drinking water? Well, let us remember that tea is extraordinarily rich in fluorides, and while the British are full of tea, their teeth are full of cavities. Why? Because the tea is full of sugar. So, of course, is the American public. They remain so, after fluoridation.[1]

The fluoridationists assert that fluorides are innocuous in the dilution in which they would appear in the reservoir. To prove this, they cite a long-term study of two cities, one of them with high fluoride water, the other with low. They announce that no significant difference was found in the health of the citizens of the two cities. But if you look up the statistics for the two cities, Bartlett and Cameron, in Texas, you will find that during the period of the study there was a 350 per cent higher death rate in the high fluoride area. Even when the statistics are adjusted for age differences, the difference still remains meaningful. The fluoridationists, therefore, support their case by deciding that death is not significant!

---

[1] In one of his newspaper columns, Dr. Fredrick Stare remarked—with apparent complacence—that the children in fluoridated cities do not have to "give up their sticky sweets." Actually, the American Dental Association has said specifically that fluoridation is not a pathway to dental health unless it is accompanied by a program of dietary education. Yet anyone who lives in a fluoridated city will tell you that the dietary education is missing, and that the fluorides are being used for what they are not—a panacea. And the evidence mounts that sugar contributes to heart disease associated with hardening of the arteries.

Animal research has shown that fluorides cause dissolving of the forming heart tissue in the embryo. Significantly, the rate of the birth of stillborn babies in New Britain, Connecticut, went up 150 per cent after fluoridation. The rate in adjacent communities without fluoridation did not change in that period.

Rappaport, an investigator at the University of Wisconsin, was struck by the fact that Mongolian idiots displayed two phenomena that long have been credited to fluorides. Alone among mentally retarded children, the Mongolian idiot is singularly resistant to tooth decay. He is also given to a type of degenerative change in the eyes ordinarily associated with extreme age in normal persons, and which is also known to be caused by fluorides. Professor Ionel Rappaport therefore studied the incidence of the birth of Mongolian idiots as it possibly relates to the amount of fluorides in the water consumed during pregnancy.[2] He found a direct relationship: the higher the level of fluorides in the water, the more Mongolian idiots born. Statistical controls indicate that there is only one chance in a thousand that this relationship is pure coincidence. Moreover, in areas without fluoride in the water, there is a direct relationship between the ages of the mothers and the birth of Mongolian idiots: they are born more frequently to older women. This relationship is accepted by science and medicine. It is accepted by fluoridationists, but when the exact same kind of mathematical analysis is applied to fluorides versus Mongolian idiots, they label the association as an example not of figures lying, but of liars figuring! At any rate, in high fluoride areas the mothers of Mongolian idiots tend to be younger women.

The whole story of fluoridation has been "backed" by "scientific" research so poorly organized, so sloppily performed, and interpreted with such bias that a doctoral candidate whose thesis reflected such disgraceful looseness could well expect to have his candidacy rejected by his University. Example: Although the diet is known to influence resistance to tooth decay, in studies of fluoridated and nonfluoridated areas there is no effort whatsoever to

[2] This research is still in progress at the University of Wisconsin.

evaluate this influence in the children. Surely the reader knows that no one can competently evaluate the influence of a significant variable in an experiment when the other variables are not controlled or evaluated.

The fluoridationists evidently feel uneasy enough about their "scientific" evidence, since they exert every effort to keep the professionals and the public from examining the details of the data that "support" their proposal. But they make even greater efforts to keep the public and the professionals from gaining access to the evidence on the other side of the picture. Example: The senior author was asked to lecture on nutrition in dentistry, at the Harvard Odontological Society. The chairman, in great embarrassment, then asked him to accept a check for services that would not be performed, on the grounds that his broadcasts had presented some of the evidence against fluoridation. The author pointed out that the canceled lecture was not on the subject of fluoridation, accepted the check, and endorsed it over to the Student Welfare Fund at the Harvard Dental School. An incredible episode in a democratic country? Yes. A less successful effort of this kind occurred in Yonkers, New York, where a local health officer "burned the wires" to the state capital in an effort to find some legal device by which he could prevent an audience of laymen in a church group from being exposed to our remarks on fluoridation. Now, please keep in mind that the remarks made in Yonkers, and in this chapter, all derive from the very same scientific literature from which the fluoridationists themselves abstract their biased evidence.

The inconsistencies of the fluoridationists are so glaring that they will not subject themselves to examination. The senior author struggled for years, unsuccessfully, to persuade fluoridationists competent in science to debate the issue with him on the air. Acceptance of the invitation could not be obtained from public health agencies such as the New York City Board of Health. A limited acceptance was obtained from the Dental Information Bureau of one of the dental societies, but only on the condition that there would be no real debate and no questions. An examination of some of the inconsistencies of the fluoridationists' position will reveal why they have turned this issue into a circus, damned the entire opposition (though it happens to include a Nobel prize winner in enzyme chemistry), and in every way try to avoid any situation where their propaganda might be examined in public by dispassionate and competent critics.

For instance, the fluoridationists train their propagandists to reject any description of fluoridation as involuntary mass medication. They liken fluoridation to the chlorination of water; and, since chlorination is not medication, they would have it follow that fluoridation likewise is not. Factually, chlorine is used to treat water, to make it pure; fluoridation is used only to treat people. Treating people and medicating water are certainly distinguishable.

The mass medication is proposed on the grounds that tooth decay afflicts over 90 per cent of the public, and water is universally consumed, constituting thereby an ideal vehicle for the treatment of a disease national in scope. Let it be noted that nervous tension, irritability, and neurosis are also nationwide. Are you willing to have tranquilizers dropped into the reservoir? Headaches are nationwide: shall we put aspirin in the reservoir? Vitamin deficiency is nationwide: shall we put vitamins in the reservoir? On this last point arises the knotty question that shook the senior author's initial acceptance of fluoridation. We were asked if we would accept the addition of vitamins to the reservoir. We rejected the proposal; too many people are allergic, and some of them might be allergic to vitamins. Water should be safe for everyone. So, our questioner asked, how can you accept fluoridation? We then searched the literature for evidence of allergy or intolerance to fluorides. The first paper we read, by Feltman, a researcher then on subsidy from the United States Public Health Service (which endorses fluoridation), reported that he had administered fluoride tablets to 1100 pregnant women. Eleven of them, or one in every hundred, showed symptoms of intolerance.

In some of them, the symptoms mounted to bloody vomiting. A New York fluoridationist, a dentist, discussing these results and aware that it is easy to stop the administration of tablets but difficult to find substitutes for fluoridated water, remarked: "Well, of course, many people exposed to fluoridated water will exaggerate the significance of vague, tenuous symptoms." We looked at this dentist with a vague, tenuous feeling of nausea, glad that we were not among his patients.

Speaking of the United States Public Health Service as endorsing fluoridation, fluoridationists cite an impressive list of other major scientific organizations who endorse their project. Only under pressure will they admit that 99 per cent of these organizations have never performed any research to learn whether fluoridation is both safe and effective. The long list constitutes a group of organizations who have faithfully followed each other's lead, and are busy congratulating each other. We learned by writing to them that some of them *never had* endorsed fluoridation.

This leads us back to the incident in Boston. The reader may be interested in the wistful comment of a member of the Harvard Odontological Society when he learned that the lecture had been cancelled. He said: "I wish it hadn't been. I would like you to have spoken on fluoridation; I'd like to hear the evidence against fluoridation." What a confession from a professional man who is supposed to guide his patients in voting on fluoridation! Yet, in the history of science we have seen many such a blatant and self-confessed example of endorsement without examination.

Here is still another example of the ramrod technique that those in control of medical groups employ. In the late 1940s, the United States Food and Drug Administration discovered certain circumstances under which lithium might become toxic. They therefore became concerned about salt substitutes containing lithium, and forbade their sale. Their reasoning? Salt substitutes are used by people with high blood pressure. Some people with high blood pressure have damaged kidneys. Damaged kidneys may fail to excrete lithium. At some point *anything* is toxic. Therefore, although lithium appears naturally in water (which is true of fluorides, and therefore is one of the defenses of fluoridation), they banned the sale of salt substitutes containing the substance. Question: What happens to a person with high blood pressure and damaged kidneys when he drinks fluorides? Will he not accumulate fluorides in exactly the same way? Are unexcreted fluorides potentially any less dangerous than unexcreted lithium? Don't ask the United States Food and Drug Administration for an answer. Don't ask a fluoridationist for an answer. We have been trying to obtain a response to this question for years. And this is only one of many inconsistencies that appear when the picture of fluoridation is examined by an open mind.

Let it be noted that the United States Food and Drug Administration nonetheless endorses fluoridation. Not only is this inconsistent with their ruling on lithium; it is directly at odds with the entire policy of the Food and Drug Administration on toxic substances in food and drink. Their general policy may be stated as requiring that any food or beverage additive not be present in quantities larger than 1/100 of the toxic dose. If the Food and Drug Administration applied this policy to fluoridation, fluorides could not be added to the reservoirs.

It is also disconcerting to find engineers and chemists in the field of water and waterworks inconsistently endorsing fluoridation when one remembers that the standards of these professionals call for a generous safety margin in the content in water of any toxic or potentially toxic substance. In other words, no superintendent of a water department would countenance raising the chlorine content of water to a level anywhere near the possibly toxic. The reader will be interested to know that the safety margin on fluoride at the one part per million level (the recommended allowance), is absolute zero; there is no margin for error.

Another inconsistency, and a very disturbing one, centers about the matter of dosage of fluorides. Such fluoridationists as the American Dental Association insist that fluorides at one part per million in the drinking water present no risk of toxicity. Unfortunately, people do not drink standardized quantities of water. With personal inclination ruling nobody can know exactly how much fluoride your child will consume. To this, the American Dental Association and other groups pushing fluoridation reply that it doesn't matter. Your child or you, they say, could drink a bathtubful of fluoridated water daily without harm. Let us pass by the point that there are people who daily drink extraordinary quantities of water. Let us instead see how the American Dental Association attempts to control dosage of fluoride when it is *not* being given in water, but in tablet form. At this point, the dentists become very, very cautious. Although each tablet contains much less than the amount of fluoride that a heavy water drinker might consume, the dentist and the public are told that fluoride tablets should be taken only in the specified dosage, and only under competent supervision. Where is the competent supervision and where is the control of dosage when the vehicle for fluorides is water? And is it not silly to guarantee that the intake of fluoride from water will never be harmful when in some diets there is frequently enough fluoride, independent of the water supply, to cause mottling of the teeth?

Apropos of mottling: on this cosmetic disfigurement the fluoridationists exhibit a schizophrenic uneasiness. Granting that mottling is a symptom of toxicity, they gloss over the fact that 17 per cent to 20 per cent of the children in fluoridated areas will exhibit mottling. In other words, they say that the disfiguring effect on the teeth of one child in every five is too slight to be significant. At least this is consistent with their attitude, previously cited, that death is not significant, for the statement means that the children have only a slight case of poisoning. (Incidentally, this "slight" mottling of the children's teeth can and does in some instances become so gross that the child is permanently disfigured). To crown this disgraceful confusion, let it be noted that *Lancet* has remarked that *systemic* poisoning from fluorides can be in progress without the dental mottling, though this is universally accepted as the "most sensitive index" of fluoride toxicity.

Not only is the public in fluoridated areas unable to determine exactly how much fluoride is going into the children from the water, and from the natural content in foods, but there is also the question of the *added* fluorides that will go into the foods in fluoridated areas, as a result of the use of such water for irrigation of crops and for the feeding of farm animals. Thus, for instance, powdered skim milk from a fluoridated area will contain an abnormal amount of fluoride, and the housewife will liquify this powder with water containing fluoride. Now add to this potential witches' brew the radioactive strontium[3] that enters food as a result of H-bomb testing and fallout, and realize that the effects of additive toxicities have not even been explored! Season this with a little penicillin and DDT added to the cow and thus to her milk, and does not the added fluoride become an epitaph to the willingness of man to rush in where angels fear to enter?

The Swiss have an aggravated problem with tooth decay. It does not occur in the valleys where there is no tourist traffic and where foods of civilization are rare, but is prevalent in the areas where transportation facilities make sugar and white flour cheap and easily available. Here the decay is so rampant that the Swiss girl often has her teeth extracted before marriage on the ground that dentures are inevitable and her husband should be spared the expense! Nonetheless, the Swiss government ruled out fluoridation, for while it is greatly concerned with the problem of tooth decay, it is even more concerned with the problem of goiter, and it does not propose to risk the known action of fluorides in aggravating the tendency to goiter. Have we no goiters in America? Is American biochemistry different from the Swiss, so that we need not fear the effect of fluoride on our thyroids? Or has the fluoridationists' propaganda been less effective with Swiss dentists and biochemists?

As reprehensible as it is that these professional do-gooders have succeeded in ramming fluoridation down the throats of millions of

[3] Suppressed evidence indicates that fluorides increase retention of strontium 90.

Americans, even more objectionable is their technique of subjecting the proposal to a referendum[4] when they cannot succeed otherwise. Surely this principle must be revolting to any thoughtful person: involuntary mass medication for a goodly minority of the public, on the basis of a majority vote that may well have resulted from exposure to pressure tactics involving biased evidence! If tomorrow 50.1 per cent of the citizens in your community should decide to add vanilla to your drinking water to make it taste better, should you be compelled to go along and swallow the stuff? Even if fluoridation were proved to be both effective and safe—and such proof, as we have seen, does not and cannot exist—how intelligent is it to medicate an entire population merely to reach the teeth of children up to the age of eight? [5]

When any proposal that involves the health of the entire community is being considered, we are surely entitled to determine whether it is the best of a number of possible solutions. On this point, fluoridation also fails to meet the criterion, for there has long been evidence (gathering dust in the libraries, to be sure) that shows clearly that tooth decay *can be controlled by diet and diet alone*—moreover, that the entire body, at any age, benefits when the diet is improved to reduce the incidence of decay. We have succeeded in reducing tooth decay as much as 60 per cent by controlled diet alone. When we have done so, the children have also shown dividends in terms of improved growth, heightened resistance to infection, and generally improved health. Here is a promise no fluoridationist can make: that the procedure benefits the entire body, and that it is beneficial to anyone over eight years of age.

Admittedly a partial measure, and demonstrably not a sound substitute for dietary education, fluoridation is not even adequate in the narrow area in which it is supposed to be effective: raising resistance to tooth decay. When the fluoridationists tell you that

[4] They now tend to avoid a referendum: too many vote fluoridation down.
[5] Fanatical pro-fluoridationists are now claiming benefit to the bones of eighty-year-olds—on the basis of evidence satisfactory to no one but themselves.

decay has dropped 60 per cent in a fluoridated area, have you ever asked to see the figures on which the percentages are based? Ask, and you will have an unpleasant surprise. The technique goes like this: Fluoridation is brought to a community where 94 per cent of the children have decayed teeth. Later, it is found that only 93 per cent of the children have decayed teeth. To the 6 per cent of the child population free of decay has been added 1 per cent for a total of 7 per cent. This, in the peculiar world of fluoridation mathematics, is interpreted as a 16 per cent improvement, 1 per cent being a sixth of 6 per cent. If the percentage of children with decayed teeth dropped to 91 per cent, 3 per cent being 50 per cent of 6 per cent, the improvement would now be denominated as a 50 per cent improvement! All this of course blinds you to the fact that after years of fluoridation nine children in every ten are still developing cavities! In their private conferences, the fluoridationists are well aware of this abuse of statistics. Some of their more responsible scientists have suggested that if they are not careful, they will wind up with 101 per cent improvement: less than no cavities!

Puzzled readers and listeners often ask us concerning the motivation behind this program. There are dark rumors about public health officials being wined and dined and sent on long sea voyages by interests who will profit by the sales of fluoride and equipment to gullible cities. There may be some venal officials and companies,[6] but essentially the behavior is typical of those persons who are determined to benefit a public that they consider to be too stupid and lethargic for any program calling for its understanding and cooperation. Hence, the public health officials' dislike of a fluoride tablet program that would involve public control of dosage and the right of voluntary acceptance or rejection. Remember that it was only a few years ago when a Food and Drug Administration lawyer, asked by a judge why the Administration proposed to limit the amount of nutrition a baker might put into white bread and also asked why the Administration did

[6] There *are* strong economic motives behind fluoridation. It's *very* profitable.

not simply insist that all ingredients be listed on the label, replied in essence that the public is too stupid to understand a label. Let *us* propose, whether the subject be limitations on the amount of nutrition in a loaf of white bread or the addition of fluorides to our drinking water: "Idiots of the world, unite!"

There have been occasions when women resistant to nutrition education have expressed their opinion obliquely by remarking: "I have two children, sitting at the *same* table eating the *same* food. One is full of tooth decay, and the other isn't. If nutrition is the prime factor, how do you explain this?"

The question reflects several faulty assumptions. Two children sitting at the same table do *not* eat the same diet. Not only does one child reject that which the other accepts, not only does one accept more and the other less of the same food, but there is a distinct difference in the requirements of and the efficiency of the utilization of food from one individual to another.[7] Moreover, in addition to the assumption that the same diet would have the same effects on two human beings, there is the assumption that the teeth are the same, and they obviously are not. As regards its teeth, the population appears to divide into two broad categories. There are "soft" teeth, in which the enamel is very susceptible to erosion and ultimate decay from the action of acids, and then there are the teeth in which the enamel seems marble hard and is most resistant to acid. The individual with the softer type of structure will, even under the influences of emotion alone, suffer tooth decay as the acidity of the mouth changes. He will be affected by the gummy starches that cling to the tooth, and by the sugar in his food, and may reap a crop of a dozen cavities under circumstances where the other type of tooth decays not at all. It is another example of the individuals who come from good eggs requiring little hygienic care, but setting a poor example for us bad eggs.

It must be emphasized that the problem of tooth decay is not solved, though it is vastly lessened by lowering of the sugar intake

[7] Ever notice the differences in the use of salt by children?

alone. Yet it must be understood that this is critical, and that excessive sugar intake contributes to evils far beyond the question of tooth decay. As we have demonstrated in previous chapters, it is perfectly possible to trace a sequence, without leaving the bounds of nutritional science, by which excessive sugar intake can be responsible for hardening of the arteries, coronary thrombosis, varicose veins, difficulties with the menstrual cycle and the premenstrual week, cystic mastitis, complications of pregnancy, impotence and infertility in the male, and even the common types of cancer of the primary and secondary sexual organs in the female.

Almost invariably, the average person who is exposed to the preceding statement will deny that his tooth decay derives from excessive sugar intake. Unfortunately, the bulk of the sugar in the ordinary diet is contained in foods, rather than in the sugar bowl itself. A case of bottles of tomato catsup contains four and a half pounds of sugar. Salad dressing is made with it. Canned and frozen foods are loaded with it. A doughnut contains five teaspoons of sugar; a single portion of apple pie may contain twelve teaspoons of sugar; serving it à la mode adds six more. A stick of chewing gum contains a half-teaspoonful of sugar, and a bottle of soda pop contains from three to five teaspoonfuls. If you realize that our intake of soda pop alone is so great that it is said that the steel used for bottle caps outweighs the steel used for automobile bodies in any given year, you will appreciate the stupidity of trying to control tooth decay by substituting fluoridation for dietary education—and thereby allowing this mountainous intake of sugar to continue its work of mischief in the body at large.[8]

The processed starches, from white flour on, also work mischief, because they cling to the teeth. The tendency of the modern diet toward these processed foods also deprives tooth and gum of the cleansing and scrubbing action of foods high in roughage and bulkage. The nutritional as well as the mechanical inadequacy of the diet therefore contributes also to the gum troubles that plague

[8] This includes loosening of teeth—greatest cause of tooth loss, by far! Thus fluoridation guarantees that all the teeth you lose will be healthy!

our population. Although the Federal Trade Commission legally restrained the tooth paste industry from advertising the statement, it is nonetheless true that four out of five Americans from the age of thirty-five on have pyorrhea or other serious disorders affecting the gums and the supporting structures of the teeth. The condition is so common that it has led to the wry joke concerning the dentist who tells his patient: "You have thirty-two perfect teeth: all I have to do is take out the gums!"

Part of the trouble that leads to gum disease starts in childhood as "bad bite." When teeth, deprived of the support of a missing tooth, drift and tilt, the biting force, which should be distributed generally, is exerted on one or two high teeth. The result is that the gum takes a beating, attempts to retreat, and the pathway to pyorrhea is open. The pounding ultimately weakens the structures supporting the teeth. The insult is superimposed on the drain of these structures that derives from the unbalanced diet initiating the decay that started the process. It is obvious, then, that pyorrhea and periodontal disease cannot be approached as a disorder of the mouth alone. It is equally obvious that fluoridation will encourage the public to continue to eat the kind of diet which (ordinarily) rotting the teeth, also attacks the integrity of the gum and the supporting structures.

Furthermore, it becomes apparent that the dentist who treats pyorrhea and periodontal disease by scraping and adjusting the bite is doing only half the job. The rest lies in repair of the diet.[9] To give you one example of the interplay of forces, physical and emotional, that may contribute to the loosening of teeth—even sound teeth—let us consider that under emotional stress the body releases cortisone, and the saliva turns acid. While the acid is busy attacking the tooth enamel, the cortisone is occupied with the withdrawal of protein from the teeth and the supporting structures. Under the emotional stress, with the consequent nervous-

---

[9] A diet low in sugar and processed starch noticeably tightens teeth in less than a week. The senior author has secured a three millimeter restoration of bone, reversing a process of resorption of the jaw bone, in three months.

ness and irritability, the sweet tooth comes into play: "Let's have a bite—I'm nervous." Now the deteriorating process is aggravated by a rise in the intake of sugar. At this point, the patient, contemplating his dental bills for tooth decay, pyorrhea, and threatened loss of sound but loose teeth, is apt to remark: "I don't understand why I'm having all this trouble—I've always been perfectly healthy." He may use the rest of his failing energy to deny the need for education in diet, and to repudiate the validity of the concept of psychosomatic disease!

Dietary recommendations for reduction of tooth decay can be generalized. Sugar intake *must* be reduced, and sugar must become a flavoring agent, quantitatively speaking, rather than a food. The diet must contain enough fruit such as apples, enough salads and whole grain breads and cereals to give tooth and gum some exercise. For advice on brushing and dental floss, consult your dentist—remembering that primitives who eat sensibly, on the basis of inherited wisdom, have little or no tooth decay or pyorrhea, although they have never heard of cleaning the teeth. But *their* foods require *chewing*.

The intake of vitamins and minerals recommended in Chapter 15 will, if added to a well-balanced diet, help to prevent trouble with the gums and the structures supporting the teeth. For those who already have these difficulties, there are nutritional therapies that involve massive doses of nutrients which support the adrenal gland and those directly important to the integrity of the gum and tooth-supporting structure. There is emphasis upon bone meal,[10] vitamin A, the vitamin-B complex, vitamin C, vitamin D, the bioflavonoids, 40-degree liver, and vitamin E. Since this is nutrition used therapeutically, self-medication is not advisable, and the reader should consult one of that small but growing group of periodontists who are learning to use nutrition as an important part of their treatment for these conditions.

There is one further simple rule that will, aside from proper

[10] The fluoride in bone meal is accompanied by the natural antidote, calcium, which is *not* used in fluoridation.

diet, prevent a good part of the troubles: Never fail to have a missing tooth replaced, whether you are five or fifty. The consequences of restoration go far beyond the mere effect on your appearance.

ANTI-TOOTH DECAY DIET

Daily Intake: One pound of vegetables, mostly green.
One-half pound of fruit.
One quart of milk.
One to two eggs.
One-quarter to one-half head of lettuce—preferably, when available, an equivalent quantity of loose leaf lettuce, chicory or escarole.
Eight ounces of orange juice, unstrained, in addition to other fruits.
Meat once daily.
Whole wheat bread and whole grain cereals exclusively.
For dessert—puddings made with milk and eggs, fruit, gelatin, dates and figs.
Sweets never more than twice a week. This classification includes pie, cake, doughnuts, candy and drinks made with artificial flavoring.

The supplements to this diet contain vitamins A, B_1, B_2, B complex factors, niacinamide, C, D, and E fortified with eight essential minerals—calcium, phosphorus, iron, copper, zinc, magnesium, manganese, and iodine. The effect of the supplements is twofold. It protects the children against variations in the natural vitamin-mineral content of the food and it simultaneously increases the efficiency of utilization while raising the vitamin-mineral intake to the optimal point without straining the capacity of the child for eating food in quantity.

This diet may be followed by both adults and children and, as the reader may surmise, will be conducive to general health as well as to dental health. The teeth may be regarded as an index of the general condition of the body. Diseased teeth, while not necessarily meaning a diseased body, are a sign of something less than good health.

FURTHER PRECAUTIONS

Certain other suggestions are useful in avoiding tooth decay.

Wash the mouth with water after eating. Easily fermented foods, like milk and citrus juice, can promote in the mouth the growth of organisms which are harmful to tooth enamel. In addition, there is reason for believing that citrus fruits, while rich in vitamin C (needed for good tooth health and good gum health) may be harmful to teeth because they contain citric acid. Take the vitamin C internally but rinse the mouth with water to remove external deposits of citric acid. Brushing the teeth and using dental floss are also sensible precautions, but they must be considered a secondary weapon against tooth decay.

The application of fluorine directly to the teeth is also helpful. In the author's experience, a 33⅓ per cent fluorine paste, applied by your dentist every three months, is more effective than the two per cent solution used more frequently. This will also help to desensitize erosions. Bone tablets, naturally containing small amounts of fluorine, are a useful childhood and pregnancy supplement.

18. Old Age: It can be treated

A remark often made by middle-aged and older Americans reflects a philosophical (if erroneous) concept that converts time from a dimension (duration) to a cause of sickness and bodily degeneration. "Well, of course I have a little arthritis—I'm growing older." In this philosophy, wrinkling of the skin, graying of the hair, cataract, and other degenerative diseases are seen as the inevitable and inescapable effects of time itself.

A glance at many seventy-year-olds will pinpoint the fallacy, for there are seventy-year-olds who are not gray, who do not have cataract or other degenerative disease, who are not wrinkled and infirm. And remember that gray hair occurs in children. As the old man who had received a diagnosis of a senile cataract remarked: "Doctor, please explain why the other eye doesn't have a cataract —is it any younger?"

It is, therefore, not strange that before one can appreciate and profit by a discussion of nutrition versus aging, one must learn to distinguish between changes measured by the yardstick of time and those that are a direct product or by-product of the aging process. You have heard it said that there are sixty-year-olds with thirty-year-old bodies, and that there are thirty-year-olds with sixty-year-old bodies. Even this concept fails to reflect the realization that the changes which we sum up in the term "sixty-year-old body" were not caused by the years themselves, though the phrase indicates that we are aware that aging may progress more or less rapidly than the calendar would warrant. In short, the calendar and the clock, in themselves, are not toxic nor are they the origin of degenerative changes and disease. It is important that this truth be grasped; otherwise, there is little point in discussing the nutritional weapons that may halt, slow down, or even reverse some of the symptoms and changes that we attribute to growing old.

Remember that the starved skeletons we found in German and Japanese concentration camps in 1945 showed many of the stigmata which in older people we unhesitatingly called "senile"—loss of visual acuity, drying and pigmentation of the skin, with loss of elasticity; drying and brittleness of the hair; loss of muscle tone and of efficiency of digestion and elimination; loss of interest in sex; and in the area of personality, that kind of self-centering and introversion which, too, we mistakenly regard as a "normal" result of aging.

If our philosophy that time itself is not aging is not accepted, the consequences can be deadly. A case history may illustrate what frequently happens when "she's growing old" becomes the phrase that prematurely and unnecessarily removes an older person from the sphere of social usefulness.

Some twenty years ago—an interval, incidentally, which will indicate that the nutritional weapons with which this chapter deals have been in our possession for a long time—the senior author was called for consultation services by a physician engaged in a debate with a group of psychiatrists. The patient was a sixty-five-year-old widow who had been displaying signs of paranoid behavior. She announced that her devoted sons were not really her sons but impostors bent on harming her. She said that her neighbors were spying upon her, and desired to harm her. Her family physician diagnosed her as suffering from "senile" cerebral atherosclerosis, and advised her sons that failure to put her in an institution would deprive her of the twenty-four-hour nursing care that she would need but they could not afford. The three psychiatrists whom they subsequently consulted confirmed the diagnosis, and polished it off by pronouncing her to be a typical case of "senile dementia."

The author noticed cracks at the corners of her mouth, parallel with the lips, and a slight bareness and shininess of the tongue. A test of the urine revealed the presence of porphyrin. This substance is found in sufferers from pellagra, and its presence usually coincides with the delirium that is one of the symptoms of this disease. Since the disturbances of the mouth pointed in the same direction, we decided that the hardening of the arteries of the brain (which could have been present) was simply a convenient hook on which the psychiatrists were hanging their diagnostic hats.

A survey of the patient's diet showed that she had been behaving in the kitchen as do many persons who find no pleasure in preparing decent meals for themselves, in the absence of their deceased spouses and their emancipated children. This history of dietary deficiency was appraised in the light of the knowledge that nutritional requirements may rise rather than fall as the human machine becomes less efficient during the years.

She was therefore treated on the basis that we were watching disturbed behavior resulting from a malnourished brain and nervous system. The delusions of persecution vanished when the lips healed, the tongue recovered its normal appearance, and the porphyrin disappeared from the urine. The woman died some six years later, from an unrelated cause, and in full possession of her faculties.

Interestingly, as her regime of vitamin injection, good nutrition, and vitamin supplements was continued, she altered her perspective on life in a way which she reflected overtly. She had been shuffling rather than walking, with her eyes fixed on the floor, and her shoulders bent forward. As the delusions faded out, she resumed her normal excellent posture. And, as she began to raise her head and look more toward the horizon physically, she did the same thing mentally. Instead of concentrating on the ground, living not one day but one minute at a time, and perhaps looking forward with anticipation to death, she began making plans for her next vacation!

A history like this indicates the importance of a correct perspective on time as duration, rather than on time as a toxic agent of degeneration. Had not this more constructive philosophy been applied, would the patient have ended her days in an old age home with symptoms worsened and her disintegration accelerated by the abominable diet so often served in such institutions?[1]

It is not the intent, in this chapter, to give the reader the impression that every old person afflicted with "senile symptoms" represents a "subclinical" stage of pellagra. Rather, our intention is:

1. To establish the realization that many of the breakdowns in physical and mental function in older persons are at least worsened, if not initiated, by poor nutrition.

2. To demonstrate that since good nutrition ordinarily prevents or mitigates what it cures or helps, this information gives us when we are young, or comparatively so, a tremendous opportunity to apply the science of modern nutrition to prolong the prime of life, retard the changes attributed to aging, and avoid premature senility.

The concept that old age and disease are part of the same equation is easy to come by when you realize that at least one in every three, at the age of forty, can anticipate in the next two decades the development of a degenerative disease such as heart trouble, arthritis, pernicious anemia, high blood pressure, and hardening of the arteries. Please keep in mind that animals fed as most of us eat also develop degenerative disease, and sometimes without waiting for old age. Please remember, too, that primitive people, who eat as we do not, escape many of these disorders. One should not ignore comments like that of a physician who, after twenty years of practice with a primitive group, announced that in those two decades he had treated cataract in very old people, inflammation of eyes from exposure of the eyes to the smoke of cooking

---

[1] It has been estimated that 4 per cent of the "senile" institutionalized population might be rescued by nutritional therapy.

fires, and injuries due to accident. But he had never seen cancer; he had never treated indigestion; he had not been confronted with the anemias; he had never known the heartbreak of struggling with multiple sclerosis or any other of the horrors that crowd our "civilization" hospitals, clinics, and medical offices: none of the disorders of civilization for which our science of medicine admits that it has neither satisfactory explanation nor efficacious treatment.

Unfortunately, many of the lessons we could apply on nutrition versus "senile" diseases are today moldering in medical libraries. Unfortunately, too, the policy of discouraging the public use of vitamin supplements has resulted in our ignoring equally valuable lessons concerning the usefulness of good nutrition in preventing what we mistakenly consider to be the "normal" changes of aging.

The story of diet versus gray hair particularly emphasizes this point. It has been established that pantothenic acid deficiency would cause early graying of the hair in young animals. The research demonstrated that the graying was accompanied by internal bleeding of the adrenal glands, and showed further that when restoration of the vitamin to the diet recolored the gray hair, the change followed repair of the adrenal glands. Today, decades later, we realize that cortisone, a product of the adrenal glands, recolors gray hair, and that pantothenic acid, in ways not yet understood, acts as a cortisone sparer. We also recognize that role for paba. It is not coincidence that paba is described as a cortisone sparer and that it, too, is listed among the vitamins which recolor gray hair. The mischief in the official attitudes toward the nutrients that affect aging is well illustrated in the case of paba. The *Journal of the American Medical Association* editorially announced that paba is not effective in recoloring gray hair. The paper "documenting" the statement reported nothing of the kind. It actually said that when gray hair is caused by calcium pantothenic acid deficiency, paba will not recolor the hair. This is quite a different statement from what the Association was saying, but nonetheless the editorial had its effect on medical men, and to this very day, some twenty years later, most physicians will tell you that the American Medical Association finds the antigray-hair vitamins worthless.

You may wonder about this academic tempest in the nutritional teapot. Why fuss about recoloring gray hair with vitamins when there is a beauty parlor on every street corner? First of all, some of the medical nutritionists who have performed research with these vitamins are convinced that gray hair is seldom if ever to be regarded as "normal," even in the context of changes that come with aging. In other words, they consider gray hair to be a visible warning of a nutritional deficiency, and regard its response to vitamin dosage as a sign that the "aging" of the pituitary gland has been halted, slowed, or even reversed. The reader will recall that we earlier described recoloring of "prematurely gray" hair as an indication that the vitamins had restored fertility to women with a history of miscarriage and stillbirth.

The same philosophy may be applied to what has been miscalled "senile pigmentation." It has been observed that the brown spots on the skin which, in the aged, are considered to be "senile" pigmentation, also appear in the severely malnourished. Moreover, they have been treated successfully in both instances with niacinamide. However, fully to capitalize upon the usefulness of good nutrition in prolonging the prime of life, we must appreciate that as the years go on the body may become less capable of extracting its requirements from food and utilizing them to best advantage. The biochemist may conjecture on the lessened efficiency of the enzyme chemistry of the body, but we need not deal with this question to reveal our present scientific inadequacies. Suffice it to say that the aging process encompasses reduced ability to absorb and utilize, and clear from the body, the by-products of the nutritional processes. Moreover, as deficiencies relative to the need increase, the inadequacies tend to accelerate functional breakdown in the glands. Since some of these glands (particularly the pituitary) are essential to absorption and utilization of food, the process becomes circular. Escape from it is possible only as the intake of nutrients is raised high enough to compensate for the inefficiency of utilization. A typical example is found in the experience of a group of aged individuals who showed slight signs of vitamin A deficiency, although the institutional diet supplied more than their "requirement" as calculated by the authorities. When they were given supplements of vitamin A, approximately doubling their intake, the symptoms of vitamin A deficiency, primarily in the skin, disappeared. The patients also became more resistant to respiratory infection, as demonstrated by the fact that the group receiving the vitamin A supplement weathered more successfully than the control group, several waves of virus infection.

The discovery that the vitamin requirements grow larger as we grow older, although the authorities insist on denying it, should not be hailed as being new. Any textbook on geriatrics will inform you that the older person does not utilize fats efficiently: he absorbs them less well and "clears" them from the blood less rapidly. Vitamins A, D, E, and K are fatty substances. However, these difficulties in absorption and utilization of vitamins in older people are not confined to the fat-soluble factors alone. Certainly protein is not metabolized in older persons as once it was and the carbohydrates are not handled as efficiently either. Yet our knowledge of nutrition is sufficient, even though we have much yet to learn about enzyme chemistry, so that we can reduce the severity and the rapidity of "aging" in any group indefinitely. We except only those unfortunates who came into the world as a product of damaged germ plasm, and who thereby have never had the potential to be excellent human machines. Even these may be helped, if only to reach their limited potentials.

For prolongation of the prime of life it is useful to remember how analogous we are to gasoline engines; the fuel that is high octane for a brand new motor is no longer such a short time later. The carbon deposits have raised the octane requirement; the valves no longer perform as efficiently as they did; the spark may be weak or erratic; and conditions are no longer optimal for the extraction of maximum energy from the fuel. Correspondingly, the diet that maintains a forty-year-old in buoyant health may be inadequate even at that age if it does not prepare the individual for the years to come when the machine will no longer be as efficient. There are three ways with which to cope with this problem:

1. One can ignore it, as the public does, and at forty continue to eat the previous lifetime diet, which may be and often is inadequate. This is the advice of those professors of nutrition whose departments have large subsidies from processed food manufacturers.

2. One can wait for signs of trouble and then change diet, and take vitamins, inadequately and incompetently, to try to compensate for only part of the pattern of poor nutrition.

3. One can change the diet toward the optimal and at forty raise the intake of nutrients as though one were dealing with the inefficient body of a seventy-year-old.

The senior author recalls a French countess who used to walk some five miles to attend his broadcasts. She was seventy-seven. Her interest? She wanted to know more about certain aspects of nutrition which would, she thought, help her to improve her sex life. She looked like a robust fifty, because through her adult life span she had selected her foods from the point of view of supporting the body and yet had not sacrificed the pleasure of the palate, because there is no compromise needed in achieving both objectives.

What kind of nutrition slows down the aging process or may reverse it? The nutrition recommended throughout this book. We repeat the regimen because it applies to almost everyone and because it cannot be emphasized too much:

1. High protein diet in frequent small meals.

2. Substantial increases in the intake of the multiple vitamins, vitamin-B complex, vitamin E, vitamin C and the bio-flavonoids, high quality protein, and within reason, unsaturated fat from wheat-germ and cottonseed oils. The supplementary intake of liver, brewer's yeast, and wheat germ should be increased.

If one is particularly interested in recoloring gray hair, the following nutrients are of special importance: Adequate complete protein in the diet; high intake of paba,[2] pantothenic acid, choline, and the other known factors of the vitamin-B complex; the trace minerals with special reference to small amounts of copper.

It goes without saying that the diet to slow the aging process should be well balanced, which in the older persons calls for a pattern of good nutrition not differing significantly from that which should be used in the childhood years of growth.

There are benefits from these steps that must be experienced to be fully appreciated. To illustrate the point, a Monsignor in the Catholic Church in his late seventies had suffered a stroke that had left him partially paralyzed and unable to speak. It was the desire of his physician to restore to him at least enough command of his body and his speech to allow him to attend the fiftieth anniversary of his ordination. We were given three months in which to accomplish this. The Monsignor attended his anniversary, and he was able to make a short address. One of the nutritional therapies we used that made this possible comprised large doses of vitamin C, the bio-flavonoids, and vitamin E. Vitamin E helps the body to absorb blood clots.

Question: Would it not be sensible at forty to raise your intake of the bio-flavonoids, vitamin C, and vitamin E, or would you prefer to wait until an alert physician identifies in you the personality changes that follow the first small stroke? At which time, of course, you will be given, not vitamin C, bio-flavonoids, or vitamin E, but doses of phenobarbital and tranquilizers, which will simply hasten your downhill course to "old age."

Thought for the dubious and brainwashed: Is it not interesting to hear people rank Gloria Swanson and Robert Cummings as "food faddist"—and then marvel (enviously) at their energy, bounce, and prolonged youth?

---

[2] This and other antigray-hair factors are logically stressed for the aged. See appendix for "antigray-hair formula."

19. What you can do to help yourself

You have read the book. We hope you are now impressed with the penalties for poor nutrition, and—more important—with your exceptional opportunity to use good diet preventively. In your hands has been placed the chance to control one of the very few environmental factors important to health and well-being, and which to some degree is controllable. But, you are probably asking: How do I apply what I have learned, so that the kitchen does not become a short route to the clinic and the hospital? Application divides itself into two phases: what you are to do in the kitchen; what you are to do in the grocery store. We must also pay attention to the fact that you very probably eat in restaurants, and must learn how to compensate for the mischief inherent, however conscientious the proprietor, in large-scale purchase and preparation of food.

In the selection of menus, there are simple rules—so simple that they appear to be innocuous—but these will have a profound effect upon your nutrition. These apply to all meals, served at home or in a restaurant. Let us summarize them.

---

1. Let no day pass without drinking 8 ounces of unstrained grapefruit or orange juice. The unstrained juices contain the bio-flavonoids

that are found in the pulp. If you don't have your own juicer, select those frozen brands which have pulp particles floating in them.

If you are intolerant of citrus fruits, make sure that it is an actual intolerance or allergy. Some of the reactions blamed on allergy to citrus fruit actually derive from the peel oil, which is highly irritative. This means that if you juice the fruit yourself, you should use the revolving type of extractor rather than the type that puts pressure on the peel.

If you are persuaded that citrus juice gets into a fight with your morning coffee, toast, or whatever, please remember that there is no such thing as food incompatibility. Foods that are good alone are good together. The "heartburn" or other evidences of intolerance that some persons blame on an internal battle between the morning glass of juice and the rest of the breakfast more often than not is the protest of the stomach against a cascade of ice-cold juice on its empty interior. The troubles people blame on incompatibility can usually be solved, therefore, by taking the breakfast first, and the juice last.

If tomato juice is used, the daily intake should be twice as much —16 ounces. The quantity would have to be four times as much with pineapple juice. In any event, it is not necessary to take all the juice, of whatever kind, at any one meal. Our objective is to provide a guarantee from such source of at least enough vitamin C to provide a generous reserve over the amount that will prevent scurvy. Whatever additional vitamin C and bio-flavonoids you obtain from the other fruits, vegetables, and salads, will constitute added protection. Those who eat in restaurants must be particularly careful not to skip the juice intake, for most restaurant cooking is extremely destructive of vitamin C.

---

2. Do not take more than two portions of food rich in starch or sugar at any one meal.

This rule is not as simple as it sounds. It directs the diet toward high protein; it prevents you from overloading with carbohydrate, and of course particularly keeps your sugar intake down; and it will dictate decided changes for the better in your dietary habits. For instance, if your meal includes bread and potato, this rule will require such a dessert as whole gelatin, since your license for starches and sugars will have expired with the potato-bread ration.

---

3. Select your breads, cereals, and baked products so far as possible from whole grains. (whole wheat, whole rye, etc.) We recognize that this rule cannot always be observed, because some persons cannot tolerate too much roughage, though it is useful in preventing constipation; and that those who do not bake at home very often find an extremely limited selection of whole grain breads, cereals, crackers, and cookies.

This rule means that you select your cereals from oatmeal, regular or instant; shredded wheat;[1] wheat germ and similar cooked and dry cereals. Avoid cereals in flake form; you can judge how much destruction the heat causes in such cereals when you realize that many of them are enriched even when they are whole grain. Enrichment should not be needed for a whole grain cereal, and the partial restoration implies a fairly total loss.

Do not feel that a cereal breakfast constitutes optimal nutrition. A portion of cereal is usually an ounce, equivalent to a slice of bread, and no one has ever suggested that a slice of bread constitutes the basis of decent nutrition at breakfast time. Those who cannot tolerate a large amount of food in the morning can convert dry or cooked cereals into better nutrition by adding a tablespoonful of wheat germ to each portion and by using concentrated nonfat milk to fortify the liquid milk used on the cereal. (Concentrated nonfat milk is made by using the amount of nonfat

[1] Brands without BHT, which the FDA permits—and the British find to be the only toxic antioxidant.

milk powder designated to make a quart of liquid milk, but adding only enough water to make three fourths of a quart. This is excellent advice for those who are watching fat calories carefully, and the fortified nonfat milk also makes a good substitute for cream in coffee.) Do not misconstrue the previous notes as an endorsement of a low fat diet, which is a superb way to develop gall stones and vitamin deficiency.

---

4. An ounce of wheat germ daily provides good diet insurance. It is a must in our dietetic scheme for anyone who can tolerate it, and most persons can. Buy it only in vacuum-packed or air-shielded brands, for wheat germ, like all good foods, spoils easily, and rancid wheat germ can actually cause a vitamin E deficiency.

The wheat germ may be taken as a cereal, added to cereal, substituted for bread crumbs in any recipe (or mixed with bread crumbs). A teaspoon and a half of wheat germ may be used in each cup of flour in practically all baked recipes. Wheat germ may also be used to fortify most loaves and hamburgers. Please note that the term "extend" was not used in place of "fortify" since "extend" implies dilution. A paper by Stare[2] indicates wheat germ has protein which is biologically very efficient, higher in concentration than meat, and very digestible. Wheat germ may also be sprinkled on ice cream, in lieu of chopped nuts, or taken with tomato juice.

---

5. An ounce of brewer's yeast daily is also recommended. This does not replace wheat germ but complements it. A quarter of a pound of brewer's yeast daily and from three to ten ounces of wheat germ are standard dosages when severe nutritional deficiency is being treated.

---

[2] This was published in the early 1940s. Stare's department at that time was largely without grants of the kind it now enjoys.

This observation is for the benefit of those who eat 100 pounds of sugar a year without question, but feel quite apprehensive if by accident they repeat a dose of two tablets of brewer's yeast. The yeast may be taken in tablet form, or in its palatable varieties added to recipes. For instance, two tablespoonfuls of brewer's yeast added to stew in the last minute of cooking will more than compensate for the losses of B vitamins in prolonged heating of meat.

6. Two portions of green salads daily. These need not be enormous and should not be confined to the monotony of lettuce and tomatoes.

They may include escarole, chicory, finocchio (fennel), Swiss chard, watercress, scallion, onion, tomato, the outer leaves of Chinese cabbage, cabbage, green endive, uncooked broccoli and cauliflower. Dressing should be varied. Mineral oil should never be used, nor should peanut oil until it is relieved of the suspicion raised in a recent report that tentatively links an unknown factor in it to cancer. All other salad oils are usable,[3] and may be rendered more nutritious by using cold pressed wheat-germ oil, 25 per cent, and salad oil, 75 per cent. This should be stored in brown bottles in the refrigerator, and never purchased in large quantities.

Salad dressing should be varied: French, Russian, herbal, Roquefort, or blue cheese. Keep monotony out of these important foods. And don't serve salads warm and limp.

7. Fried foods should be deep fat fried in a thermostatically controlled fry pan.

Many of these thermostats will hold at a given temperature, but it may not be the temperature indicated on the dial. It is therefore

[3] Cottonseed oil is nutritionally preferred.

necessary to recalibrate, so that you know at what temperature you are really cooking. This can be done with an accurate deep fat thermometer. Without such accurate temperature control, deep fat fried foods may be undercooked and oversoaked with fat, or overcooked and present the risk of combustion products that are at best disturbing to digestion (see appendix for Decomposition Points of Fats chart).

The subject of fried foods brings up the current fad that has plunged the American public into a highly dangerous effort to substitute vegetable fats for animal fats. For reasons too technical to fall within the scope of this book, a high vegetable fat diet represents a completely uncharted experiment and unpredictable results, but among the possible consequences can be "collagen diseases" of the type for which medicine has neither explanation or satisfactory treatment. As partial explanation, let us note that rancidity of vegetable fats can occur within the human cell, too.[4]

---

8. Include in the weekly menu three portions of seafood; both fish and shellfish.

If you are interested in preventing hardening of the arteries (and who is not?), this suggestion makes a lot more sense than tampering with the quantity or type of fat in the diet. In satisfying the requirement for protein foods, use at least one portion of liver a week. The calf's liver that the public prizes is the lowest in value. Pork liver over-all is the most desirable and cheapest; lamb liver is next; beef and chicken liver follow. The chicken liver can be chopped in the usual way; the other forms need not be served only as broiled liver. In hamburger and meat loaf, 10 per cent of liver may be incorporated without changing taste enough to run into idiosyncrasies of the palate.

[4] This may result, if vitamin E intake is low, in production of free radicals like those created by irradiation, which can be responsible for premature aging.

9. At each meal take an animal protein.

This means a selection among eggs, milk, cheese, meat, fish, and fowl. If the budget permits only one portion of these more expensive foods daily, split that portion among the meals. By so doing, you make the inferior protein of the other foods more effective.

10. For adults, two portions of a dairy food daily are desirable.

This may be milk in any form, such as yogurt, ordinary milk (homogenized if you are intolerant of fats) buttermilk, etc. Since an intake of uncooked protein seems to have important protective value, and practically all our protein foods are ordinarily cooked, consume *certified raw milk* daily if you can manage to obtain it (See Chapter 13).

An ounce of cheese substitutes for a glass of milk. The natural cheeses are preferable to the processed, for the reason that the processed cheeses are cooked to achieve a flavor, regardless of the original quality of the cheese. A natural cheese, if it is to be flavorful, must be of good quality to start with. The naturally yellow cheeses (Cheddar and the ilk) tend toward higher calcium value than the white. Pot cheese is preferable to cottage cheese. All such statements are relative: the majority of dairy products are good food. "Cheese spread" is a term that allows the manufacturer to evade the more rigid legal requirements for composition of cheese, permitting the sale of water and other diluents at cheese prices.

Do not ignore the dairy food requirement. Despite certain claims that milk and milk products are being overeulogized, responsible scientists find that the brittle skeleton of the older American can be traced to a lifetime of suboptimal calcium intake, and the ideal intake simply cannot be achieved from food without the use of appropriate dairy products.[5]

[5] This is one of the reasons for using a mineral supplement.

---

11. If wheat germ is not used, include two slices of whole grain bread in each meal.

This may be reduced to one slice per meal if wheat germ is employed. This means whole wheat bread, whole rye bread, or whole corn bread or sticks or muffins. It does not mean enriched white bread, unless it contains added wheat germ; nor does it mean cracked wheat bread, ordinary commercial rye bread, ordinary pumpernickel, French or Italian breads. Anyone who portrays enriched white bread as being equivalent to whole grain is turning his back, advertently or inadvertently, on the inadequacy of the enrichment. The vitamin B_6 and the vitamin E (among many other factors) of which bread should be our good source are removed from white bread and are *not* restored in enrichment.

With you who are "normal" in your reaction to food, we are almost done. Add to these simple rules in selecting and preparing food a reminder: use your vitamin-mineral supplements as instructed in Chapter 15, and you will have a pattern of nutrition that will satisfy the requirements even of those whose body chemistries outrage the "authorities" who, as we have seen, have set up minimum daily requirements on the basis of a mythical and misleading "average" determined by methods that demand unquestioning acceptance of conjecture posing as the axiomatic.

It is assumed in this chapter that the housewife is aware of the rules for normal protection of the diet; that she knows, for example, that her cooking water should be saved and used for soup stock, gravies, sauces, and vegetable juice cocktails. We assume that you know that vegetable juices are desirable to use if you do not overdo them. We assume that you know that iodized salt is preferable to plain table salt; even better is sea salt (which is more valuable than the FDA is willing to admit).[6] We assume likewise that you are aware that there are good mineral waters pro-

---

[6] Sea salt is a "faddist" food in the FDA lexicon. This would vastly astonish India and Greece, where sea salt has been used for centuries.

duced naturally in this country that carry health benefits with them.

But what of those who cannot eat some of these recommended foods? "I'm allergic—half these things I can't eat!" they will probably wail.

Although there are perhaps 42 million people in this "healthy and well-fed" country who have allergies, or otherwise react adversely to good foods, it is obviously impossible to write a general book on diet for the normal person and simultaneously pay more than lip service to the specialized needs of the minority. However, the following recommendations will very often help to rescue an allergic person from the vicious circle where allergic reactions force the use of a restricted diet which, in turn, creates deficiencies that make the allergies worse, not better.

Allergy to citrus fruits and other good sources of vitamin C can be partially compensated for by the use of 250 milligrams of vitamin C daily, in tablet form. To compensate fully would call for a supplement of the bio-flavonoids. However, these are usually derived from citrus fruits. While allergy to citrus fruit does *not* mean allergy to vitamin C, it may mean that the bio-flavonoids will not be tolerated. In this case, a supplement of rutin can be substituted: 200 milligrams of rutin are used daily or from 800 to 1,000 milligrams of the bio-flavonoids would be desirable.

If allergy interferes with the intake of protein foods, several devices can be employed. There are preparations of predigested protein called protein hydrolysates, which represent the protein so treated that it is no longer specific, with the result that it is much less likely to stir an allergic reaction even in an individual who is allergic to the particular source of the food. Highly allergic individuals who have been given such predigested protein accompanied by the vitamin-B complex from a tolerated source—rice polishings if not liver or yeast—have sometimes recovered from their food allergies in a period of one or two years.

Allergy to milk and milk products calls for the use of a calcium supplement, since optimal intake of calcium without dairy products is impossible. A supplement yielding half a gram of calcium will compensate for the inability to drink 2 glassfuls of milk or to use 2 ounces of cheese. The preferred type of supplement would be one that supplies phosphorus as well as calcium. Dicalcium phosphate is an example. In pregnancy, because of the large amounts of phosphorus yielded by the high protein diet, a supplement such as calcium gluconate may help to avoid the penalties that will come if the phosphorus intake is boosted still higher by use of *that* type of calcium supplement. These penalties include severe cramping of the leg muscles.

Since liver possesses unique values, substitutes are never adequate. A device allowing at least some liver values to enter the diet for those allergic to the food consists of overbroiling chicken liver until it is actually hard,[7] scraping it into a powder, and administering it in any vehicle in which it is palatable, even applesauce or ice cream. The use of rice polishings, concentrated yeast, or wheat germ for those allergic to liver or wheat germ can be compensated for by the use of whole rye in bread or in cracker form. Corn allergy, though it shuts out many foods with corn starch as well as baked products made primarily with corn, presents no such nutritional problem as does an allergy to wheat. In other words, corn is easily replaceable with any whole grain; wheat is not. Therefore, when allergy forbids the use of whole wheat and whole rye as well as wheat germ, a deliberate effort must be made to raise the intake of organ meats and other B complex sources such as yeast, liver, and rice polishings, and to increase the intake of vitamin E with supplements. Frequently, those who are allergic both to wheat and wheat germ are able to tolerate wheat-germ oil. Incidentally, while this is not a required supplement in the program presented by this book, a teaspoonful and a half of wheat-germ oil daily does yield demonstrable benefits, particularly for the middle-aged and aged.[8]

Fat intolerance, while not strictly in the field of allergy, does

[7] This denatures the protein—but some values remain.
[8] Wheat germ oil is not a substitute for wheat germ.

present problems that interfere with proper nutrition. Homogenized milk, homogenized fats, whipped butter, and whipped margarine are usually better tolerated by those who are fat intolerant. Vegetable fats are usually better tolerated than animal fats. Since certain vitamins of the B complex are directly involved in fat utilization, it is wise for such persons to select a supplement that supplies a significant amount of choline (at least 1000 milligrams in the daily dose), inositol (500 milligrams), pyridoxine (10 milligrams) and B_{12} (5 micrograms).

Lecithin is a supplement that has excellent tonic benefits for most persons, and has particular importance for those who need help in utilizing fats. One or two tablespoonfuls of lecithin crystals daily will be helpful, either in capsule form or in crystal form, sprinkled on cereal, or stirred in juices.

It should be noted here that these nutrients that help in the utilization of fat are administered medicinally to persons with hardening of the arteries, gall bladder trouble, and liver disease. Accordingly, those who are fat-intolerant may derive benefits from the use of these supplements far beyond better utilization of fats.

Intolerance to bulkage and roughage presents a serious threat to the adequacy of a person's diet, because a bland diet may be low in both vitamins and minerals. However, the basic supplements outlined in this book will serve to protect such an individual from these deficiencies.

Now let us look into the Cornucopia of Plenty which is the modern grocery store, remembering that 50 per cent of what it has to offer is carbohydrates deficient in vitamins important to human health. Let us imagine that we are shopping together, so that you may watch the application of the nutritional principles that have been discussed in this book, and realize again that eating to meet the needs of the body does not cost more and may cost less; does not sacrifice the enjoyment of eating but contributes to it.

VEGETABLE AND FRUIT DEPARTMENT

To select fresh spinach in invidious distinction to the canned and the frozen is to fall prey to the propaganda of fanatics. The "fresh" spinach was fresh when harvested, say, in Magic Valley, Texas. But it has been shipped perhaps some 2,000 miles. It has gone from producer to railroad to produce exchange to wholesaler and to the retail counter. Here it is displayed usually without refrigeration, and by the time that you buy it, it may be five or six days old. Preferable will be the spinach which has been frozen within hours of harvesting.

Further, the canners and the freezers make an effort to protect you against an excessive dose of poisonous insecticides. There are quality control departments operating in the major freezing and canning factories. Although there is no one to inspect fresh produce at the smaller farm, conscientious processors actually have discarded hundreds of thousands of pounds of heavily sprayed vegetables, and this is true also of the packers of baby foods. So long as our government justifies the insanity of the "legal" residue of such poisons as DDT in our foods, on purely economic grounds —they actually call these insecticides "economic poisons"—just so long will the canned and frozen foods from major packers always be a better choice than the fresh. Of course blanching causes some loss of mineral value in frozen foods; and failure to control refrigeration temperatures in transportation and in the cabinets in the stores will likewise contribute to vitamin losses. But unless you raise your own vegetables, and so know what you are eating, the canned and the frozen vegetables and fruits are a good choice.

Unfortunately, frozen and canned fruits are often packed in heavy sugar syrup. To reduce dental bills, this syrup should be discarded.[9] The vitamin-mineral loss so incurred will more than be compensated for by the regular use of your dietary supplements.

[9] At least as much sugar will have permeated the food.

When selecting frozen foods from the store cabinets, choose the packages close to the walls of the freezers, for in the cabinet type of freezer the coldest area is there. You may have noticed that the contents of packages from the middle of the cabinet are often thawed. This slushiness does not create danger but does contribute to loss of both vitamins and flavor.

The frozen fruit juices are at least as good food as the fresh that you might squeeze at home.

FRESH AND FROZEN MEATS
AND PREPARED FROZEN FOODS AND DINNERS

There is no basis for distinction between frozen meat and fresh, unless the wrapping on the frozen meat has not properly protected it against the discoloration that comes with "freezer burn." This affects flavor more than nutritional value. The purchase, however, of foods such as frozen hamburger is an act of faith: it is like eating blackberry jam at a picnic without watching to see if the seeds move. When frozen meat is cooked in large pieces, such as roasts, preliminary thawing is necessary, and the prudent housewife will do this in the refrigerator rather than at room temperature.

Frozen fish is good food, too, though its origin in the sea does not protect you, as some people have supposed, against the insecticides to which cattle have been exposed. Sprays are used in the wholesale fish market, as well as on the farm.

Such foods as frozen fish sticks must be examined critically, for the proportion of bread crumbs to fish in some brands approaches larceny. Some of the frozen "TV dinners" are excellent and some abominable. Most of them do not provide an adequate portion of the protein food, but the better ones are at least as good as the individual with limited facilities might be able to prepare at home.

A very important element in the use of frozen foods is the facility for home storage. Combination refrigerators and freezers may be perfectly adequate, but some are not. It must be remembered that frozen food is best preserved with temperature at zero, and in many of the combination units it is impossible to reach that level in the freezer, or it demands overchilling the refrigerator section to keep the freezer compartment cold enough.

The cabinet type freezer, as the previous discussion indicates, is inferior to the upright, since in the upright the cold surfaces are everywhere—above and below the food—and wherever the food is placed it is bathed in sufficient cold. The upright freezer, contrary to popular opinion, does not lose significant amounts of cold air when the door is open. Contrary to popular opinion, too, a freezer is worthwhile for a city family. The ability to purchase foods in season, rather than to be at the mercy of sky-rocketing prices as market supply goes down, can alone result in a substantial yearly saving.

The efficiency of a freezer, like the efficiency of the freezing compartment in a combination unit, should not be taken for granted. Both should be checked with a reliable thermometer. Losses of vitamins in prolonged storage of frozen foods are insignificant at zero degrees and disastrous at 10 degrees above. Therefore, the ice cube compartment in a refrigerator should not be used for more than a few hours for storage of frozen food. It simply cannot create the required low temperature.

Canned meat foods are nutritious, but it must be remembered that prolonged cooking is often required of the manufacturer by the Department of Agriculture. The inevitable denaturing of the protein should be compensated for by the use of uncooked protein: certified raw milk, oysters, clams and desiccated liver. The vitamin loss should be offset by the use of the supplements. When there are ingredients in a canned meat product other than meat, the sequence of the ingredients on the label no longer tells you which are in higher concentrations. Thus, formerly corned beef hash where potatoes and water are first on the list of ingredients and meat last would represent a purchase less desirable than a brand where the meat content is listed before the water. Now the labels—legally—are anonymous.[10]

Margins of profit on meat are extremely low, and the giant chain stores enjoy very little advantage in their purchasing as compared with the corner butcher store. Indeed, some chains use their meat departments as crowd bringers, and must lose hundreds of thousands of dollars a year on the prices that they charge in that department. When meat or fish or fowl are consistently priced remarkably below market averages in any individual store, let the buyer beware. On meats of equal quality, a price differential of 10¢ per pound is highly improbable, unless the seller is losing money. Heeding this advice will prevent you from watching a piece of corned beef lose 75 per cent of its original weight in cooking: proof positive that you purchased an illegal amount of brine, masquerading as beef.

The housewife's shopping habits in the meat department have produced a group of butchers with ulcers. She purchases on the apparent assumption that the animal comprises pot roast, filet mignon, porterhouse, sirloin, and T-bone cuts. Since these are only a part of the edible carcass, the housewife finds herself bidding against her neighbor for the dozen "desirable" cuts. The butcher, in business to make a living, is compelled, in self-defense and in deference to the law of supply and demand, to raise the prices of the popular cuts. This means that there are approximately 100 cuts of perfectly good meat available, ignored by the housewife and marked down by the butcher, so that he may sell the entire carcass. It is true that the American housewife finally discovered that beef neck is perfectly good meat at a low cost, and that when ground into hamburgers with lamb neck mixed in, it produces a less costly hamburger that is juicier and more palatable.

The housewife has decided that liver, by some unwritten statute, can be served but once a week, and that calf's liver is a status

[10] This ruling by the FDA clashes with their suggestion that the consumer should read labels for his own protection.

symbol, which it may be. We have already noted that it is the lowest of all forms of liver in total nutritional value, though of course a good food. Pork liver, the cheapest, being least wanted, is the most nutritious. In short, the woman with a desire to bring home maximum nutrition for the dollar might shop more intelligently in the meat department than she does now and her family will still enjoy their meals and be better fed.

THE CEREAL DEPARTMENT

The American public would suffer no nutritional deprivation whatsoever if 90 per cent of the dry cereals on the market were suddenly to vanish. Priced beyond conscience, these "foods" often represent, like the maraschino cherry, a triumph of the embalmer's art. Although they make no nutritional sense, or economic sense, the housewife has somehow been persuaded that a one-ounce serving of a typical product constitutes a breakfast. In the advertising of these cereals, the nutritional assays given are usually based primarily on what is obtained from the milk one is supposed to add.

There has been a spate of high protein cereals in recent years. They appear to be made from the good nutritional material that is removed from the other cereals made by the same manufacturers. Since, like the less nourishing flake cereals, they are subjected to intensive roasting and since excessive heat applied to a protein food may be fully as undesirable as improper cooking of vitamin-rich foods, it would seem that the four or five cents you spend for a portion of these cereals might better be used to buy cheese or an egg.

This is not to say that there are no cereals worth buying and eating. Oatmeal, Shredded Wheat, Familia, Wheat Chex, Wheatena, and wheat germ itself are among those that constitute good nutrition.

THE SWEETENING DEPARTMENT

Aside from honey, which has a high sugar content but also contains some vitamins and minerals, there is no form of sugar that represents good nutrition or deserves a place in the *food* cabinet. Sugar should be employed only as a *flavoring* agent. This applies to yellow and brown sugar as much as it does to white. Raw sugar has no discernible advantages, and unless packaged by a reputable processer, may be filthy. The fact that yellow and brown sugars have traces of a mineral or two does not alter the fact that they contribute to tooth decay as much as white sugar does, and increase the need for vitamins without supplying them. The pancake syrups fall into the same classification. Honey in the comb offers some advantages. The vitamin content of honey in the comb is higher by about 35 per cent than commercial clarified honey, the reason being that honey is clarified by filtering it through charcoal, an excellent technique for removing vitamins. It makes the honey clear enough so that the label on the bottle can be read from the back, but the objective seems dubious.

Other than honey, the only sweetening agents on the market that yield some appreciable nutritional value are molasses and dehydrated banana flakes. The story of molasses has been badly distorted by government agencies collaborating closely with the propaganda departments of the large sugar refiners. Light molasses has less nutritional value than dark. Blackstrap molasses is the dregs left after the extraction of the last possible bit of sugar and ordinary molasses. While blackstrap molasses is certainly not the miracle food it is represented to be by certain food propagandists, it is not the contaminated and unnutritious substance that it is pictured to be by some others. The vitamins that should be in sugar are in the blackstrap. An assay of blackstrap at Yale University School of Medicine showed a very sizable vitamin content, as well as a rich supply of iron and calcium, much more than is contained in molasses sold for human consumption. The health book industry has also clouded the issue by exaggerating the virtues of blackstrap and selling it to those who wish to avoid excessive sugar intake. Despite claims to the contrary, blackstrap contains a sizable amount of sugar.

If the housewife can find clean blackstrap molasses (there are canned varieties on the market for human consumption) she is justified in mixing this with her regular molasses (25 per cent blackstrap, 75 per cent regular). In so doing, she is reversing the effect of processing, and she is also not inflicting on her family the rather strong molasses taste of blackstrap. In some baked products, blackstrap is quite palatable, undiluted. In any event, its rich supply of iron, at least fifteen times as great as ordinary molasses, should be gratefully received by American women, in whom nutritional anemia is appallingly frequent.

THE BREAD DEPARTMENT

Bread should be our good staple source of added vitamin E and B_6. It will be if you emerge from the bread department with only the following types:

Whole wheat bread.

Whole rye bread (sometimes available, more often packed in cans).

White bread that has been enriched not only with vitamins but with wheat germ.

Muffins and sticks made from whole, undegerminated corn meal.

Whole wheat cookies and crackers.

Whole rye crackers.

Have you been concerned about cholesterol? Do you know what vitamins help to metabolize fats? They are the vitamins present in whole wheat but removed from enriched white bread. And what do you smear on the bread? Cholesterol, in the form of butter. Let us be sensible!

The so-called Jewish rye bread and its variations are not Jewish, not rye, and hardly bread. They comprise 55 per cent processed white flour combined with 45 per cent processed rye flour. Commercial pumpernickel represents such bread, fermented and colored with burnt sugar. The term on the label, "burnt sugar" or "caramel coloring," is the clue; whole grain does not need cosmetic coloring. Cracked wheat bread may run as high as 70 per cent ordinary white flour. The breads mixed with vegetables are deserved by the people who buy them. The so-called "Cornell bread" is an excellent formulation. The French and Italian breads are ordinary white bread made with water instead of milk. Bagels are made from white flour, and are boiled before they are baked, thus doubly insuring that they will be vitamin-free.

Melba toast, ounce for ounce, has *more* calorie value than bread. Reducing breads won't reduce you; nothing that you eat reduces you.

If you have never tried baking at home, believe us that the delightful aroma of home-baked bread will keep a man closer to hearth and home than gallons of Chanel No. 5. There are many excellent recipes for home-baked bread, yielding nutritional values equaled by very few commercial products.

Years ago, there was a woman who baked whole wheat bread for her sick son, who had received no benefit from medical treatment. Her whole wheat bread ultimately became the basis for a giant business. And when her commercial bakery had prospered in selling the bread that had cured her boy, what do you think their next product was?—white bread, lacking in the nutrients that had made the difference between sickness and health for her youngster!

THE INSECTICIDE PROBLEM

Our government permits the use of deadly poisons on our foodstuffs as a method of pest control, and allows the farmer and the processor to pass along certain residues of these poisons. Thus, it is legal for vegetables to contain 5 parts per million of DDT, although autopsies have shown us that the stuff remains in the body.

Add radioactive strontium 90 and penicillin in milk, tetracycline and other antibiotics in chicken and meat, and we arrive at a diet that seems designed to test the capacity of the human body for taking punishment. Although the tests conducted for the toxicity of these various contaminants in our food, as well as that of the hundreds of food additives in use, are conducted on each substance *individually*, it is possible that some of these chemicals in *combination* acquire an added degree of toxicity. A striking example of such *additive* toxicity is the interaction between fluoride, an approved ingredient in our drinking water, and iodine; the fluoride prevents the thyroid gland from taking advantage of the iodine, with goiter as a result. Another is the postulated interaction between fluoride and strontium 90. And these are only the beginnings of the problem.

What protection have we? One can wash vegetables, but insecticides are made to be somewhat tenacious; if they are not, the farmer resprays after each rainfall.

One should pursue the best possible nutrition, even though the good foods themselves are vehicles for insecticides and other toxic intruders; but at least with the good foods, the body has the advantage of a supply of the agents that help to throw off the effect of these toxic agents, to degrade them, to render them less toxic or even harmless. Thus, it well may be that whole wheat contains more strontium 90 than white flour; the processing of flour, in removing anything that might support life, also removes the strontium. But the eater of white bread still gets strontium in the milk used in the bread and does not have the protection of the natural vitamin-B complex that helps the body to resist radiation. This is not cited as a specific safeguard but as an example of the fallacy in the reasoning that would have us eat overprocessed foods to avoid by-products of fallout.

AND NOW A FEW POINTERS FOR THOSE WHO EAT OUT
AND PASS OUT

The restaurant chef faces almost inescapable losses of nutritional
value in the large-scale preparation of foods. Unless restaurants
can be persuaded to use small pressure cookers for short order
preparation of leafy vegetables (we have been trying for years to
persuade them), and thereby eliminate the use of the steam table,
losses of vitamin C, for example, can approximate 90 per cent.
While it is true that this vitamin is unusually susceptible to destruction, it is likewise true that any procedure which degrades 90
per cent of the vitamin C value in a food must destroy significant
amounts of other vitamins. A simple suggestion results: if the restaurant in which you eat has steam tables for vegetables, go to
lunch and dinner as early as possible, and never cheat on the rule
that calls for two portions of green salad daily, for it is the vitamin
content of the raw vegetables that will in part compensate for
what happened to the cooked. For this same reason, the restaurant eater must not skip the daily water-glassful of citrus juice.

What many restaurants serve as whole wheat bread is actually a
form of white bread. To the deficit in vitamin-B complex factors
caused by restaurant breads and sweet desserts must be added the
considerable losses of B vitamins in the prolonged cooking of
meat and other protein foods. Here the supplements suggested in
Chapter 15 are protective, but it is also intelligent to emphasize
such organ meats as liver in your selection. To avoid the losses in
prolonged cookery, pass by the stews, roasts, and meat loaves and
concentrate on broiled meats and similar short orders. In some
cases the vitamins lost may be secondary to the probability that
the protein is rendered less digestible by the long cooking.

Most restaurant desserts are well worth by-passing. Fruit, with
the sweet syrup left uneaten, cheesecake (if not too sweet), and
assorted cheeses represent intelligent selections. Gelatin desserts
in restaurants are more likely than not to be 85 per cent sugar.

The restaurant eater who has food allergies should attempt to secure the cooperation of the manager: if he is a regular patron, this may be possible. Many commercial recipes contain unlikely ingredients, some of which can cause, for those who are sensitive, headaches, colds, constipation, and diarrhea, as well as the more conventional allergic reactions: hives, dermatitis, sinus trouble, and asthma. If you, the sufferer, do not make such an effort to avoid unnecessary trouble, the restaurant really cannot be held responsible.

AIR POLLUTION

Wits have pondered in wartime on the difficulty of distinguishing between urban air and a gas attack. Certainly none of us needs reminders of the deaths in Donora, Pennsylvania, or the preoccupation with smog in California. In the past, only the hay fever sufferer "did anything" about it—with filters, air conditioners, or flight. Now none of us can ignore the tons of soot, dust, dirt, jute, kapok, bacteria, gases, pollen, viruses, spores, and sulfuric and other acids embellished with exhaust-carcinogens which daily we breathe, as a reminder that man is one of the few living creatures to befoul his own environment.

It has been said that lethargy was a good girl, though she had her moments—and this is true of the average person, who is stirred into anxiety by sporadic newspaper campaigns against air pollution, and lapses into inertia when the stimulus is ended. Yet, other than action at city, state, and Federal level, other than voluntary compliance at industrial level, there are at least two contributions that the average citizen can make to clean air, in his own behalf. Simplest of measures is a mineral oil spray which brings dust down to the floor, and keeps it there. Several such products are available. More effective is an electrostatic dust precipitator. These are available as portable units, consoles, and "built-ins," the latter designed for permanent installation in a new house, often as an adjunct to an air conditioning system.

While air conditioning of itself somewhat cleans air, it is highly inefficient, resting its action on repeated recirculation of air, thereby lessening outer contamination; and the use of filters. The best of these will stop perhaps 5 to 8 per cent of the particles in air, allowing all else through. In reverse is the efficiency of the electrostatic dust precipitator, which removes at least 98 per cent of the particulate matter in air, by the simple technique of giving it an electrical charge, and drawing it to a charged plate. Since it takes only five or six grains of pollen to start a hay fever attack, it is obvious that air conditioning will help, but is only a gesture.

An investment in air conditioning *plus* electrostatic dirt precipitation is an investment in better health. In longer life for the aged, too.

20. The power of body over mind

In reading Chapter 11, the reader realized, we are sure, that at least two types of vitamin deficiency and a condition of poor utilization of carbohydrate are capable of causing symptoms perfectly mimicking those of neurosis or psychosis. However, emotional disorders are not only simulated by nutritional deficiency or malutilization. There are a number of physical disturbances which—not recognized as such, or thrust into the psychiatric realm by "diagnosis by exclusion," may also subject a person to psychoanalysis, psychotherapy, or shock treatment. These physical conditions range from food allergy to postviral-infection depression. They include cancer, multiple sclerosis, and a variant of epilepsy, among other diseases. If the physician does not have a high index of suspicion, it is possible that many of these disorders—serious as they are—may go unrecognized, sometimes until it is too late. In one study, 115 patients had been diagnosed as being emotionally disturbed, and were found eventually to have physical illness. This discovery resulted in the cure of 45, the improvement of 36, no response in three, and the death of 31, 25 of whom—remember that they had been told that they were neurotic!—died from cancer.

It has been said that the layman who indulges in self-medication has an idiot for a physician and a fool for a patient. The same criticism cannot be directed to the average person who tries intelligently to appraise his state of health or lack of it, and to keep his own index of suspicion high enough to protect himself without becoming a hypochondriac. The last is ironic, for some of the individuals who have been abused by faulty diagnosis which assigned them to psychiatric treatment in the presence of an unrecognized physical disease were initially labeled as hypochondriacs.

What happens when the index of suspicion is not high may be appraised from a recent article in *Reader's Digest* on the subject of influenza. Although the article was written in usual *Digest* style —which is to say that in a pedestrian way it concentrated a great deal of information into its highly readable prose—there was in the article no evidence that the author had been apprised of two aftermaths of influenza which have been recognized for many years. Pediatricians will tell you that an attack of measles, influenza, or certain other virus infections in children may be followed by an alteration in behavior which bespeaks an impact of the virus upon the brain and the nervous system. Normally well-behaved children may become aggressive, asocial, hostile, liars, and thieves. In adults, the postviral state is fully capable of imitating both neurosis and psychosis. In the early 1950s, the senior author was struck by the similarity of the "emotional" symptoms which occurred in a group of about fifteen adults who had all suffered, a few months before, a severe "virus infection." This undoubtedly was one of the influenza variants. The emotional symptoms began, usually, soon after the respiratory symptoms had faded away. Initially, they were blamed on the fatigue which is almost inevitable after a severe upper respiratory sickness. As time went on, the fatigue was embellished by anxiety, completely unprovoked; by depression, descending to the level of suicidal thoughts; by lack of zest, apathy, fitful sleep, and gloomy forebodings about the future. By the time that these symptoms were in full flower, enough time had passed so that the patients no longer associated them with the respiratory infection immediately preceding the first of the "emotional" troubles. When the emotional symptoms reached their height, they were so mixed that the patient himself could no longer decide what was particularly troubling him. He complained of feeling very low and wretched, had very little energy, very little appetite, and—to put it briefly—presented a condition so closely simulating the complaints of the person with a genuinely psychiatric depression that one can hardly be astonished that the majority of these patients wound up in psychotherapy or psychoanalysis.

There are four characteristics of this postviral syndrome that make it possible—without elaborate tests—to recognize it, as distinct from disturbances of a purely emotional nature.

Depression is characteristic in the postviral state, but may be hidden. In other words, the patient may go to a doctor because he is tired, because his sex drive is down, because he has insomnia, is low and wretched—and does not realize that his illness closely resembles a state of depression. The physician who is cautious will recognize that the patient usually has not been prone to attacks of depression, in the past, and that this "emotional" illness has struck him like a thunderbolt. He will also observe that the life situation of the patient does not provide any obvious excuse for depression. He will also note, if his investigation is careful, that some days, weeks, or even months before these symptoms struck, the patient had a brief illness which was characterized by a general lack of well-being and by fever. Sometimes this illness will be spoken of merely as a "nasty cold." Particularly suspicious in the "nasty cold" that strikes out of season: in the summertime.

There is an obvious effect of the virus on the functioning of the body and the total personality, though, once again, these symptoms will be indistinguishable from those caused by a depression of purely emotional origin. The patient may complain that he is unable to organize his tasks as well as ordinarily he could. The housewife will say that she is literally unable to function properly when she goes shopping. The teacher will state that he is in trouble in trying to organize his lectures. The patients complain that small decisions worry them, that memory is tricky, and appointments are forgotten. They soon arrive at a feeling of being inadequate, apprehensive, and tense.

Any physical ailments predating the viral infection are likely to be magnified by it. Toothaches become worse; allergies worsen; indigestion and skin rashes will flare. The patient's typical comment concerning all this is: "Since I had that cold I have never been well." Once the virus origin has been recognized, it becomes apparent that the infection has somehow dropped the resistance of the body to illnesses of all kinds.

In rare instances, a major mental disorder, such as schizophrenia, appears as an aftermath of an attack of influenza. Obviously the influenza does not create this problem, but possibly triggers the loaded gun.

Medical recognition of this disorder is largely missing. There was one paper by Dr. Desmond O'Neil, in *Medical World*, March, 1959, in which Dr. O'Neil confessed that he learned to recognize the postviral syndrome only because he himself had had it. The physician points out that the best way to "treat" this disorder is to prevent it, but this of course would imply the availability of a flu vaccine of genuine effectiveness—which, to the knowledge of the authors, has not yet been developed. Dr. O'Neil remarks in his paper that he treats his patients with a stimulant and with injections of vitamin B_{12}. However, the senior author's research, in collaboration with the medical men to whose attention he called this largely unknown disorder, has indicated that while vitamin B_{12}, because of its general tonic effect, may be slightly helpful, there are nutrients which have a more specific effect. These include vitamin E, concentrated wheat-germ oil, and factors of the vitamin-B complex. Here again we see an indication that the dietetic history of the individual may have a very profound effect upon his reaction to a given infection, for what nutrition helps, it ordinarily helps to prevent.

Interestingly enough, although the recommendation of vitamin E in the postviral syndrome would probably elicit mockery by the "consensus," the fact remains that the senior author suggested the use of this vitamin to the physicians treating the condition, for the good reason that at the National Institute of Health, a few years ago, vitamin E was found in vitro (not in the body) to attenuate or weaken the influenza virus. Likewise, a deficiency of vitamin E in the hen results in symptoms in the chicks indistinguishable from those of encephalitis. Since this is a condition of the brain, there is more logic to the use of vitamin E in the postviral syndrome than would appear to the cynical eye.

One of our colleagues, Dr. Harry Swartz, some years ago remarked that the incidence of allergy in children confined for "juvenile delinquency" is far greater than that which would be anticipated in a random sampling of the general child population. He also pointed out in several of his textbooks on allergy that an allergic reaction in the brain can have impacts on behavior, for the very good reason that swelling which is confined in the bony skull must exert pressure. Dr. Swartz's awareness of the contribution of allergy to behavioral disturbances and "mental disorder" was not widely shared, however, until recently, when (in two reports to the First International Congress of Social Psychiatry) physicians spoke of failure to recognize food sensitivity as a widespread cause of illness which may appear to be, in some cases, purely psychiatric-like depression. It is interesting to see the language used by one of these physicians, who obviously realized that the "consensus" was not likely to look with favor upon this unorthodox theory. He acknowledged that psychiatrists and other physicians have generally "given first place" to psychogenic factors in the cause of mental illness, and that it sounded unorthodox therefore to suggest that environmental factors—foods and their chemical contaminants—may by allergic reaction involving the central nervous system be as important as purely emotional stress in the production of mental and functional disorders. He pointed out that when a symptom can be relieved by elimination of a specific food, reproduced by administration of the food, and again relieved by a subsequent withdrawal of the food, it is logical to assume that allergy is the cause of the symptom. He cited a case history of a thirty-one-year-old woman suffering from depression, who did not respond to psychotherapy or to any of the mood-changing drugs. It was discovered that administration of eggs, tea, rice, salmon, wheat, milk, peas, potato, butter, and cheese induced symptoms ranging from depression and fatigue to colds, itching, muscle cramps, stiff neck, and headache. Another case was that of a child with insomnia, nail-biting, bedwetting, compulsive masturbation, tremor of the hands, stammering, quarrelsomeness, and inability to concentrate at school. Elimination of processed carbohydrates—the cereal grains—brought "immediate improvement." Not only was the boy "as bad as ever" when the foods were reintroduced, but the doctor indicated that an outburst of the pattern of "delinquent behavior" could always be traced with certainty to the boy's inadvertently breaking his diet. Another report, at the same meeting, pointed to allergy to many popular foods causing in some individuals acute and chronic syndromes which included fatigue, nervousness, insomnia, depression, and mental confusion. From the foregoing, it is obvious that an allergic individual requires exhaustive investigation by an allergist before his "emotional" disturbances are definitely so labeled. Since the conventional skin test may be fallacious, it is here perhaps helpful to suggest that the reader consult the textbook, *The Pulse Test,* by Dr. Arthur F. Coca, M.D.[1] This test is based on the simple premise that your pulse rate is accelerated by the foods and substances to which you are allergic. The technique offers the possibility of identifying allergies which sometimes are not diagnosed with certainty by other means. The reader will note that Dr. Coca, in the list of symptoms which he assigns to allergy, includes nervousness, nervous and emotional instability (neurasthenia), dizziness, depression, and other symptoms ordinarily relegated to the purely emotional.

At the height of pellagra, when delirium is present, a chemical is found in the urine—porphyrin—which disappears as sanity is

[1] Published by Lyle Stuart.

regained. However, this chemical has been found in the urine of over 1 per cent of the patients entering a large psychiatric institution. The implications of this finding are that as many as five thousand people may have been institutionalized because of this disorder, porphyria. It usually begins in the early years, the twenties and thirties, and is more frequent in women. Abdominal pain is often present. Anxiety, nervousness, outbursts of hysteria, and depression are characteristic of the people suffering from this metabolic aberration. Physicians studying the problem suggest that in patients with psychic or neurological disturbances where there is also unexplained pain in the abdominal area, the simple test of the urine for porphyrin should always be done.

When the adrenal gland misbehaves, producing inadequate amounts of the hormones from the cortex, the symptoms which follow—before recognizable Addison's disease appears—may include irritability, weakness, fatigue, loss of appetite, diarrhea, and nervousness: symptoms which, once again, can be responsible for mislabeling of the patient as a neurotic, hypochondriac, or even psychotic. This disorder of course can be treated by appropriate hormone and nutritional therapies.

Another glandular disorder which may be masked as "neurosis" is underactivity of the thyroid gland. Disoriented and confused behavior may be the early symptoms. Unfortunately, hypothyroidism is more common than many physicians realize (we have already quoted one authority as indicating that perhaps some 3 per cent of the adult population suffer from it) and the physical symptoms that clearly label hypothyroidism as being present are very often missing at the stage where behavior is disturbed. These remarks can be repeated in terms also of overactivity of the thyroid gland.

A vitamin B_{12} deficiency, untreated, will of course ultimately lead to pernicious anemia. However, the blood is less sensitive to this deficiency than is the brain and the nervous system. The result is—and this is not hypothetical, but as actually happened to some patients—that it is possible for a sufferer from vitamin B_{12} deficiency to be subjected to shock therapy for a condition that is actually a product of malutilization of a vitamin. Depression, slow thinking, defects of memory and attention span, paranoid behavior, and outright psychosis may be the presenting symptoms that are the mark of vitamin B_{12} deficiency. It may be months before the blood clearly reveals what is actually happening, but there are tests that can be made long before that, which will positively identify the patient as suffering with the preliminary stages of pernicious anemia.

Multiple sclerosis, which is clearly recognizable in its advanced stages, sometimes appears—particularly in women—in a mild form, which almost inevitably leads to the patient being labeled a hypochondriac. She complains about intense fatigue, aches, pains, dizziness, weakness, and a feeling of inadequacy in coping with her everyday responsibilities. After a few years, multiple sclerosis in a recognizable form finally appears. Of course, at this point, the resources of modern medicine are infinitesimal. There *is* a nutritional therapy with which the senior author has experimented, in collaboration with his medical colleagues, over a period of many years, in the course of which we have worked with more than 300 sufferers with multiple sclerosis, in many of whom significant benefits were derived. Information concerning this and other therapeutic applications of nutrition mentioned in this text are available to the physician only. The senior author may be addressed in care of this publisher.

Though the average person thinks of epilepsy as producing "fits" or convulsions, there are atypical types which sometimes are responsible for assaulted behavior, "juvenile delinquency," nervousness, irritability, headaches, "bad temper"; and such atypical epilepsies frequently yield to the medications used for grand mal and petit mal epilepsy, or to nutritional therapies, or to a combination of the two. Eliminating sugar, coffee, and cola drinks has proved helpful.

As vitamin B_{12} deficiency may exert its effects on the nervous system before the blood shows signs of pernicious anemia, so may iron deficiency show itself only in nervousness and fatigability, which are likely to be labeled as "emotional." Women are more subject to this, because of the loss of iron in the menstrual, and here one sees an interesting example of the vicious circle that can develop in nutrition. The intense and prolonged menstrual may very often be the product of a diet low in vitamin-B complex and protein. The deficient diet thereby contributes to a cause of iron deficiency, in excessive loss of blood; and iron deficiency itself will contribute to prolongation of the menstrual. It is obvious that the ounce of prevention in nutrition is particularly valuable.

There are iron-dependent enzymes in the body, important ones, which are more sensitive to iron deficiency than is the blood. This explains the "emotional" symptoms, which may be caused by deficiency in iron when there is no evidence of iron deficiency in lowered hemoglobin.

Confusing symptoms which may suggest the purely emotional can, oddly enough, be caused by a "bad bite." Such disturbances of the lower jaw can cause pain in the head, stiffness of the neck, and even intestinal symptoms resembling those of peptic ulcer. Obviously, when the physician cannot find physical evidence of any disease to warrant the symptoms, he is likely to label the sufferer as a neurotic.

A warning should be spelled out against self-diagnosis, presenting here a pretty problem to the authors in that we wish to encourage a high index of suspicion on the part of the layman where the physician's index is unfortunately low, and yet not contribute to hypochondriacal behavior. Persons with genuine emotional disturbances will go to great lengths to avoid both accurate diagnosis and psychological treatment. There remains in the mind of the public some stigma about psychiatric disorders. One is almost persuaded that the average person would rather be accused of a positive Wasserman (the presence of syphillis) than to be accused of neurosis. Indeed, some individuals who have been diagnosed as being neurotic have actually "retreated into cure"—all symptoms disappearing—when threatened with psychological treatment.

We therefore do not wish to encourage the emotionally disturbed to go through repeated physical examinations in an effort to evade psychotherapy. One should not "shop" from physician to physician in an effort to find a comforting diagnosis: in this instance, a diagnosis of a physical disorder to replace one of an emotional disorder. The real answer to this problem lies in the old-fashioned "family doctor," the one who knew the entire history of the family. Unfortunately, he appears to be a fossil. In any case, one good, thorough, *complete*[2] physical examination by a physician whose indexes of suspicion are sufficiently high will save some persons from institutionalization, or unneeded psychotherapy or psychoanalysis.

[2] Including a sugar-tolerance test.

APPENDIX

Carbohydrates: Caution!

Because a high intake of sugar is a pathway to disturbances of the nervous system, digestive disorders, and the unhappy troubles that come with vitamin-B complex deficiency—to say nothing of rotting teeth—the thesis of this section is: *Don't* stay as sweet as you are!

Ultimately, all carbohydrate is sugar. When you take sugar straight, or pleasantly masquerading as candy, dessert, or a hundred other delectables which will be listed for you, you are taking carbohydrate straight. When you eat starchy foods it is like taking a carbohydrate highball; starches are chemically composed of many sugar groups linked together. During and after digestion, these links are severed and the complex starches fall apart to make simple sugars. The process of splitting starch into sugar begins in the mouth by action of an enzyme in saliva. This is why you are advised to chew bread, cereals, and other starchy foods very thoroughly and why it is not good to drink water through a mouthful of food. A rinsing of the mouth after any meal is advisable for many reasons, among them the fact that when the enzymes of saliva change starch into sugar, acidity is created which may be responsible for tooth decay.

It is impossible and probably not very wise to avoid carbohydrate foods entirely, but the carbohydrate intake of the average person is almost invariably too high. These foods, unfortunately for our well-being, are cheap, habit-forming, high in calorie value but devoid of the vitamins needed to burn those calories, and very nice to taste. One of the dangers of a high-carbohydrate intake is that the sweet or starchy foods are filling and too frequently lower the intake of other, needed foods. It has been found that a high carbohydrate diet lengthens convalescence in respiratory infections and predisposes the individual to conditions such as the common cold and sinus trouble.

Physiologically, it is best to eat carbohydrates that furnish body-building elements—vitamins, minerals, protein—as well as calories. This means, eat whole grain cereals, breads, cornmeal, barley, buckwheat, and rye, and brown rice in preference to white. It also means minimizing the use of white sugar and its products—candy, syrup, sugary drinks, jelly, jam, and other similar stomach-filling but body-starving concoctions. A famous physician who practices the science of nutrition has seriously proposed that a law be passed forbidding the sale of sweet foods and drinks within a quarter of a mile of any school!

RULES FOR EATING CARBOHYDRATES

Do not serve more than two foods rich in sugar or starches at the same meal. When you serve bread and potatoes, your starch license has expired for that meal. Dinner that includes peas, bread, potatoes, sugar, cake, and after-coffee mints should also include a vitamin-B complex capsule, a dose of bicarbonate of soda, and the address of the nearest specialist in arthritis and degenerative diseases!

Avoid eating insufficiently baked hot breads. If you must eat them, chew them thoroughly. The rumor that hot breads are indigestible appears to be superstition, and so is the mistaken belief that day-old bread is somehow more nutritious and digestible than fresh. No food gains nutritional value by standing.

Do not eat any carbohydrate foods that are soggy in texture because of improper frying.

When you eat starchy foods, drink milk and eat fruits and vegetables with them.

Above all, keep your total intake of sugar very low. No matter what advertising tells you, do not regard candy as a food, never eat it between meals or on an empty stomach, and always follow it with a glass of water. During World War II, if you remember, the English people were deprived of sugar. According to Lord Woolton, English food czar, this deprivation was a great health benefit for the English. A further advantage to health in the austerity program was the national law that gave the English whole grain bread. As a matter of record, the growing suspicion that people generally have come to attach to the absorbent white cotton optimistically called "modern white bread" has led to nutritional improvement of certain brands. Cornell University, among others, has urged a formula that combines generous amounts of soy and dry skim milk to improve the protein and vitamin value of devitalized white flour. There are also unbleached white breads to which milk and wheat germ have been added. Ironically, our government will not permit these better loaves to be called "bread" or "white bread." Presumably, they are too nutritious!

Sugar, however, is the great white menace. It is so palatable, so stable, so concentrated, so digestible, so "pure." It lacks only one virtue, for it will not support life.

Carbohydrate Content of Popular Foods

NOTE: For those who do not realize the vast amount of sugar concealed in food, thereby making many meals a little "sugar tolerance test," the following sugar assays will be revealing.

Approximate Refined Carbohydrate Content of Popular Foods Expressed in Amounts Equivalent to Teaspoonfuls of Sugar
100 gm. = 20 teaspoonfuls = 3½ oz. = 400 calories

FOOD	AMOUNT, gm.	SERVING	SUGAR EQUIVALENT, Tsp. Sugar
CANDY			
Chewing gum		1c stick	⅓
Chocolate fudge	30	(15 to 1 lb.) 1½ inches sq.	4
Chocolate cream	13	35 to lb.	2
Hershey Bar	60	5c size	7
Lifesaver		1 usual size	⅓
CAKE			
Angel	45	1 piece (1/12 large cake)	6
Chocolate	100	2 layer with icing (1/12 cake)	15
Cream puff (iced)	80	1 average custard filled	5
Doughnut, plain	40	3 inches in diameter	4
Sponge	50	1/10 of average cake	6
COOKIES			
Brownies	20	2 x 2 x ¾ inches	3
Gingersnaps	6	1 medium	1
Macaroons	25	1 large or 2 small	3

FOOD	AMOUNT, *gm.*	SERVING	SUGAR EQUIVALENT, *Tsp. Sugar*
CUSTARDS			
Custard, baked		½ cup	4
Gelatin		½ cup	4
Junket		⅛ quart	3
ICE CREAM			
Ice cream		⅛ quart	5 to 6
Water ice		⅛ quart	6 to 8
PIE			
Apple		⅙ of med. pie	12
Cherry		⅙ of med. pie	14
Custard, coconut		⅙ of med. pie	10
Pumpkin		⅙ of med. pie	10
SAUCE			
Chocolate	30	1 tsp. thick heaping	4½
Marshmallow	7.6	1 aver. (60 to 1 lb.)	1½
SPREADS			
Honey	20	1 tablespoon level or 1 heaping tsp.	3
Jam	20	1 tbsp. level or 1 heaping tsp.	3
Jelly	20	1 tbsp. level or 1 heaping tsp.	2½
Marmalade	20	1 tbsp. level or 1 heaping tsp.	3
MILK DRINKS			
Chocolate (all milk)		1 cup, 5 oz. milk	6
Cocoa (all milk)		1 cup, 5 oz. milk	4
Cocomalt (all milk)		1 glass, 8 oz. milk	4
SOFT DRINKS			
Coca Cola	180	1 bottle, 6 oz.	4⅓
Ginger ale	180	6 oz. glass	4⅓

FOOD	AMOUNT, gm.	SERVING	SUGAR EQUIVALENT, Tsp. Sugar
COOKED FRUITS			
Apple sauce (no sugar)	100	½ cup scant	2
Peaches, canned in syrup	10	2 halves, 1 tbsp. juice	3½
Prunes, stewed, sweetened	100	4 to 5 med. 2 tbsp. juice	8
Rhubarb, stewed	100	½ cup sweetened	8
DRIED FRUITS			
Apricots	30	4 to 6 halves	4
Dates	30	3 to 4 stoned	4½
Figs	30	1½ to 2 small	4
Prunes	30	3 to 4 med.	4
Raisins	30	¼ cup	4
FRUITS AND FRUIT JUICES			
Fruit cocktail	120	½ cup, scant	5
Grapefruit juice unsweetened	100	½ cup, scant	2⅕
Grape juice commercial	100	½ cup, scant	3⅔
Orange juice	100	½ cup, scant	2
Pineapple juice unsweetened	100	½ cup, scant	2⅗

Fats for Fuel

No diet, not even one designed to reduce overweight, should be completely devoid of fats. The human body needs fat to provide fuel, to help utilize the fat-soluble vitamins, to protect nerves, and support internal organs. Fat also serves as a reserve supply for emergencies. If you skip a meal, either through necessity or deliberation, you do your body an injustice for it never skips its needs. A reserve supply of fat comes in very handy at this time, for, in the absence of nourishment, your body feeds on itself.

A diet that is too low in fats produces great irritability, as you must know if you have ever attempted a starvation diet. The reason for this is that the nerve sheaths lose their protective cushions—hence, "raw" nerves, exposed to the impact of irritations. Faddists in diet who resort to fasting in order to lose weight rapidly run into other difficulties as well. When the body is driven to feeding on its own fat, the fat burns with what is called a "smoky flame" and results in a dangerous condition of acidosis. By this is meant true acidosis, which can sometimes be fatal, not the word employed by lay advertisers who claim that it will respond to this or that mild medication.

Fats also supply a flavor to make foods taste better, and eating should be fun. They give a satisfying quality to meals because they slow up digestion, making meals "stick to the ribs." Too much fat, however, retards digestion excessively. This is why too many fat-rich foods in one meal make you feel lethargic. Fats are the natural carriers of some vitamins, too. Some fats—wheat-germ oil or corn oil, for instance—contain fatty acids which may aid in the digestion of other fatty substances.

Do not be indiscriminately harsh on all fried foods, for some may be eaten in moderation without causing distress. Frying has actually been found *less* destructive to certain vitamins than broil-ing but fried foods are somewhat more difficult to digest and should, therefore, be omitted for children or for adults who are tired or ill.

In the process of frying, fat is heated to a temperature that is sometimes high enough to break it down, producing decomposition elements that are highly irritating. There have been reports that overheating fats, or fats carried to the smoking point too often, can cause cancer in animals. Therefore, it is important to select fats that have not been cooked to the decomposition point.

Decomposition Points of Fats

	Centigrade	Fahrenheit
Olive oil	175°	347°
Butter	208°	406°
Leaf lard	214-221°	417-430°
Hydrogenated fats	219-232°	426-450°
Cottonseed and corn oils	222-232°	432-450°

These figures do not mean that you must discard butter for frying. Simply adjust your frying temperature to suit the characteristics of the particular fat you are using but have it as hot as possible—without decomposition—before putting the food in. This way, you sear the food and prevent the loss of juices and the absorption of fat. After the food is seared, reduce the heat. Starchy foods fare better in frying than do proteins. The frying of proteins nearly always lowers their digestibility.

Be careful to avoid using rancid fats, for they interfere with the utilization of vitamin E. Always refrigerate fats, salad oils, and fatty foods, but remember that even refrigeration will not protect these foods against rancidity forever. This is why you may keep beef in a food freezer for a year or longer, while frozen pork, which is fattier, can be stored for only a few months.

Fats for your Furnace

Fat metabolism—as the reader knows after examining the discussion of the low-fat, low-cholesterol diet in Chapter 4—is still not fully understood. It may be that the body has a fixed requirement for both types of fat—unsaturated and saturated. It may be that adults have the capacity to synthesize some of the required fats but that children do not. Inasmuch as certain of the unsaturated fatty acids must be available if the body is to manufacture the saturated ones it may require, a portion of the total fat intake should come from oils that are rich in polyunsaturated fatty acids. However, if more than 20 per cent of the total fat intake is taken from such polyunsaturated fatty acids, the requirement for vitamin E is raised—and may not be met, for two reasons: some of the fats do not contain enough vitamin E; the processing or heating of some destroys at least a part of the vitamin E content. Vitamin E assays of vegetable oils are frequently misleading, since the form of vitamin E most active in the human body is not necessarily the form of vitamin E most richly supplied by the particular fat, which may contain a sizable amount of the other types. The vitamin E value of corn oil, for instance, is quite deceptive, if stated quantitatively. Qualitatively, corn oil does not supply very much of the active form of vitamin E. The recommended type of vegetable oil is cottonseed oil; but the addition of wheat-germ oil to other types of vegetable oil will serve to bring up their values both in polyunsaturated fats and in vitamin E. In the low-carbohydrate reducing diet, which has been a longtime subject for research by the senior author, it has been shown that obtaining 20 per cent of the total fat intake from polyunsaturated fat has an influence in persuading the body to burn its depot fats. How this comes about, nobody knows, but the effect is obvious. This does not mean that consuming polyunsaturated fat as an *addition* to an already adequate diet will have any effect in seducing the body into burning the material in bulges and other undesirable storage places. It is a substitution of polyunsaturated fat for 20 per cent of the saturated fat content of the low-carbohydrate diet that does the trick.

It has long been known that the eczemas displayed by newborn babies sometimes derive from a deficiency in polyunsaturated fat in the pregnant woman's diet. The responses of these children to a few teaspoonfuls of wheat-germ oil or cottonseed oil daily is sometimes dramatic.

Although some medical men prescribe low-fat diets with great freedom, particularly for gall bladder syndrome and in the effort to avoid hardening of the arteries, it must be remembered that the human organism has a requirement for fat; that a low-fat diet may interfere with the activity of a number of essential hormones, which are fat soluble; and with the utilization of a number of vitamins that dissolve in fat. Likewise, a low-fat diet may be deficient in those vitamins which are borne by fats. In the case of gall bladder syndrome, a low-fat diet is actually irrational. The purpose of the treatment of functional gall bladder trouble, where stones are not present (which would justify surgery) should be to encourage the production of freely flowing bile fluid. The effect of a low-fat diet, however, is to "thicken" the bile fluid, so that ultimately such a diet proves not only to be but palliative, but actually may lead to the atrophy of the gall bladder, which then will demand surgery. It is likewise noteworthy that some 57 per cent of the patients who have their gall bladders removed recover all their original symptoms after the operation. This has led the senior author to take a somewhat jaundiced view of low-fat diets in gall bladder syndrome and, indeed, in many other disorders. It is popular to restrict fats in the diet of the child with acne, for instance. In our experience, this may actually lead to increased oiliness of the face, and dermatologists will sometimes discover that the administration of vitamin B_6 is more effective in reducing the oiliness than is tampering with the diet.

In choosing and using fats, therefore, remember the rule of "not too much, not too little," and remember that this group of dietary factors warrants the same intelligent attention as is demanded by the vitamins, protein, and other factors.

Table of Protein Foods

Complete Proteins

Meat

When meat is expensive, the protein value of one ounce of meat may be replaced by:

- 2 tablespoonfuls of cottage cheese
- (1) 1-inch cube of solid cheese
- (1) 1½-inch cube of cream cheese
- 1 ounce of fish
- 1 ounce of fowl
- 2 shrimp
- 1 cup of milk soup
- 1½ teaspoons of soybean[1] flour
- 1 egg
- 1 glass of milk
- ½ cup of custard
- ⅘ ounce nonfat milk powder

Incomplete Proteins

(Serve substantial portions)

Dried

- Beans, Lima
- Beans, marrow
- Lentils
- Peas, chick
- Peas, yellow split

Fresh

- Beans, green
- Beans, Lima
- Beans, wax
- Corn, yellow
- Peas, green
- Rice, brown
- Sprouts, Brussels
- Wheat, rye, barley, whole

[1] *Special Note on Soybeans:* Unheated, soybeans are not complete proteins. Heated they are complete, but the quality of the protein is not quite equivalent to that of dairy products, meat, fish or fowl. Animals depending on soybeans alone for proteins do not grow and reproduce as satisfactorily as those on meat. However, soy protein is far superior to that of other vegetables, and they are good food in many ways.

Vitamins: Their functions and sources

This section comprises a comprehensive survey and discussion of those all-important microscopic substances, the vitamins. You will learn what they are, where they exist, and how vital they are to the healthy functioning of your body.

In order to realize the importance of buying foods rich in these vitamins it is essential that you understand what happens when an animal or human being is deficient in them; it is also edifying to know for what medicinal purposes they are given to patients by physicians. It is hoped that the knowledge you gain here will help you remember the urgent necessity for intelligent food shopping and preparation; for vitamins must be shielded from alkalies, light, air, and excessive heat if they are to be profitable to your well-being.

VITAMIN A

Guardian of your eyes, teeth, bones, skin, soft tissues

Although green growing things are the original source of all the vitamin A in the world, this essential vitamin does not exist *per se* in any vegetable. This may seem to be a contradiction until we learn that the source substance in edible green leaves, fruits, and vegetables is *carotene*, the mother substance from which your liver manufactures the true vitamin A. It therefore follows that when we eat domestic animal liver, fish roe, eggs, and dairy foods —all of which are high in true vitamin A—we are actually eating *carotene*, which has very kindly been assimilated and transformed into the true vitamin by the creatures of earth and sea.

Vitamin-A deficiency reveals itself in many ways. It dries the skin. It delays the formation of the visual purple in the eyes, thereby causing difficulty in adjusting vision to changes in the intensity of light—as, for example, going from a light room into darkness, or vice versa. The soft tissues of the body need the vitamin—those of the nose, mouth, throat, digestive tract, and the male and female genital organs. Other signs of vitamin-A deficiency are soft enamel and many cavities in the teeth; inflammation or pimples at points where hair comes through the skin, especially on the upper back, thighs, and legs; susceptibility to colds, sinus trouble, ear infections, tonsilitis, bronchitis, and similar respiratory infections. A deficiency may predispose an individual to kidney stones and may be a contributory cause of certain allergies.

You will begin to understand why physicians use large doses of vitamin A to help break a cold, to treat certain skin disorders and disturbances of the eyesight, to help guard against return of kidney stones, and in treating some disturbances of the soft tissues.

In nutrition, as in all else, we are highly individualistic. Not all of us convert our *carotene* (from vegetables) into vitamin A in adequate percentages. Some persons change only 25 per cent of their carotene into the true vitamins; diabetics change it inefficiently and must be fed sufficient quantities of the true vitamin, from animal sources, or they may remain deficient even though their diet is high in vegetables and fruit.

Some diseases that interfere with utilization of carotene also block utilization of true vitamin A. In liver disease, gall bladder disturbances, and other ailments that include disturbance of fat metabolism, both carotene and vitamin-A utilization may be impaired. In such cases, true vitamin A in concentrated form, *accompanied by bile salts and lecithin,* may be better utilized, and the diet must be kept as high in fats as tolerance permits.

When extra vitamin A is given to industrial workers who labor under bright lights, they become much more efficient in their work and complain less of eyestrain and headaches. These workers also find that their colds are less frequent and far less severe. It must be pointed out, however, that vitamin A alone is often not enough to correct conditions of eyestrain and chronic colds.

Other vitamins and certain minerals are also involved, which is why multiple supplements are preferable to single vitamins or arbitrary combinations. In order to utilize vitamin A properly, the body needs bile salts. (This is true of any fat-soluble vitamin—A, D, E, K.) If the diet is deficient in fat or the body deficient in bile salt production, the efficacy of vitamin capsules is decreased. Individuals who do not seem to gain heightened resistance to colds through the use of multiple supplements sometimes do so when the vitamins are administered in unconcentrated cod liver oil. The answer to this puzzle is found in the oil's *fat* content, which is not present in the fish-liver *concentrate* ordinarily used in a capsule.

Vitamin A is destroyed rather easily in cooking and there are considerable losses in canning. Freezing of foods, however, sacrifices only a slight amount. Losses in dried foods may be high. A fresh apricot contains 50 per cent more vitamin A than its dehydrated counterpart.

A word about your requirements: Although the government believes that 5,000 units of vitamin A daily is sufficient for an active man or woman, 6,000 for a pregnant woman, and 8,000 for a nursing mother, research has convinced many authorities that these amounts do not represent a sufficient margin of safety even for the "average" person. For those who are not "average" such minimal intake may actually result in serious deficiency. Dr. H. C. Sherman of Columbia University has reported that increased intake of the vitamin—four times the maintenance intake—adds considerably to the life span of animals, literally extending their prime of life. We therefore agree that 15,000 units of vitamin A daily are likely to raise individual resistance to respiratory infections and tooth decay. The higher amount also provides protection to eyes and soft tissues. Pro rata, in terms of body weight the same daily intake holds for school-age children and may be used to calculate the requirements of infants and preschool children.

Try to obtain generous amounts of vitamin A in your diet from both animal and vegetable sources. You may raise your intake to ideal amounts without increasing calories by using multiple supplements. Consult the chart on foods and their vitamin contents at the end of this section. Regular consumption of recommended foods should yield at least 10,000 units of vitamin A daily. When you "feel a cold coming on," large doses of additional vitamin A may be used to throw it off. Don't wait until the cold breaks in all its miserable fury; reach for extra vitamin A at the first sniffle.

VITAMIN B

"Group insurance" for your nerves and energy!

Vitamin B was the first of all the vitamins to be discovered and, at the beginning, was believed to be a single substance. A quarter of a century of intensive research later, the original substance was divided into two parts, one of which was vitamin B_1 as it remains today. The second part, named vitamin B_2, was soon discovered to be divisible also, and the scientists began to realize that they had in their hands a very complex situation indeed. Eagerly probing the secrets of this amazing vitamin-B complex, the chemists soon extracted and synthesized an orange powder which we call vitamin B_2.

Having gone so far, the scientists ventured further and soon triumphantly brought to recognition Vitamin B_6, which was finally synthesized as pyridoxin, a vitamin of many marvels.

Next in the romantic saga of the B complex came niacin (nicotinic acid), which was found effective in treating pellagra. Ironically, nicotinic acid was first manufactured around the time of the Civil War, before vitamins were known. A reaction product of nicotine, the therapeutically precious factor of niacin remained a laboratory curiosity while thousands of people died of pellagra.

Still more treasures were to come from the remarkable B complex, and our lives are now enriched by the factors choline, biotin, para-amino-benzoic acid, pantothenic acid, the extrinsic factor, and many others. Some of these have been synthesized and some have not. To put the unsynthesized ones into a capsule, therefore, it is necessary to use natural sources such as yeast, liver, rice polishings, wheat germ, or milk whey.

Each of the B vitamins has a separate and distinct function in the body. Although some of these functions overlap, one vitamin cannot replace another. These vitamins are always found together in the same foods, but in varying proportions. Since they are always found together, you cannot be deficient in only *one* of them. Therefore—even though symptoms may, on the surface, indicate a vitamin-B_1 deficiency alone—it is not wise to take only that vitamin. Full results will be obtained only by using the entire vitamin-B complex to provide supplies of all the vitamins of the B group, which you may need, and the absence of which probably counteracts the effect of the vitamin B_1 you are getting.

To the nutritionist, many of the disturbing symptoms of that period of life we call "middle age" are based on vitamin-B complex deficiency. Certain of our customary food habits contribute unnecessarily and destructively to these deficiencies. We perpetuate deficiency, for example, when we eat processed carbohydrates from which vitamin-B factors are removed. If the food you eat has been deprived of the B vitamins, you are asking your body to burn sugar, rice, flour, and similar foods without wicks. It is an unfair demand, for your body cannot and will not do so. The result is that you fill the furnace (your body) with fuel (carbohydrates) which will not burn fully. Your furnace then will be filled with the smoke of partial burning. That is its technical description. In daily living, this "smokiness" translates into nervousness, indigestion, constipation, or any of a thousand common disorders.

It follows, therefore, since every mouthful of carbohydrate requires a certain amount of vitamin B_1 and vitamin-B complex to help burn it, that eating too much starch or sugar can create a deficiency. Every calorie you consume must be released (burned) before you can utilize it. Calories from carbohydrates—and that means sugar and starch—cannot be released without the vitamins of the B complex. Unprocessed carbohydrates—whole wheat, brown rice, whole buckwheat, whole corn, whole barley—contain the needed vitamins. Their overprocessed counterparts—white rice, white flour, and white sugar—will not. Although "enriched" flour contains three important vitamins of the B complex group, we consider it less than sensible to remove fifteen vitamins and replace three. This, however, is what we accept from the baking industry.

Remembering always that the entire B complex is necessary in the diet, let us examine the various components of this group in close-up:

Vitamin B₁

Known also as *thiamine chloride*, this vitamin is specifically necessary for growth, normal heart function, circulation, blood building, appetite, digestion, and functioning of the nervous system.

Persons deficient in vitamin B_1 develop neurasthenia (nervous breakdown), apathy, lethargy, oversensitivity to pain or noise, uncertainty of memory, loss of morale, digestive disturbances, faulty metabolism of starches and sugars, constipation, nausea, lack of appetite, and excessively rapid beating of the heart—which is sometimes followed by excessively slow beating. With these disturbances may also come abnormally low activity of the thyroid gland and practically no resistance to fatigue. Irritability and loss of resistance to suggestion are among the phenomena of a vitamin-B_1 deficiency in human beings.

If you simply will not eat wheat germ, whole wheat, and whole rye bread and cereals—or cannot, because you are not allowed bulkage—use the B complex in supplementary form. Adult intake of B_1 should not be less than 10 mg. daily.

Vitamin B₂

Vitamin B_2 (or G—or riboflavin) is needed for the soft tissues of the body, where it helps the cells to exchange oxygen. It is, therefore, used with vitamin B_1 to help the "burning" of starches and sugars. It is important to the eyes, where oxygen transfers are vital; and because riboflavin is sensitive to light, the vitamin also functions specifically to aid vision.

Disturbances of digestion, faulty blood building, burning of the eyes and lids, cracking of the corners of the lips, impaired lactation in nursing mothers, skin disorders, and cataract are among the deficiency symptoms produced by lack of riboflavin. Large doses of this vitamin have been reported to reduce the "sweet tooth" of children and adults, to raise resistance to athlete's foot and similar fungus infections, and to bring relief to sufferers of neurodermatitis, atopic eczema, and allergy. Riboflavin is found in liver, somewhat less richly in lean meat, in milk, and in yeast. At least five milligrams of riboflavin daily in *addition* to normal intake in food is the author's personal habit.

Vitamin B_6

The other name for this vitamin is pyridoxin, and it is important to the skin, to the utilization of fats and protein, the building of blood, and the function of the nerves and muscles. This is one of the most promising of all the vitamins and it is almost certain that continuing research will discover more marvels than are now known. It has already been seen to accomplish near miracles —restoring function to paralyzed legs (where nerves were involved in the pathology); shrinking enlarged hearts, and relieving distressed intestinal tracts after a lifetime of misery for dyspepsia sufferers. Doctors have reported that pellagra patients do not recover their full strength until given vitamin B_6. Surgeons administer the vitamin before operations to avoid postoperative nausea from ether and many obstetricians find that the nausea of pregnancy can sometimes be interrupted with vitamin B_6.

Because of the effects of this vitamin on muscle tone, it is frequently used in the treatment of multiple sclerosis and numerous other nerve and muscle disorders, which increasingly trouble our generation. It is also helpful for its effects on the centers of the autonomous nervous system, which control rhythm and fine movements. Hence, vitamin B_6, vitamin E, and other food factors are used in the treatment of cerebral palsy, Parkinson's disease (senile palsy), epilepsy, and similar disorders where there is faulty transmission of nerve impulses to the muscular system. It has been found helpful in the treatment of adolescent acne, as well.

Vitamin B_6 has the effect of conserving protein and is therefore administered when there are losses of protein, as in kidney disease. While oral use of the vitamin is possible and occasionally helpful, many of its uses are best introduced by injection. Vitamin B_6 is incorporated in some of the multiple vitamin capsules available on the market, and it is sensible to supplement diet with a minimum of 5 milligrams daily. Again, this supplementary intake might not be necessary if our more popular foods were not robbed of it in the course of processing.

Vitamin B_{12}

This vitamin, supplied in the diet by milk and liver, was originally called the "animal protein factor," indicating that it is not obtainable from vegetable sources. Vitamin B_{12} appears to be the specific externally derived preventive for pernicious anemia. It is the only vitamin that contains a mineral (cobalt) as part of its molecule. Its action differs from that of folic acid in combating pernicious anemia in that it protects the body against the degeneration of the nerves that frequently accompanies the disease. Vitamin B_{12} is available by injection and in a form which may be taken orally. An amazingly minute dosage is sufficient to produce benefits in pernicious anemia, stimulate retarded growth in children, aid in the treatment of bronchial asthma, help recovery in certain skin disorders, and serve as a general "tonic" for adults. Dosages as small as 5 to 25 micrograms are effective and a wise procedure.

Niacin

Known also as nicotinic acid, niacinamide, nicotinamide, nicotinic acid amide, niacin is needed, like the other B vitamins, for normal liver function; for the functioning of the nervous system and the brain; by the soft tissues—from mouth to reproductive organs; by the skin; for circulation, and for burning of starches and sugars.

Niacin deficiency upsets the higher centers of the brain, causes nerve disorders ranging from simple neurasthenia to outright insanity. In the presence of a deficiency, the brain disturbances include loss of a sense of humor, uncertainty of memory, negative behavior, and delusions. The tongue may appear purple or bright red, bare and shiny. The gums become swollen and angry and rise on the teeth. The skin breaks out.

Although we speak of niacin and niacinamide as being synonymous, the average vitamin supplement contains niacinamide rather than niacin. This is because the amide does not dilate the blood vessels and stimulate circulation as noticeably as does niacin. The manufacturers of vitamins protect you against feeling excessively warm after taking their capsules.

In medical treatment, however, physicians use niacin to stimulate circulation in conditions ranging from simple cold feet to disturbances of hearing and even migraine headache. He also uses niacinamide to treat nervous disorders, skin diseases, disturbances of the mouth and gums (such as trench mouth), liver disorders, and chronic digestive upsets. The American Medical Association has remarked that "the health of the mouth in many supposedly normal individuals is improved by dosages of niacinamide." A daily intake of a minimum of 35 to 100 milligrams is good protection.

Para-amino-benzoic Acid

This is a tongue-twister, and so we have given it the professional nickname of paba. Back in 1942, the government decided that paba was a vitamin and criticized any vitamin-B complex preparation that did not supply it. The following year, however, Uncle Sam's bureau reversed its opinion, claiming that paba is not only not a vitamin but is not a drug either, which reduces it to being merely a chemical—in the opinion of the government.

This writer is convinced, federal authority notwithstanding, that paba is legitimately a vitamin; that it has a profound beneficial effect on glandular function, and that the human being has a definite requirement for it. Physicians have used it successfully, with other B complex vitamins, in recoloring of prematurely gray hair. It has been prescribed in the treatment of sterility in women. It has been found to help the body retain salicylic acid and is used in the treatment of rheumatic fever, Rocky Mountain spotted fever, and similar disorders. One authority has reported that paba helps to reduce the activity of an overactive thyroid gland, and it has been used to reduce the size of a simple goiter. An eminent research group has evidence to show that paba helps to normalize the function of the pituitary gland, which explains its helpfulness in the treatment of sterility and in the management of those types of arthritis—such as rheumatoid arthritis—where pituitary misbehavior is definitely known to be involved.

Inositol

At this writing, not too much is known about inositol and the role it plays in body chemistry. It is believed, however, that it is needed by the hair, muscles, and liver—for it is known to be essential in the proper digestion of fats. It is also important in helping the body to utilize vitamin E, with which it may combine chemically in the digestive tract. Inositol is essential to the functioning of the brain, and is richly found in the heart muscle. Certain mental disorders may arise from malutilization of the vitamin, for these disorders—as well as retarded mentality—have been helpfully treated with inositol. Physicians also use this little known vitamin in the treatment of diabetes, arteriosclerosis, gall bladder trouble, intolerance to fats, multiple sclerosis, muscular dystrophy, cerebral palsy, and other disorders affecting nerve-muscle function.

Inositol, like paba, is processed out of many popular foods.

Choline

Generously provided by organ meats and eggs, choline is essential to normal metabolism of fats. It is needed by the kidneys, for lactation, and for liver function. It is required by the thymus gland and is important to the kidneys and spleen.

Choline deficiency impairs liver and kidney function, causing hemorrhaging of the kidneys; it produces intolerance to fats and fatty degeneration of the liver, and may result in a blocking of the transmission of nerve impulses to the muscles. For these reasons, physicians are prescribing choline in large amounts in the treatment of diabetes, gall bladder trouble, intolerance to fats, and numerous other disorders. Choline is also used in the treatment of muscular dystrophy, glaucoma, and arteriosclerosis. It is more effective when accompanied by inositol and other vitamins that affect fat utilization.

Calcium Pantothenate

Available commercially, this vitamin is a growth essential, important to the skin, and needed by the adrenal gland. It also affects the functioning of the entire digestive tract. Although symptoms of deficiency in this vitamin are not clearly known, it is known that animals lacking the factor develop gray hair, toughening of the skin, skin disease, constipation, granulation of the eyelids, destruction of adrenal tissue, and digestive disorders. Pantothenic acid deficiency also prevents the animal from building antibodies in its blood, thus decreasing resistance to infection.

Physicians use calcium pantothenate as they use other vitamin-B complex factors—in the treatment of digestive disturbances[1] (especially in cases where the stomach empties too slowly) and occasionally as an adjunct in the treatment of anemias. Since the vitamin favorably affects the adrenal gland, it is used in the treatment of rheumatoid arthritis and other conditions showing depressed adrenal function.

[1] Including regional ileitis.

This factor is, like so many others, processed out of many popular foods. It will be found in protective amounts in good multiple supplement capsules.

Folic Acid

Essential to normal size and amounts of red blood cells in the blood, folic acid is also necessary to liver function, where part of blood manufacture takes place. Folic acid is also interrelated with gland function; chicks deficient in this vitamin respond to female hormone treatment only one fortieth as much as chicks well supplied with it. Folic acid deficiency contributes to digestive disturbances and liver dysfunction and may also contribute to pernicious anemia and lowered hydrochloric acid production. Physicians are therefore using folic acid in the treatment of anemias and intolerance to fats.

Vegetables subjected to room temperatures lose a considerable portion of their folic acid values.

Biotin

This vitamin is an enormously potent stimulant to the growth of cells and is therefore, undoubtedly important in general growth. Deficiency is known to produce a type of anemia, complicated with a skin disease. Biotin is among the host of vitamins removed from processed foods. Daily supplements supply us with added biotin, for it is intrinsically a part of any source of concentrated vitamin-B complex. We can obtain added quantities of it by the use of brewer's yeast and wheat germ.

VITAMIN C

Especially if you're restless—or pregnant!

Vitamin C is an excellent example of the "Factor of Demand," one of the elements in life which determine our need for vitamins and for other food elements. If you work very hard, "normal" nutrition—normal, that is, for the average person—becomes inadequate for you. During the middle ages, soldiers developed the hemorrhages of scurvy in their legs; the blacksmith suffered with scurvy of the right arm. These, respectively, were the points of stress. The sailor fell prey to a total scurvy, because he was active with all his muscles.

Thus it is that a pregnant woman may develop varicose veins. Not only is she carrying extra weight and walking for exercise (both of these constitute hard work) but her unborn child imposes a greatly increased demand for vitamin C. Unless the expectant mother's intake is appreciably higher than "normal," her supply becomes exhausted and, in protest, her legs develop varicosities.[2]

Of all the vitamins, C is the easiest to obtain in assured amounts from natural foods, for citrus juice or whole fruit is always rich in it. One of the most important functions of the vitamin is in its material aid to the body in the manufacture of "collagen," the "glue" that holds the cells of the body together. An early sign of vitamin-C deficiency is bleeding gums; another is a tendency of the small blood vessels in other parts of the body to break on slight strain. This breaking is called *petechia*. One of the clinical tests for vitamin-C deficiency is binding the arm and counting the number of petechial hemorrhages exhibited. If too many appear, the patient is sent home with a high citrus fruit diet.

The United States Department of Agriculture states that there are probably thousands of people in this country suffering from an *unrecognized* vitamin-C deficiency. Restlessness and irritability in infants and children, "spring fever" in adults, or a run-down feeling at any time of the year may mark the deficiency. Without one outward symptom of trouble, a person may be in a state of deficiency more dangerous than scurvy itself, says the Department, which warns that such a condition—undetected and unchal-

[2] There are other nutritional factors involved: roughage, vitamin-B complex, vitamin E.

lenged—can damage teeth and bones and weaken the blood system to the point where it can no longer resist or fight infections.

The precise role of vitamin C in building resistance to shock and infection is not yet clearly understood, nor is its function in helping the body to create immunity. We do know that an animal extravagantly nourished with the vitamin will throw off the effects of a dose of poison that quickly kills an animal less well nourished with the vitamin. This, even though the succumbing animal is not deficient in the true sense of the word. It dies by poison although not a single sign of scurvy itself is displayed.

Loss of appetite marks a C deficiency, and so do a disinclination to activity, a congestion and sponginess of the gums, and an anemia that does not respond to liver or iron feeding. Infants low in vitamin C have poor muscle function, lack of appetite, anemia, cessation in weight gain or actual loss of weight, susceptibility to infection, intestinal disturbances, and a tendency toward frequent crying.

Because of increased requirements, deficiency may occur frequently in pregnancy, tuberculosis, osteomyelitis, overactive thyroid states, rheumatic fever, pneumonia, and other diseases in which high fever depletes the body store of the vitamin. For, although obtainable with comparative ease, the vitamin is poorly stored by the body. Ulcers, both peptic and varicose, require high vitamin-C intake to guard against delayed healing; yet the peptic ulcer diet is often deficient in this vitamin.

In many persons, utilization of vitamin C is very poor. Cases have been known in which a full pint of orange juice daily did not bring a response in patients known to be deficient. This means that a high intake of vitamin C is necessary on two counts: because saturation of the body with C is believed to be the ideal state and because such a precautionary intake *overcomes* the danger of poor utilization.[3]

[3] It is also effective against some disorders refractory to lower doses—slipped disc, as an example.

The ideal vitamin-C intake for adults is set at up to 150 milligrams (one milligram equals 20 units). Generally, this means 20 units (or one milligram) per pound of body weight. Very active people will need more, children proportionately less. An ounce of orange juice supplies 15 milligrams, or 300 units.

Allergies to fruits—particularly to those rich in vitamin C—are frequent. Those who are in this position, as well as those who have limited budgets, must turn to other sources for this vitamin. In using the vitamin-C chart, therefore, you need not despair if citrus fruits are beyond your capacity or your purse. Depend on cabbage, preferably served as cole slaw, green and red peppers, and the recommended fresh green leaves. Tomato juice, although only half as rich in vitamin C as citrus juice, is still a good source and may be used by those allergic to citrus fruits. Drink twice as much.

Among other requirements, vitamin C is specifically needed by the adrenal gland. When a shock of any kind stimulates this gland into producing its hormones, the reserves of vitamin C present there would be exhausted in as little as five seconds. If the blood does not generously and promptly resupply the vitamin, both you and your adrenal gland will suffer. It is a vitamin that appears to have the property, in large doses, of stimulating latent tuberculosis into revealing itself. A very large intake of the vitamin may, therefore, be undesirable in those cases of bronchial asthma which portend latent tuberculosis. This is for your physician to decide, but it should be remembered that vitamin A offsets this action. Because vitamin C has a diuretic effect, it is useful in congestive heart disease and other conditions that prompt the physician to promote fluid excretion. Concentrated vitamin C is sometimes very effective in relieving the symptoms of food and inhalant allergies. It protects against—and relieves—ivy poisoning and prickly heat.

In conclusion, and at the risk of repetition, be sure to maintain high intake of vitamin C unless pathological conditions say otherwise. Feed your children raw fruit in lieu of candy; give them fruit juices (followed by a little water) instead of soda pop; buy fresh orange juice rather than soda at the corner drug store; make a habit of slaws and salads. You and your family will emerge with prettier complexions, healthier nails, tougher gums, better blood, and improved resistance. Isn't that inducement enough?

Remember, too, that C does *not* stand for Cooking—it is temperamental and volatile; too much or too long subjection to heat destroys it. Use such raw foods as your stomach will tolerate. It should not object to the nourishing goodness of foods *au naturel*.

Bio-Flavonoids

Bio-flavonoids aid vitamin C in its roles in the body. Where vitamin C may be protective against allergy, bio-flavonoids protect against the type of violent allergic reaction called anaphylaxis, which can be fatal. Vitamin C affects the larger blood vessels; bio-flavonoids increase the strength and decrease the permeability of the smaller vessels. For this reason, they are used in treating high blood pressure and to help guard against strokes, and are useful in diabetes, in helping avoid eye hemorrhage, and in the treatment of glaucoma, swelling of the ankles, and allergies. The factor is supplied in the diet by grapefruit, oranges, grapes, liver, and asparagus. It requires two grapefruits or four large oranges to yield a truly satisfactory daily intake of this factor, however, and so not less than 200 mg. of bio-flavonoids should be provided by tablets used supplementarily. Bio-flavonoid concentrates are available.

VITAMINS D, E, AND K

For glorious glands

VITAMIN D

Actually, no foods will offer a safe supply of vitamin D. Daily intake of 400 units will be adequate for child or adult. (Note: an *infant's* intake of vitamin D should not *exceed* 400 units.) This amount may be derived from:

1. A few hours of summer sunshine on the body daily.
2. Alphabet capsules or syrups containing natural fish-liver oil concentrates.
3. A sun lamp of the carbon arc type, or one of the quartz tube type. (These give the full quota of "bands" of sunlight that create vitamin D; other types may give fewer "bands.")

Vitamin D is not used only to *prevent* rickets. The preventive dosage—1,000 units daily—may rise to as high as 50,000 units or more daily to *cure* active rickets. The vitamin is sometimes helpful in acne, together with B_6 and superimposed on supplementing with alphabet vitamins. It is most important to dentition. Breast-fed babies need just as much vitamin D as formula-fed; premature babies need twice as much, and expectant and nursing mothers may need as much as 2,000 units daily.[4]

High dosage of synthetic vitamin D is sometimes very helpful in arthritis. In this use, the vitamin is employed in such high dosage that it is acting as a chemical rather than as a vitamin. The amount may run from 50,000 to 200,000 units daily, or even higher. It should be administered only under a physician's direction, because this vitamin—especially in such large quantities—is sometimes toxic. Individuals with heart trouble complicating the arthritis should be particularly careful in this use of vitamin D, for the nausea it may cause would be dangerous to a cardiac patient.

Other uses for vitamin D include the treatment of psoriasis, tetany, myopia (near-sightedness) and disturbances in the parathyroid glands. Remember that vitamin D (and, for that matter, all other vitamins) cannot perform its work without minerals—primarily calcium and phosphorus, secondarily magnesium and iron.

[4] Except in excessively rare instances of sensitivity to the vitamin.

VITAMIN E

In the research laboratory, animals in which a vitamin-E deficiency is induced develop wasting and weakness of muscle tissue, disorders of the reproductive glands, sterility, miscarriages, stillbirths, and spontaneous abortions.

In humans as well, habitual miscarriage or spontaneous abortion has been traced to vitamin-E deficiency. The vitamin is concerned with the firmness of the hold taken by the placenta upon the wall of the womb; apparently E deficiency either weakens the placental grip or allows it to penetrate too deeply, thus weakening the wall itself. In either event, miscarriage will result.

We therefore find physicians prescribing vitamin E for women who have a record of miscarriages, and for men who show evidence of testicular degeneration evidenced by impaired fertility. They prescribe the vitamin for wasting of muscles; during menopause; and in liver disturbances accompanied by intolerance to fats. We have observed tremendous benefits from treatment with vitamin E in heart disease, and the writer's medical colleagues report usefulness for the vitamin in the treatments for cerebral palsy, senile palsy (Parkinson's disease), Mongolian idiocy, hydrocephalus, epilepsy, chorea (St. Vitus). Vitamin E is also used for "nervous" disorders and mental diseases of many types and is often helpful where shock treatment has failed.

Like the B group, vitamin E is really a complex. It contains alpha tocopherol and the beta and gamma tocopherols. Of these, the alpha form is more effective and is the form in which the vitamin is most commonly offered in concentrates. Alphabet capsules should contain either alpha tocopherol or mixed tocopherols, for two reasons: it helps to stabilize the other vitamins chemically; and, secondly, vitamin E is interrelated with the other vitamins.

Vitamin E is fat soluble, as are vitamins A, D, and K. This means that disturbances in fat metabolism may interfere with the individual's utilization of the vitamin. It also means that insufficient production of bile salts may produce a deficiency in a fat-soluble vitamin. This explains why so many women have miscarriages as possible signs of vitamin-E deficiency despite the fact that the vitamin is very widespread in foods and fairly stable in cooking processes. Incidentally, a large part of the deficiency incidence may be traced to the devitalization of civilized man's (and woman's) bread, which has lost its wheat germ, the best source of vitamin E in foods. Wheat germ—or vitamin E—has not generally been restored to enriched bread, an omission that may have its effect on generations to come. There seems indeed to be a destiny that shapes our beginnings as well as our ends, for nature made the child's life line dependent upon a substance derived from the "birthplace" of new life in wheat. That is what wheat germ is.

Since, therefore, vitamin E is removed from many popular foods, the author supplements his own diet with alpha tocopherol, 100 mgs. plus multiple vitamin supplements—and adds more to the diet by use of wheat-germ oil in salad dressings, by using wheat germ, whole grains, and eating bread reinforced with the germ.

While still promising no miracles, it is suggested that you add to the intake of vitamin E in your family's diet. It may be that menopause will be subsequently less trying to the female members, and neuropathic disorders less of a threat to all.

VITAMIN K

Vitamin K is essential for the production of prothrombin, a substance which aids the blood in clotting. It is, therefore, important to liver function, the liver being involved in the manufacture of blood. It is also essential to the proper utilization of vitamin E.

Vitamin K is fat soluble, requiring a good fat intake and bile salts to metabolize it. Consequently, such diseases as obstructive jaundice interfere with utilization of the vitamin. When obstructive jaundice was operated upon in the past, the vitamin K deficiency inherent in the disease would cause prolonged bleeding and, in too many cases, death in the operating room. In liver disease, obstructive jaundice, and other similar conditions, therefore, the doctor orders vitamin K, especially if an operation is scheduled. An injection of the vitamin is sometimes given in labor; it may also be given to a newborn baby. The vitamin-K activity in the blood of a brand new infant is rather unsatisfactory until the first week passes. This means that if a baby less than a week old is cut or injured, bleeding is prolonged. In this connection it is interesting to recall that the Hebrew religion taboos operations upon a child until it has lived through its first week.

New evidence indicates that supplements of vitamin K will help to protect the liver and blood of those who work with lead or other heavy metals, or those who must regularly take cinchophen or salicylates (such as aspirin).

Vitamin K has been used successfully in the treatment of coronary thrombosis, which seems paradoxical when it is remembered that this is a blood-clotting vitamin and that coronary heart disease results from the formation of a clot. It has been shown, however, that in some cases of this cardiac disorder, the hemorrhage is within the wall of the artery. Vitamin K would help to stop the hemorrhage and thereby rectify the trouble at its source. Thus, in two groups of patients with acute attacks of coronary thrombosis, the mortality in the group given low doses of vitamin K was 38 per cent; in the group given high doses of the vitamin, it was less than 4 per cent.

Many green leaves, some fats, and egg yolk supply vitamin K. Intestinal bacteria synthesize it.

Conditions Under Which Vitamin-Mineral Intake Must Be Raised

(Assembled from medical reports)

I. *Interference with food intake*

Gastrointestinal diseases as
   Acute gastroenteritis
   Gallbladder disease
   Peptic ulcer
   Diarrheal diseases
Food allergy
Mental disorders as
   Neurasthenia
   Psychoneurosis
Operations and anesthesia
Infectious diseases associated with lack of appetite
Loss of teeth
Heart failure (nausea, vomiting)
Pulmonary disease (vomiting due to cough)
Toxemia of pregnancy (nausea and vomiting)
Visceral pain (as in renal colic, and angina that produces nausea
   and vomiting)
Neurologic disorders which interfere with self-feeding
Migraine

II. *Interference with absorption*

Diarrheal diseases as
   Ulcerative and mucous colitis
   Intestinal parasites
   Intestinal tuberculosis
   Sprue
Gastrointestinal fistulas
Diseases of liver and gallbladder
Lack of hydrochloric acid

III. *Interference with utilization*

Liver disease
Diabetes mellitus
Chronic alcoholism

IV. *Increased requirement*

Abnormal activity, as associated with prolonged strenuous physical exertion, with lack of sufficient sleep or rest

Fever

Hyperthyroidism or other instances of high glandular activity

Pregnancy and lactation

V. *Increased excretion*

Biliary or gastrointestinal fistula

Perspiration

Loss of protein in nephritis and nephrosis

Long-continued excessive fluid intake as in urinary tract infections

VI. *Therapeutic measures*

Therapeutic diets, as in
   Sippy regimen
   Gallbladder disease
   Antiobesity diets
Antacids
Mineral oil
Diuretics

In each of the conditions named above, supplementing of the diet with concentrated vitamins and minerals is essential. The physician should be consulted.

One great cause of deficiency is not named here: That is the factor of *faulty utilization in the absence of disease: the individual does not utilize foods well because of congenital inability to do so.* From the author's experience with tens of thousands of individuals who respond dramatically to concentrates (*after years on very good diet*), faulty utilization must be very common, for on no other ground can this response be explained. It is particularly interesting to observe the reaction of older persons who are given vitamin-mineral concentrates. They do not respond to improved diet—or they have no time to wait for its gradual accumulation of benefits; but the concentrates bring to many middle-aged and aged individuals something approximating a new lease on life.

FOODS AND THEIR VITAMIN CONTENT

The following charts list the more highly nutritious foods, richest in vitamins and minerals. In using these charts, remember that the foods under Group I are usually higher in vitamin-mineral values than those under Group II. Consequently, you might serve and eat larger portions of Group II foods than of those in Group I. All the foods in both groups are nutritious, however, and the list is intended as a useful guide for shopping. If one food is more expensive than the other and they are listed in the same group under the specific vitamin, let price and taste be your criteria.

The omission of a food does not mean that it has no value. It means only that it is not a *rich* source of vitamins and minerals. Such unlisted foods do have distinct usefulness. For example, whole gelatin desserts have no vitamin content at all of themselves, yet the use of gelatin—aside from its value as a source of some protein acids—permits you to serve fruits and vegetables in appetizing forms, thereby raising the vitamin-mineral content of your diet.

When you prepare food for the table, please observe the cooking instructions which are given in Chapter 19.

Intelligent use of these charts will happily result in lowering your food bills while improving your nutrition.

VITAMIN A

(*Carotene—Provitamin A*)

Light helps destroy vitamin A, and air devitalizes it. Shield your foods!

Functions: Needed for growth, eyes, skin, nose, throat, ears, lungs, reproduction, energy, resistance against infection.

Vegetables

Beans, green string
Beet tops
Broccoli
Cabbage leaves (as greens)
Carrots
Chard leaves
Chicory
Collards
Dandelion greens
Endive, green
Escarole

Green soybeans
Kale
Lettuce, loose green leaf
Mustard greens
Peas, green
Peppers, red
Potatoes, sweet
Squash, yellow
Tomatoes and juice, red
Turnip tops
Watercress

Artichokes
Cabbage, Chinese
Cabbage, green head
Celery, green
Corn, yellow

Lettuce, green head
Okra
Peppers, green
Sprouts, Brussels
Tomatoes, green

Animal products

Butter
Cheese
Cream
Eggs

Fish-liver oils
Fish roe
Liver, any kind

(*Fish-liver oils are very rich in true vitamin A.*)

Fat, beef
Fat, poultry
Ice cream
Kidney

Milk, whole
Oysters
Salmon, red

Grains and Seeds

Cornmeal, yellow

Soybeans

Fruits

Apricots
Avocados
Mangoes

Papayas
Peaches, yellow
Prunes

GROUP II

Bananas	Oranges—yellow juiced
Canteloupe	Pineapple
Cherries	

VITAMIN B_1

(Thiamin)

Functions: Needed for growth, starch and sugar utilization, appetite, nerves, intestinal action, energy.

Grains and Seeds

GROUP I

Beans	Peanut butter, raw
Barley, whole	Peanuts, raw (Va. Reds)
Bran	Peas, cow
Buckwheat	Rice, brown
Cercals, whole grain	Rice, polishings
Cereals, whole (Breakfast)	Rye, whole
Corn, whole	Soybean, flour
Cornmeal, whole yellow	Wheat germ
Hominy, whole grain	Wheat, whole
Oats	

GROUP II

Almonds	Peanuts, roasted
Brazil nuts	Peanut butter, roasted (Va. Reds)
Chestnuts	Pecans
Hazelnuts	Walnuts

(Milling methods that remove the grain germ also remove B vitamins.)

Animal Products

GROUP I

Chicken	Liver
Heart	Oysters
Kidney	Pork, lean

GROUP II

Bacon, rare	Eggs
Beef	Milk
Brains	

Vegetables

GROUP I

Artichokes	Kale
Beans, green string	Peas, green
Beans, Lima	Potatoes, sweet
Beet greens	Potatoes, white
Broccoli	Soybeans, fresh
Cabbage	Spinach
Carrots	Sprouts, Brussels
Collards	Turnip greens
Corn, sweet yellow	Yeast

GROUP II

Asparagus	Mustard greens
Dandelion greens	Okra
Eggplant	Tomatoes
Kohlrabi	Turnip
Lettuce	Watercress

(Vitamin B dissolves in water. Save and serve your cooking water in soup or gravy.)

Fruits

Avocados	Oranges
Bananas	Pears
Canteloupe	Pineapple
Citrus fruits	Raisins
Dates	Raspberries, red
Figs	Watermelon
Grapes	

(Excessive cooking, high temperatures, and air are all destructive to vitamins.)

VITAMIN B₂ (G)

(Riboflavin)

Functions: Needed for life span, skin, eyes, digestion, energy.

Animal Products

Visceral meats, such as liver, are very rich in vitamin B_2 (G) as well as other vitamins.

GROUP I

Cheese	Kidney
Eggs	Liver
Heart	Milk (whole, skim, evaporated)

GROUP II

Bacon	Pork
Ham	Veal
Mutton	

Fruits

GROUP I

Avocados	Peaches
Grapefruit	Pears
Mangoes	

GROUP II

Apples	Guavas
Bananas	Melons
Figs	Raisins

Vegetables

Light destroys vitamin G. Cook carefully to preserve this vitamin in these delicious vegetables.

Beet greens	Kale
Broccoli	Leaves, other green
Collards	Lettuce, green
Dandelion greens	Mustard greens
Endive	Peas, green
Escarole	

Grains and Seeds

Yeast and grains are perfect complements—as found in whole grain bread.

Peanuts	Soybeans
Pecans	Wheat germ
Rice polishings	

VITAMIN B$_6$

(*Pyridoxine*)

Functions: Needed for skin, blood, nerves, muscles, utilization of
fats.

Cabbage	Liver
Egg yolk	Meat
Fish	Milk
Grains, whole	Rice polishings
Kidney	Wheat germ
Legumes	Yeast

VITAMIN B$_{12}$

Functions: Needed for nerves; preventive for pernicious anemia.

Liver	Milk

NIACIN

(*Nicotinic acid, Niacinamide*)
Vitamin P-P

Functions: Needed for liver, nervous system, brain, soft tissues,
skin, circulation, and for burning of starches and sugars.

Bran	Meat, lean
Eggs	Peanuts
Fish	Wheat germ
Heart	Whey
Kidney	Yeast, dried
Liver	

INOSITOL

Functions: Needed for hair, muscles, liver, brain, heart.

Beef brain	Milk
Beef heart	Nuts
Fruits	Vegetables
Grains, whole	Yeast
Meat	

CHOLINE

Functions: Needed for kidneys, liver, spleen, thymus gland, lactation.

Brain
Egg yolk
Fish
Fruits
Grains, whole
Heart
Kidney
Meat
Milk
Pancreas
Soybeans
Sweetbreads
Tongue
Vegetables, root
Wheat germ
Yeast

PANTOTHENIC ACID

(*Calcium pantothenate*)

Functions: Needed for growth, skin, digestion, adrenal glands.

Beef, lean
Bran, rice
Broccoli
Cabbage
Corn
Egg yolk
Liver
Milk
Molasses
Oats, rolled
Peanuts
Peas
Potatoes
Salmon
Wheat germ
Whey
Yeast, dried

FOLIC ACID

(*Pteroylglutamic acid*)

Functions: Needed for red blood cells, liver, glands.

Eggs
Fowl
Fruits
Grains, whole
Meat
Oysters
Vegetables
Wheat germ

VITAMIN K

Functions: Needed for liver, blood clotting.

Bran, Rice
Cabbage
Kale
Liver

Carrot greens
Cauliflower
Egg yolk
Hempseed

Spinach
Soybean oil
Tomatoes

VITAMIN C

(*Ascorbic acid*)

Freshness is important in vitamin-C foods.

Functions: Needed for healing, teeth, gums, bones, joints, eyes, energy.

Fruits

This vitamin is very sensitive to heat. Whenever possible, eat your fruits uncooked.

GROUP I

Fruit juices, all fresh
Fruits and juices, canned citrus
Grapefruit
Guava, fresh
Lemons

Limes
Mangoes
Oranges
Strawberries
Tangerines

GROUP II

Bananas
Blueberries
Cherries
Cranberries
Loganberries

Melons
Peaches
Persimmons
Pineapple and juice, canned
Raspberries

Animal Products

Brains, rare
Clams, raw

Liver, rare
Oysters, raw

Vegetables

Vitamin C dissolves in water. Quick-cook these vegetables and save and serve the cooking water.

GROUP I

Asparagus
Cabbage
Carrots

Kohlrabi
Leeks
Mustard greens

Collards
Dandelion greens
Endive
Escarole
Kale

Peppers
Tomatoes, whole and juice
Turnip greens
Watercress

GROUP II

Beets
Broccoli
Cauliflower
Cucumbers
Grains and Seeds, sprouted
Horse Radish
Lettuce

Onions
Parsnips
Radishes, red
Rutabagas
Sauerkraut, fresh
Spinach
Sprouts, Brussels

BIO-FLAVONOIDS

Functions: Needed to aid vitamin C.

Asparagus
Grapefruit
Grapes

Liver
Oranges

VITAMIN D

(*Calciferol*)

Functions: Needed for digestion, bones, teeth, energy.

NOTE: No food is naturally an adequate source of vitamin D, although it is present in concentrated liver derivatives. Nature intended that man shall obtain this vitamin through the action of sunlight on the skin. Properly designed sun lamps may be used where natural sunshine is not available.

GROUP I
Fish-liver oils (tablets, capsules)

GROUP II

Beef liver
Butter
Cereals, fortified or
  irradiated
Cheese
Chicken liver

Cream
Eggs
Milk, fortified or
  irradiated
Salmon

VITAMIN E

Functions: Needed for fertility, reproduction.

Grains, whole

Wheat germ, undefatted

MINERALS: The mineral content of foods will be found in the following section devoted to minerals, their sources, functions, and requirements.

MEASURING VITAMINS

In order to become familiar with the weights used to measure vitamins, study the following table. If you learn it well, no vitamin manufacturer can fool you by stating the potency of his capsules in the smallest unit of weight, which bulks largest in numerical figures.

Vitamin weights

One gamma equals one microgram, mcg.
One microgram equals $\frac{1}{1000}$ of a milligram, mg.
One milligram equals $\frac{1}{1000}$ of a gram, gm.
One gram equals approximately $\frac{1}{30}$ of an ounce, oz.

Gammas (or micrograms) and milligrams are the common weight measurement terms used when synthesized vitamins are weighed. If a manufacturer tells you he has 200 gamma of B_6 in his capsule, it sounds like a lot more than ⅕ of a milligram, but it is actually the same amount. Read labels carefully.

Although this is only a cursory introduction to the vast subject of vitamins, which are described in detail above, it might be well to itemize here the known vitamins available commercially in concentrated form, along with ideal supplementary adult intake daily:

Vitamins and Ideal Supplementary Intake, Adult

Vitamin A	15,000 units
Vitamin B_1	10 mg.
Vitamin B_2	5 mg.
Vitamin B_6	10 mg.
Choline	500 mg.
Niacinamide	30-50 mg.
Para-amino-benzoic acid	30 mg.
Calcium Pantothenate	30 mg.
Vitamin C (ascorbic acid)	150 mg.
Vitamin E (alpha tocopherol)	30-100 mg.
Bio-flavonoids	200 mg.
Inositol	500 mg.
B_{12}	5 mcg.

NOTE: Where allergy to citrus fruits exists, it is possible that the bio-flavonoids, often extracted from such fruits, may likewise touch off sensitivity. In this case, rutin can be substituted. The minimum quantity of rutin that should be used as a supplement is 60 mg.

The Antigray Hair Formula

The latest research shows that the daily vitamin-supplementing formula should be constituted as follows:

Para-amino-benzoic-acid	30 mg.
Calcium Pantothenate	30 mg.
Choline	2 grams (2000 mg.)

in a natural B-Complex base fortified with additional B vitamins.

Minerals (Required): Their functions and sources

CALCIUM

Builds bones and teeth; regulates heart rhythm; controls neuro-muscular irritability; helps blood to clot; important to the skin, and helps prevent rickets and softening of the bones in adults. Balanced high calcium diets are sometimes helpful for under-weight persons, insomniacs, and in some types of neurasthenia, as well as in certain skin disorders and dental decay. Calcium metabolism is controlled by vitamins A, B complex, C, and D; viosterol alone is not enough; phosphorus and iron are needed to assist assimilation.

Best sources: Milk. This is not only the richest source of calcium, but also supplies lactose (milk sugar), which provides the acid medium in which calcium is best absorbed. Equally good sources are yellow cheeses. For the most part, vegetables are poor sources. The deficiencies in this mineral are nationwide.

Requirements: For adults, about 1 gram daily. For growing children, about 1½ grams daily. For expectant mothers, about 2 grams daily. A quart of milk supplies one gram; so do four to six ounces of yellow cheese.

PHOSPHORUS

Builds bones and teeth; important in brain function, nerve and muscle activity; sugar metabolism, and vitamin utilization. This mineral's most important indirect function is its relationship to calcium metabolism.

Best sources: Meat and poultry, eggs, yellow cheeses.

Requirements: Slightly more than calcium. It is the American public's high-phosphorus, low-milk diet that gives the average person in this country the all-too-common calcium deficiency. A wise precaution is to increase the intake of dairy foods or to use a calcium supplement.

IRON

Vitally important to the formation of hemoglobin, therefore important to transport of oxygen and metabolism of food materials in the cells. Without iron, you would need three hundred quarts of blood to absorb oxygen; with it, you need only six quarts. Copper or a trace of certain rare minerals is needed for the best utilization of iron in blood building. The metabolism of vitamin A depends on hemin iron, and so a good supply of the mineral is indirectly important to teeth and bones. Not all anemias come from iron deficiency, although it is responsible for many.

Best sources: Pork liver, beef liver, many other kinds of liver; molasses, apricots, eggs, oysters, pancreas, sweetbreads, other organ meats.

Requirements: 15 mg. daily. See discussion on "Anemia."

SPECIAL NOTE: If you use a properly formulated multiple vitamin-mineral capsule you will not need any additional sources of iron and need not be concerned with your supply of copper, iodine, or trace minerals such as zinc, magnesium, and manganese.

SULPHUR

This mineral is a constituent of protein and vegetable matter and is an important ingredient of the hair and nails, making mandatory a higher intake of meat and eggs for those whose brittle nails or hair do not respond to vitamin-mineral supplements. Sulphur is also an ingredient of vitamin B_1, insulin, and bile salts. Inability to excrete sulphur properly is an early indication of kidney disease. Neither colloidal nor inorganic sulphur can be utilized by the body, and injections of sulphur in any form will cause excretion of more sulphur than the amount injected. Only the sulphur-containing protein acids can be utilized by man as a source of sulphur. Do not, therefore, be misled by the extravagant claims of purveyors of inorganic or colloidal sulphur medicines, spring waters, and the like.

Best sources: Wheat germ, lentils, cheese, lean beef, peanuts, clams, eggs.

Requirements: In excess of 1 gram daily.

SODIUM CHLORIDE

Common table salt is the mineral most directly used but least understood by the public. Life cannot be maintained without sufficient salt, and no one should attempt a salt-free diet unless he has been specifically directed by his physician. By the same token, salt tablets should be used as supplements only under a physician's direction. While it is true that they are useful to those who perspire heavily and have, combined with vitamin C, helped steel workers avoid heat prostration, an excessive salt intake can cause serious disturbances.

The human body requires an intake of at least 10 grams (⅓ oz.) of salt daily, although twice this amount is used by Europeans. Vegetarians especially need ample salt. The food sources of sodium chloride that follow are high in the mineral. The list is given for the convenience of those whose physicians have prescribed salt-free diets.

Best sources: Caviar, rye krisp, butter, clams, cream cheese, American cheese, rye bread, Boston brown bread, oysters, graham crackers, whole wheat bread, white bread, molasses, condensed milk, dates, white fish, turnips, greens, escarole, banana, fresh coconut.

NOTE: Many of these foods are inferior sources of other nutrients.

POTASSIUM

Fortunately, this is a mineral in which none of us is normally deficient, for it is particularly important during periods of rapid growth. The child requires more potassium and less sodium than the adult. Like calcium, potassium curtails neuromuscular irritability. There have been reports that potassium chloride may be helpful in hay fever and other allergies.

Best sources: Dry lima beans, meat, fish, olives, molasses, dried beans, dried prunes, dried figs, dried peas, lentils, dried currants, raisins, almonds.

IODINE

Vital to the production of thyroid hormones; sometimes useful when thyroid is overactive or in the presence of goiter. This mineral also affects hair coloring and texture. To answer a frequent question, iodine deficiencies spring from diets that are low in this mineral, or because the soil from which the food came did not contain iodine. It is therefore wise to use iodized salt unless you are taking a mineral supplement that includes iodine.

FLUORIDES

A highly toxic substance added to drinking water, which licenses the continued eating of foods which then no longer cause tooth decay, but continue to destroy the supporting structures of the teeth. Vigorously if covertly recommended by manufacturers of white sugar, white flour, and other foods which cause tooth decay.

ZINC

Important in several chemical reactions of the body. Since it is part of insulin and interrelated with vitamin B_1 metabolism, it helps in the digestion of carbohydrates and also in protein metabolism. The zinc content of the body of a diabetic is much lower than that of a normal person. In leukemia, also, the zinc content of the white blood cells is low. Whether this is cause or effect has not yet been established.

Best sources: No good listing exists, although the recommendations are beans, lentils, liver, oysters, pancreas, peas, spinach, and watercress.

NOTE: It has recently been declared that zinc deficiency is possible. The symptoms resemble those of thiamine deficiency.

Requirements: Ten mg. daily. It must be noted here that the mineral supplements offered to the public, so far as zinc is concerned, are formulated capriciously, for the zinc content is usually $\frac{1}{15}$ the quantity of iron these capsules supply, yet the human zinc requirement is actually larger than that for iron.

MAGNESIUM

This mineral is the balance wheel for calcium metabolism. It is interrelated with vitamin C metabolism to a degree that renders the vitamin useless without it. Magnesium also exerts a quieting action on neuromuscular irritability, promotes elimination, and is important to bones and teeth.

Best sources: Beans, bran, Brussels sprouts, chard, clams, corn, nuts, oatmeal, peas, prunes, raisins, spinach, whole grains, honey.

Requirements: 2.70 mg. daily.

MANGANESE

Essential for proper functioning of the mammary glands. Together with calcium and many vitamins, this mineral is important in lactation. It is interrelated with vitamin B_1 metabolism and is necessary to reproduction, glandular function, tissue respiration, and the utilization of vitamin E. It is interesting to note that animals deficient in this mineral are lacking in maternal instinct.

Best sources: Bananas, beans, bran, celery, liver, oatmeal, onions, pancreas, peas, filberts, chestnuts, walnuts, whole grains.

Requirements: 1 mg. daily.

ALUMINUM

This mineral is included in our discussion only to throw the light of reason on the irrational faddist claim that aluminum may cause cancer. Disregard these claims; they represent propaganda against aluminum cooking utensils and come from faddists, quacks, or possibly manufacturers of other kinds of cooking utensils. Mayo Clinic's Dr. Russell Wilder says: "Many physicians are giving hydrated alumina as an antacid in the treatment of ulcer of the stomach and the duodenum. This treatment has been popular for many years, and so far as I know has never aroused any suspicion of provoking cancer in the stomach. The amount of aluminum given by this means exceeds by many hundred times what would be obtainable from the cooking of foods in aluminum vessels."

Classification of fresh vegetables and fresh fruits

According to percentage of carbohydrate content

VEGETABLES

3%

Asparagus
Beans, string (tiny)
Beet greens
Broccoli
Cabbage
Cabbage, Chinese
Cauliflower
Celery
Cucumber
Eggplant
Endive
Lettuce
Marrow
Mustard greens
Okra
Pepper, green
Radish
Sauerkraut
Sorrel
Spinach
Sprouts, Brussels
Squash, summer
Tomato
Watercress

6%

Artichokes—French
Beans, string (mature)
Beet
Carrot
Celeriac
Dandelion greens

FRUITS

5%

Avocado
Cantaloupe
Honeydew
Rhubarb
Watermelon

10%

Blackberry
Cranberry
Gooseberry
Grapefruit
Lemon
Lime
Orange
Papaya
Peach
Pineapple
Prune, fresh
Strawberry
Tangerine

15%

Apple
Apricot
Blueberry
Cherry
Currant
Grape
Guava
Huckleberry
Nectarine
Pawpaw

Kale
Kohlrabi
Leeks
Onions
Parsley
Peas (tiny)
Pumpkin
Rutabaga
Squash
Turnip

15%
Parsnip
Peas (mature)
Salsify

20%
Beans, shelled
Corn
Garlic
Horse-Radish root
Potato

Pear
Plum
Quince
Raspberry

20%
Banana
Fig, fresh
Grape Juice

Menu suggestions

This section is included as a "sampler" of the kind of menus you can feed your family in order to give them nutritional advantages without sacrificing variety, interest, or savor. It is not suggested that you weary your housemates with a repetition of these same 14 daily menus; but that, having introduced them to eating habits that are sensible as well as satisfying, you will continue with improvised meals of your own planning, which will follow the pattern of good nutrition.

You will note that luncheon and dinner menus seldom include a first course. From the nutritional point of view, one is not necessary. When family preference makes first courses desirable, they may be added.

For salads not specified as green salads, the author assumes that a generous amount of greens will be used as a base, not just as garnish.

Vegetables should be used in season, as should fresh fruits. If frozen or canned fruit is used for breakfast, drain it and reserve the sweet juice for a dessert or dessert-salad rather than add the extra carbohydrate to breakfast.

The luncheons given in the menus complete a well-balanced day's meal along with breakfast and dinner, but they are patterns rather than rules and need not be followed literally. For example, when eggs are indicated they may be used in any form, but should be included in the meal.

It is assumed that absent members of the family will make an effort to balance lunch with breakfast and dinner. School children who carry their lunches can of course be provided with properly balanced noontime meals.

Breakfast	*Lunch*	*Dinner*
SUNDAY		
Stewed Figs and Cream	Quick Rarebit on Whole Wheat Toast Triangles	Citrus Fruit Cup
Frizzled Beef and Scrambled Eggs	Finger Salad	Chicken Fricassee— Whole Wheat Biscuits
Whole Wheat Coffee Ring	Pineapple Chunks Cookies	Crab Apple Jelly Okra—Squash
Beverage	Milk	Mixed Green Salad
		Fruit Gelatin— Whipped Cream
		Beverage
MONDAY		
Citrus Juice	Banana and Peanut Butter Salad on Shredded Greens	Ragout of Heart
Soft Cooked Eggs		Mashed Potatoes
Whole Wheat Toast and Apple Butter	Jelly Sandwich— Whole Wheat Bread	Wax Beans
Beverage		Red Cabbage, Apple, Celery Salad on Chicory
	Milk	Boysenberries
		Beverage
TUESDAY		
Citrus Juice	Deviled Egg Salad	Veal Chops
Pettijohn Cereal— Brown Sugar	Whole Rye Toast	Mexican Corn
	Fresh Fruit	Spinach
Beverage	Milk	Fresh Fruit Salad
		Whole Wheat Crackers and Cheese
		Beverage
WEDNESDAY		
Fresh Pears	Liverwurst or Salami Sandwich—Whole Wheat Bread	Beef Stew—with Vegetables
Fried Eggs and Bacon		Cole Slaw
Whole Wheat Toast	Green Salad	Hot Whole Wheat Rolls
Marmalade	Baked Apples	Citrus Fruit Cup
Beverage	Cocoa	Oatmeal Cookies
		Beverage

Breakfast	*Lunch*	*Dinner*
THURSDAY		
Citrus Juice	Eggs Cooked in	Boiled Tongue—
Hot Cornmeal	Tomato Sauce	Horse-Radish
Honey	Whole Wheat Bread	Creamed Potatoes
Beverage	Watercress	Broccoli
	Fresh Fruit	Mixed Green Salad
	Milk	Gingerbread—
		Applesauce
		Beverage
FRIDAY		
Citrus Juice	Creamed Tuna Fish—	Baked Fish Turbot
Codfish Cakes	Whole Wheat	Cauliflower
Whole Wheat Rolls—	Toast	Mixed Vegetables
Jelly	Waldorf Salad	Raw Spinach,
Beverage	Milk	Romaine, Green
		Pepper Salad,
		French Dressing
		Strawberry Shortcake
		—Whipped Cream
		Beverage
SATURDAY		
Citrus Juice	Soup—Whole Wheat	Frankfurters—Baked
Poached Eggs on	Crackers	Beans
Whole Wheat Toast	Peanut Butter, Bacon,	Buttered Kale
Apple Butter	and Romaine Sand-	Brown Bread and
Beverage	wich—Whole	Honey
	Wheat Bread	Peach and Cottage
	Fresh Fruit	Cheese Salad
	Milk	Beverage
SUNDAY		
Minted or Honeyed	Fresh Fruit Salad	Baked Ham—
Grapefruit	Assorted Cheese Tray	Cranberry Sauce
Scrambled Eggs	Whole Wheat	Candied Sweet
Smoked Salmon	Crackers	Potatoes
Cream Cheese	Whole Rye Bread	Buttered Kale
Whole Wheat Rolls	Milk	Green Salad
and Jelly		Chocolate Nut Sundae
Beverage		Beverage

Breakfast	*Lunch*	*Dinner*
MONDAY		
Citrus Juice	Cottage Cheese,	Veal Fricassee
Oatmeal	Green Pepper, and	Brown Rice
Honey	Watercress Salad	Asparagus Tips
Beverage	Deviled Ham Sand-	Vinaigrette (gen-
	wich—Whole	erous Greens)
	Wheat Bread	Baked Custard
	Fresh Fruit	Beverage
TUESDAY		
Baked Apples	Sliced Pineapple,	Pan Fried Liver and
Fried Eggs and Bacon	Grated Carrot, and	Bacon
Whole Rye Toast	Raisin Salad	Baked Potatoes
Orange Marmalade	Peanut-butter Sand-	Turnip Greens
Beverage	wich—Whole	Mixed Green Salad—
	Wheat Bread	French Dressing
	Milk	Citrus Fruit Cup
		Nut Cake
		Beverage
WEDNESDAY		
Citrus Juice	Toasted Deviled Ham	Cheese Souffle
Buckwheat (Whole)	and Cheese Sand-	String Beans
Griddle Cakes and	wich—Whole	Cole Slaw with Cel-
Syrup	Wheat Bread	ery Seeds on Greens
Sausage	Fresh Fruit	Apple Brown Betty
Beverage	Nut Cake	Beverage
	Milk	
THURSDAY		
Grapes	Soup	Roast Pork—Apple
Eggs Poached in Milk	Whole Wheat	Sauce
Whole Wheat Toast	Crackers	Pan Browned Potatoes
Beverage	Pear Waldorf Salad	Broccoli Broil
	Milk	Mixed Green Salad
		Orange Surprise
		Beverage

Breakfast	Lunch	Dinner
FRIDAY		
Citrus Juice	Tuna Fish Salad	Baked Halibut-Egg
Jelly Omelet	Whole Wheat Rolls	Sauce-Slivered Al-
Cinnamon Toast	Fresh Fruit	monds
Beverage	Milk	Lima Beans
		Stewed Tomatoes
		Mixed Vegetable
		Salad-Roquefort
		Dressing
		Sliced Peaches
		Cookies
		Beverage
SATURDAY		
Citrus Juice	Cream Cheese and	Tomato Juice
Hot Ralston	Green Pepper	Hawaiian Hamburg
Molasses Butter	Sandwich—Whole	Peas and Carrots
Beverage	Wheat Bread	Wilted Greens
	Fresh Fruit	Raisin Rice Pudding
	Cookies	and Cream
		Beverage

influence of religion on, 22
low salt, 39-40
900-calorie, 119, 120, 121
no large-scale survey, 14
reducing, neuroses resulting from, 138-139
results of study, 14-15
study of, in pregnancy, 15
through history, 15-16
wheat germ in, 276, 283
diet, individual: *see also* diet
antithyroid factors, 112-113
calcium, 104-105
calories, 98-99
deficiency diseases, 83-84, 107-108
frequent small meals, 114
functions of food, 98
glutamic acid, 107
iodine, 112-113
low blood sugar, mental ills, 159-162
need for particular nutrient, 106
phosphorus, 105
thiourea, 113
vitamins, 99-104, 105-116
vitamin A, 113
digitalis, 33, 39, 44
disorientation and glutamic acid, 154
Doles, H. McGuire, 30
Donora, smog, 295
drugs, anticlotting, 30, 31
Dupuytren's contracture, 211
dystrophy, muscle, 35-36

eggs
declared dangerous, 48, 49, 50
in menstrual disturbances, 69
useful in arthritis, 207
value as food, 45, 55
Eisenhower, Dwight D., 30
electroencephalograph, 7
endrocrinologist, 169-172, 187
England, diet gains during World War II, 310-311
enzymes, raw milk, 192-193
epilepsy and glutamic acid, 155-156
Eskimos, 47, 52
estrogen, destroyed by well-nourished liver, 109
ether anesthesia, 6

faddism, faddists, 13, 18-19, 23, 34, 45, 82, 91, 124, 204, 227

Familia, 289
fats
acne, and vitamin B₆, 318-319
animal, declared dangerous, 47, 48, 49, 50
cholesterol, 44-55
cottonseed, 317-318; after forty, 272-273
decomposition points, 316
frying, 278-279, 315-316
as fuel, 315-316
gall bladder syndrome, 318
intolerance of, 283-284
low, diet, danger of, 277
metabolism of, 317
polyunsaturated, 43-44, 124, 273-274, 317
rancidity, 51; and vitamin E, 316
refrigeration of, 316
requirements of vitamin E, raised by polyunsaturates, 317
wheat germ oil, 317-318; after forty, 272-273
Federal Trade Commission, 261
Feltman, researcher, U. S. Public Health Service, 252-253
fertility: *see* sterility and fertility
First International Congress of Social Psychiatry, 301
Fleming, Alexander, Dr., 5-6
flour, white, products in diet, 206
fluoridation, fluorides, 357
and aggravation of goiter, 256
American Dental Association, inconsistency on control of dosage, 254-255
barred, by Swiss, 256
Bartlett and Cameron, comparison, 249
diet, value of, 257
dissolves forming embryo heart tissue, 250
Grand Rapids, 248-249
inadequacy of, 257-258
individuals, differences in teeth, 259
Mongolian idiots, 250
mottling, 255
multiplication of dosage, 256
New Britain, stillbirths, 250
paste applications, 264
statistics, eccentricities of, on fluoridation, 258
strontium, radioactive, 256
stupidity of public? 258-259
sugar, 248, 260, 260n, 261-262

About the Authors

CARLTON FREDERICKS, Ph.D.

Carlton Fredericks is a graduate of the University of Alabama, and a Phi Beta Kappa. He took the master's and the Ph.D. degrees at New York University School of Education. He taught nutrition to nursing students at N.Y.U.; to the public in the adult extension divisions of Brooklyn College and the City College of the City University of New York; and as Associate Professor at Fairleigh Dickinson University. He has also taught nutrition as a member of the postgraduate faculty of a major dental society.

Although Dr. Fredericks has specialized in nutrition for more than thirty years, his degree is in the field of public health education, and his broadcasts and books, while preoccupied with nutrition, have dealt with many aspects of the public health problems of modern man.

As staff nutritionist with a medical sanitarium and a medical group practice, Dr. Fredericks found many examples of the therapeutic use of nutrition that would not have been necessary if the science of nutrition had been applied early and prophylactically.

This is the philosophy he has applied in his broadcasts on nutrition, which have been heard throughout the United States and much of the civilized world.

The service rendered the public in these broadcasts brought to Dr. Fredericks an award from a foreign foundation, an honorary degree from a Canadian college, and citations from medical institutions and practitioners.

Dr. Fredericks is a member of the International College of Nutrition (Founding Fellow); President of the New York Chapter, American Nutrition Society; American Chemical Society; Association of Vitamin Chemists; A.A.A.S.; American Academy of Dental Medicine.

He is the editor of "Health and Nutrition News," a monthly publication, and the author of *Nutrition, Your Key to Good Health,* which is a revised edition of *Eat, Live and Be Merry; The Carlton Fredericks Cook Book for Good Nutrition; Dr. Carlton Fredericks' Low-Carbohydrate Diet.*

HERBERT BAILEY

Herbert Bailey is a veteran reporter who has worked for newspapers in North Carolina, Nashville, and Chicago. During the past fifteen years, he has contributed significant medical articles to leading magazines, among them are *Pageant, Collier's, Better Homes and Gardens, Argosy,* and *Science Digest.* He is credited with bringing national attention to the first large-scale successful and practical use of atomic energy in medicine—a force which has saved or prolonged countless thousands of lives. Also, Mr. Bailey wrote about the first clinical trials of hydrocortisone in the treatment of arthritis and other diseases. He first acquainted the American public with ultra sound, which has been used for many years in Europe and elsewhere for treating various diseases. He directed the world's attention to one of our greatest medical heroes—Dr. Emil Grubbé, who first used X-ray in the treatment of cancer on January 29, 1896. As a result of the author's efforts, Dr. Grubbé was finally accorded the recognition due him by the medical profession.

Mr. Bailey is the author of several books on medical subjects, among them, *Your Key to a Healthy Heart:* The Suppressed Record of vitamin E, a definitive work which conclusively demonstrates the value of vitamin E in the prevention and/or control of heart disease. He is the founder of Man's Frontiers, an organization devoted to explorations of the unknown and the dissemination of information on generally suppressed subjects.